# Cybersecurity, AI Collaboration, and Software Practice for Healthcare

Hanh Le
https://orcid.org/0009-0007-8172-0809
*University of the Cumberlands, USA*

IGI Global
Scientific Publishing
Publishing Tomorrow's Research Today

Vice President of Editorial — Melissa Wagner
Director of Acquisitions — Mikaela Felty
Director of Book Development — Jocelynn Hessler
Production Manager — Mike Brehm
Cover Design — Jose Rosado

Published in the United States of America by
IGI Global Scientific Publishing
701 East Chocolate Avenue
Hershey, PA, 17033, USA
Tel: 717-533-8845 | Fax: 717-533-7115
Website: https://www.igi-global.com E-mail: cust@igi-global.com



Library of Congress Cataloging-in-Publication Data

LCCN: 2026032936 (CIP Data Pending)
ISBN13: 9798337391199
EISBN13: 9798337391212

British Cataloguing in Publication Data
A Cataloguing in Publication record for this book is available from the British Library.

# Table of Contents

# Detailed Table of Contents


*Abu Sulman, University of Agriculture, Faisalabad, Pakistan*
*Maria Shafaqat, School of Natural Sciences, University of Kent, Canterbury, UK*
*Muhammad Saad Naeem, University of Agriculture, Faisalabad, Pakistan*
*Anam Hanif, University of Agriculture, Faisalabad, Pakistan*
*Fahad Ahmad, University of Agriculture, Faisalabad, Pakistan*
*Zubair Murtaza, Canterbury Christ Church University, UK*
*Izza Noor, University of Agriculture, Faisalabad, Pakistan*
*Sabira Sultana, Department of Eastern Medicine, Faculty of Medical Sciences, Government College University, Faisalabad, Pakistan*
*Adnan Afzal, Government College University, Faisalabad, Pakistan*
*Babar Khan, Centre for Biotechnology and Microbiology (CB&M), University of Swat, Pakistan*

The use of artificial intelligence (AI) in healthcare software systems has enhanced the necessity of safe and reliable human-AI integration. Although AI technologies improve the support of clinical decisions and efficiency of operations, a number of cybersecurity, governance, and software engineering issues arise. The chapter explores the concept of secure human-AI collaboration in healthcare by critically reviewing cybersecurity threats unique to AI-enabled systems such as data-centric security threats, model-level security threats and human interaction security threats. It also covers the issue of governance and regulatory factors influencing accountability, ethical supervision, and adherence to healthcare AI adoption. There is focus on safe software engineering which instills safety, privacy, and hardening across the system life cycle. Chapter offers researchers and practitioners with guided insights in the ways to design, govern, and maintain secure AI-driven healthcare systems helping to facilitate successful human-AI collaboration by introducing a socio-technical perspective.

This study analyses five decades of research at the intersection of computing, informatics, and organisational studies to trace trends in qualitative (e.g., discourse analysis, ethnography) and quantitative (e.g., experimental design, statistical modelling) methods. Emphasizing methodological pluralism, it bridges positivist and constructivist paradigms using a pragmatism-triangulation-bibliometrics framework (co-citation, co-word analysis) to map the evolution of computational research. It identifies emerging domains, such as AI ethics, reinforcement learning, and experimental designs for new technologies. Findings highlight how interdisciplinary methods are shaped by innovations from machine learning to quantum computing. Recommendations emphasise sustainable technology, ethical AI, and hybrid methods that balance both academic rigour and real-world relevance.

*Afsheen Mansoor, Shaheed Zulfiqar Ali Bhutto Medical University, Islamabad, Pakistan*
*Emaan Mansoor, Islamic International Dental College, Riphah International University, Islamabad, Pakistan*
*Ezza Mansoor, Islamic International Dental College, Riphah International University, Islamabad, Pakistan*
*Efrah Mansoor, Islamic International Dental College, Riphah International University, Islamabad, Pakistan*
*Mobeen Ghulam Ahmed, Department of Pharmacology, Faculty of Pharmaceutical Sciences, Government College University, Faisalabad, Pakistan*
*Adnan Afzal, Government College University, Faisalabad, Pakistan*
*Imrana Amir, Department of Zoology, University of Mianwali, Mianwali, Pakistan*
*Hafiz Aamir Ali Kharl, Narcotics Forensic Laboratory, Anti-Narcotics Force, Ministry of Interior and Narcotics Control, Islamabad, Pakistan*
*Muhammad Nouman Arif, Department of Pharmacy, Iqra University H-9 Campus, Islamabad, Pakistan*
*Amina Arif, Department of Basic and Applied Chemistry, Faculty of Sciences and Technology (FOST), University of Central Punjab, Pakistan*
*Hira Bukhat, University of Mianwali, Mianwali, Pakistan*

Healthcare software is one of the places where artificial intelligence is being employed as an effort to assist the decision, diagnoses, and healthcare efficiency in healthcare operations among others. Nevertheless, AI pipelines are also new cyber threats because they use sensitive data and inter-connect clinical systems and their models. This chapter examines design of cyber-resilient artificial intelligence (AI) pipelines of healthcare software with a full AI software lifecycle of growing datasets and data pre-processing to model development, validation and deployment to clinical use. It highlights some of the most significant threats such as data poisoning, adversarial attacks and system compromise, and technical, governance and ethical methods to additionally ensure the system resilience. The focus is put on patient safety, regulatory compliance and trust, seen through the AI-enabled clinical environments lens.

connections is the biggest obstacle to electronic healthcare. Due to its efficiency and dependability, blockchain—a distributed, immutable ledger or database—is having more popularity in a number of industries, like medical applications. Its benefits include immutability, better security, and decentralization. This chapter provides a realistic assessment of blockchain's advancement in healthcare with the goal of examining the advantages and difficulties of adopting blockchain technology in medicine 4.0.



Artificial intelligence (AI) is increasingly embedded in healthcare, promising improvements in diagnosis, efficiency, and cost, but it faces rising cybersecurity risks, regulatory challenges, and trust issues following data breaches. Despite financial losses, cybersecurity remains a compliance cost rather than a strategic investment. This chapter introduces a new view by considering cybersecurity as key to trust and cost-effectiveness in AI healthcare. Using health, cybersecurity, and AI governance research, it presents an Economic Evaluation Framework for Cybersecure AI (EECAI) that applies cost-benefit, cost-effectiveness, and return-on-security-investment analyses to evaluate secure AI deployment. The chapter shows how cybersecurity investments deliver measurable economic, clinical, and organizational value, emphasizing cybersecurity as a trust-building asset rather than a cost. It offers key insights for healthcare managers, developers, and policymakers to sustain safe, viable AI healthcare.



The health care systems are increasing both emotional and operational pressures that affect the clinical workforce's well-being and patient care quality. Compassion, which has always been seen as the symbol of the healthcare practice, tends to worsen when the workload pressure was high, time runs out, and the complexity of the administration was overwhelming. Simultaneously, artificial intelligence was being deployed more often in clinical decision support, workflow organization, and communication. This change provides possibilities and threats to the continuity of human contact in care settings. The principles of emotional intelligence used to inform the application of AI towards the practices that would safeguard the role of

# Preface

Healthcare is experiencing an unprecedented transformation driven by advances in artificial intelligence (AI), digital health technologies, software engineering, cloud computing, and interconnected healthcare ecosystems. These innovations offer significant opportunities to improve clinical decision-making, operational efficiency, patient engagement, and healthcare outcomes. However, they also introduce new cybersecurity threats, privacy concerns, governance challenges, and ethical responsibilities. As healthcare systems become increasingly dependent on intelligent software and data-driven technologies, ensuring security, trust, and resilience has become as important as achieving innovation and performance.

This book, *Cybersecurity, AI Collaboration, and Software Practice for Healthcare*, explores the intersection of three rapidly converging domains: human–AI collaboration, healthcare cybersecurity, and secure software engineering practices. Together, these domains form the foundation of trustworthy digital healthcare systems that support clinicians, protect patients, and maintain confidence in technology-enabled care.

Several key themes guide this volume.

First, the book emphasizes secure and trustworthy human–AI collaboration, recognizing that healthcare decisions require a balance between machine intelligence and human expertise. AI systems are increasingly supporting diagnosis, treatment planning, patient engagement, and administrative workflows. Their successful integration depends on transparency, explainability, trust, accountability, and meaningful human oversight.

Second, the book examines cybersecurity risk management and cyber resilience in healthcare environments. Healthcare organizations face growing threats from ransomware, data breaches, medical device vulnerabilities, and attacks on critical infrastructure. Understanding these risks and implementing effective defense strategies are essential for safeguarding patient safety and operational continuity.

Third, the volume highlights the importance of privacy-preserving AI and data protection. As healthcare increasingly relies on large-scale data analytics and machine learning, protecting sensitive patient information remains paramount. Emerging approaches such as federated learning, collaborative AI, privacy-enhancing technologies, and secure data-sharing frameworks offer new pathways for innovation while maintaining confidentiality and regulatory compliance.

Fourth, the book explores secure software engineering practices for healthcare applications. Security must be embedded throughout the software lifecycle—from requirements engineering and system design to deployment, monitoring, and maintenance. The concept of secure-by-design and privacy-by-design is particularly important in environments where software directly influences patient care and clinical outcomes.

Fifth, contributors address governance, ethics, and regulatory compliance, emphasizing the need for frameworks that ensure fairness, transparency, accountability, and responsible AI adoption. Effective governance provides the mechanisms needed to manage risks, build trust, and align technological innovation with societal and healthcare values.

The book also examines several emerging areas shaping the future of healthcare technology. These include telemedicine and connected healthcare security, medical Internet of Things (IoT) protection, blockchain-enabled healthcare systems, AI-driven cybersecurity defenses, quantum-resilient security strategies, and Healthcare 4.0 ecosystems. These technologies are redefining the delivery of healthcare services, creating new opportunities and challenges for cybersecurity and software practice.

An equally important theme is the recognition that technology should remain fundamentally human-centered. The volume, therefore, considers the roles of emotional intelligence, compassionate design, workforce wellbeing, and patient trust in the development and deployment of healthcare technologies. Successful digital transformation depends not only on technical excellence but also on the design of systems that support clinicians and improve patient experiences.

Finally, this book emphasizes the necessity of adaptive cyber governance across the entire journey from code to clinic. Secure healthcare systems require continuous oversight, monitoring, risk assessment, and improvement throughout their lifecycle. Building resilient healthcare ecosystems demands collaboration among software engineers, cybersecurity professionals, healthcare practitioners, researchers, policymakers, and organizational leaders.

The chapters assembled in this volume provide multidisciplinary perspectives on these challenges and opportunities. Collectively, they demonstrate that the future of healthcare will be shaped not merely by advances in AI or software alone, but by the ability to integrate innovation with security, privacy, trust, and responsible governance.

This book is intended for researchers, practitioners, healthcare leaders, software engineers, cybersecurity professionals, policymakers, and students seeking to understand and contribute to the development of secure, trustworthy, and intelligent healthcare systems. We hope it serves as both a scholarly reference and a practical guide for navigating the evolving landscape of healthcare technology and for building resilient, ethical, patient-centered, and trustworthy digital health ecosystems.

This book is organized into twenty-two chapters that collectively examine the evolving relationship between artificial intelligence, cybersecurity, governance, privacy, and software engineering in healthcare. The chapters are arranged to guide readers from the foundational concepts of trustworthy human–AI collaboration and cyber governance, through cybersecurity threats and resilient system design, to privacy-preserving AI architectures, emerging digital health technologies, and the broader economic, ethical, and human-centered implications of healthcare transformation.

## Chapter 1: Secure Human–AI Collaboration in Healthcare Software Systems, Cybersecurity Risks, Governance, and Software Engineering Practices

The use of artificial intelligence (AI) in healthcare software systems has enhanced the necessity of safe and reliable human-AI integration. Although AI technologies improve the support of clinical decisions and efficiency of operations, a number of cybersecurity, governance, and software engineering issues arise. The chapter explores the concept of secure human-AI collaboration in healthcare by critically reviewing cybersecurity threats unique to AI-enabled systems such as data-centric security threats, model-level security threats and human interaction security threats. It also covers the issue of governance and regulatory factors influencing accountability, ethical supervision, and adherence to healthcare AI adoption. There is focus on safe software engineering which instills safety, privacy, and hardening across the system life cycle. Chapter offers researchers and practitioners with guided insights in the ways to design, govern, and maintain secure AI-driven healthcare systems helping to facilitate successful human-AI collaboration by introducing a socio-technical perspective.

## Chapter 2: Designing Human–AI Collaborative Workflows in Healthcare: Roles, Trust, and Clinical Decision Support

Artificial intelligence (AI) is progressively revolutionizing healthcare systems by facilitating more data-driven, efficient, and precise clinical decision-making. This study examines the design and execution of human–AI collaborative workflows in healthcare, emphasizing roles, trust, and clinical decision support systems. It analyzes the integration of AI technologies into clinical settings via efficient workflow design, user-centric system development, and organizational preparedness. The discourse underscores the synergistic functions of physicians and AI systems, accentuating the significance of clinical acumen, elucidative algorithms, and transparent decision-support mechanisms. The study examines the ethical, technical, and organizational problems related to AI use in healthcare environments. The results indicate that effective human–AI collaboration necessitates robust governance structures, workforce training, and ongoing system assessment to guarantee dependable, safe, and patient-centered healthcare provision.

## Chapter 3: Explainability-as-a-Defense (XaaD) for Secure Healthcare AI

The rapid adoption of AI in healthcare has made the clinical functionality more convenient at the expense of exposing multifaceted cybersecurity risks which are difficult to detect using the traditional perimeter-based approach to security. Although explainable AI is fully deployed with intent to achieve transparency and regulation compliance, the prospects of explainable AI as a native security control have not been pursued. The chapter is a presentation of Explainability-as-a-Defense (XaaD) a framework which transforms the results of AI explanations into continuous behavioral fingerprints to perform proactive cybersecurity monitoring. A XaaD architecture that takes advantage of a layered architecture with explainability generation, drift detection, and human-in-the-loop validation is proposed, which is shown in the example of a clinical decision support, medical chatbots, IoMT analytics, and federated learning. XaaD re-imagines explainability as a post-hoc interpretability condition into an active form of defensive health care AI performance of trust.

## Chapter 4: Trends and Convergence in Healthcare Cybersecurity Literature

This study analyses five decades of research at the intersection of computing, informatics, and organisational studies to trace trends in qualitative (e.g., discourse analysis, ethnography) and quantitative (e.g., experimental design, statistical modelling) methods. Emphasizing methodological pluralism, it bridges positivist and constructivist paradigms using a pragmatism-triangulation-bibliometrics framework (co-citation, co-word analysis) to map the evolution of computational research. It identifies emerging domains, such as AI ethics, reinforcement learning, and experimental designs for new technologies. Findings highlight how interdisciplinary methods are shaped by innovations from machine learning to quantum computing. Recommendations emphasise sustainable technology, ethical AI, and hybrid methods that balance both academic rigour and real-world relevance.

## Chapter 5: Designing Cyber-Resilient AI Pipelines for Healthcare Software from Data Ingestion to Clinical Deployment

Healthcare software is one of the places where artificial intelligence is being employed as an effort to assist the decision, diagnoses, and healthcare efficiency in healthcare operations among others. Nevertheless, AI pipelines are also new cyber threats because they use sensitive data and inter-connect clinical systems and their models. This chapter examines design of cyber-resilient artificial intelligence (AI) pipelines of healthcare software with a full AI software lifecycle of growing datasets and data pre-processing to model development, validation and deployment to clinical use. It highlights some of the most significant threats such as data poisoning, adversarial attacks and system compromise, and technical, governance and ethical methods to additionally ensure the system resilience. The focus is put on patient safety, regulatory compliance and trust, seen through the AI-enabled clinical environments lens.

## Chapter 6: Ransomware Threats in Healthcare Systems Encryption-Based Attacks and Defensive Strategies

The healthcare systems have become the most common target of ransomware attacks worldwide. The data consists of invaluable patient information, clinical processes and the unrelenting susceptibility of medical systems. It offers an extensive review of ransomware as a healthcare environment threat, its anatomy (starting with initial infection and behavioral development), cryptographic file encryption algorithms, and a deep examination of double extortion models complexity. The chapter analyzes the ransomware infection of healthcare-specific vulnerabilities such as Internet of Medical Things devices, Electronic Health Record systems, PACS imaging archives and HL7 clinical data interfaces. The main contribution is developing a complete defensive approach and Governance, Risk, and Compliance framework mapping ransomware countermeasures within the frameworks of the HIPAA Security Rule, NIST Cybersecurity Framework 2.0, and ISO 27001:2022 standard. The chapter also ends by providing practical suggestions to the cybersecurity teams, compliance officers, and clinical governance stakeholders.

## Chapter 7: Benefits, Difficulties, and Healthcare 4.0 Effects of Blockchain Technology in Medicine

Machine optimization for a variety of industrial applications is now possible because to the development of AI methods and their translation into intelligent automated processes using the Internet of Things (IoT). One noteworthy development that occurred was the healthcare industry's tremendous advancement, which paved the way for the development of Health 4.0. The IoT, Internet of Services (IoS), Medical Cyber-Physical Systems (CPS), Health Cloud, Health Fog, and other cutting-edge technologies are all part of this new age. Securing all medical devices with internet connections is the biggest obstacle to electronic healthcare. Due to its efficiency and dependability, blockchain—a distributed, immutable ledger or database—is having more popularity in a number of industries, like medical applications. Its benefits include immutability, better security, and decentralization. This chapter provides a realistic assessment of blockchain's advancement in healthcare with the goal of examining the advantages and difficulties of adopting blockchain technology in medicine 4.0.

## Chapter 8: The Economics of Trust: Evaluating the Cost-Effectiveness of Cybersecure AI Systems in Healthcare Delivery

Artificial intelligence (AI) is increasingly embedded in healthcare, promising improvements in diagnosis, efficiency, and cost, but it faces rising cybersecurity risks, regulatory challenges, and trust issues following data breaches. Despite financial losses, cybersecurity remains a compliance cost rather than a strategic investment. This chapter introduces a new view by considering cybersecurity as key to trust and cost-effectiveness in AI healthcare. Using health, cybersecurity, and AI governance research, it presents an Economic Evaluation Framework for Cybersecure AI (EECAI) that applies cost-benefit, cost-effectiveness, and return-on-security-investment analyses to evaluate secure AI deployment. The chapter shows how cybersecurity investments deliver measurable economic, clinical, and organizational value, emphasizing cybersecurity as a trust-building asset rather than a cost. It offers key insights for healthcare managers, developers, and policymakers to sustain safe, viable AI healthcare.

## Chapter 9: Designing for Compassion through Emotional and Artificial Intelligence to Enhance Workforce Wellbeing in Healthcare

The health care systems are increasing both emotional and operational pressures that affect the clinical workforce's well-being and patient care quality. Compassion, which has always been seen as the symbol of the healthcare practice, tends to worsen when the workload pressure was high, time runs out, and the complexity of the administration was overwhelming. Simultaneously, artificial intelligence was being deployed more often in clinical decision support, workflow organization, and communication. This change provides possibilities and threats to the continuity of human contact in care settings. The principles of emotional intelligence used to inform the application of AI towards the practices that would safeguard the role of clinicians, relational sensitivity, and psychological resilience. The chapter draws on the idea of Compassion-Centered Hybrid Intelligence (CCHI), which was a model that integrates both emotional intelligence and artificial intelligence to enhance compassionate practice and support the well-being of the workforce.

Collectively, the chapters provide a multidisciplinary perspective on the design, governance, security, and deployment of AI-enabled healthcare systems. By integrating insights from cybersecurity, artificial intelligence, software engineering, healthcare informatics, governance, economics, and ethics, this volume offers a comprehensive roadmap for developing healthcare technologies that are secure, resilient, privacy-preserving, trustworthy, and patient- and clinician-centered.

**Hanh Le**
*University of the Cumberlands, USA*

# Acknowledgement

This book is the culmination of years of inquiry, discipline, reflection, and lived experience. Although my name appears on the cover, this work is the product of a much larger community that has shaped, challenged, and supported me along the way. I am deeply grateful to the colleagues and collaborators who sharpened my thinking. Your encouragement, intellectual rigor, and generosity of spirit made this work possible.

I am especially thankful for my family. Your patience during long nights of writing, your understanding during seasons of absence, and your unwavering belief in me provided the quiet foundation upon which this work was built. Academic achievements are often measured in publications and credentials, but behind every milestone stands a family that sacrifices, supports, and sustains.

I dedicate this book to my beloved mother and father, who are no longer here to see its completion. Their lives were marked by perseverance, humility, and quiet strength. From them, I learned the value of hard work, the dignity of integrity, and the transformative impact of education. Their sacrifices created opportunities they themselves never had, and every accomplishment I achieve rests upon that foundation.

Mom and Dad, though you are no longer physically present, your lessons guide me daily. Your resilience echoes in every challenge I overcome, and your love lives in every page of this work. This book is a tribute to you and to the enduring power of family.

With gratitude, love, and remembrance.

# Chapter 1
# Secure Human-AI Collaboration in Healthcare Software Systems:
## Cybersecurity Risks, Governance, and Software Engineering Practices

**Abu Sulman**
http://orcid.org/0009-0008-7194-5219
*University of Agriculture, Faisalabad, Pakistan*

**Maria Shafaqat**
*School of Natural Sciences, University of Kent, Canterbury, UK*

**Muhammad Saad Naeem**
*University of Agriculture, Faisalabad, Pakistan*

**Anam Hanif**
*University of Agriculture, Faisalabad, Pakistan*

**Fahad Ahmad**
*University of Agriculture, Faisalabad, Pakistan*

**Zubair Murtaza**
*Canterbury Christ Church University, UK*

**Izza Noor**
*University of Agriculture, Faisalabad, Pakistan*

**Sabira Sultana**
*Department of Eastern Medicine, Faculty of Medical Sciences, Government College University, Faisalabad, Pakistan*

**Adnan Afzal**
http://orcid.org/0009-0001-4359-5695
*Government College University, Faisalabad, Pakistan*

**Babar Khan**
*Centre for Biotechnology and Microbiology (CB&M), University of Swat, Pakistan*

DOI: 10.4018/979-8-3373-9119-9.ch001

## ABSTRACT

*The use of artificial intelligence (AI) in healthcare software systems has enhanced the necessity of safe and reliable human-AI integration. Although AI technologies improve the support of clinical decisions and efficiency of operations, a number of cybersecurity, governance, and software engineering issues arise. The chapter explores the concept of secure human-AI collaboration in healthcare by critically reviewing cybersecurity threats unique to AI-enabled systems such as data-centric security threats, model-level security threats and human interaction security threats. It also covers the issue of governance and regulatory factors influencing accountability, ethical supervision, and adherence to healthcare AI adoption. There is focus on safe software engineering which instills safety, privacy, and hardening across the system life cycle. Chapter offers researchers and practitioners with guided insights in the ways to design, govern, and maintain secure AI-driven healthcare systems helping to facilitate successful human-AI collaboration by introducing a socio-technical perspective.*

## SECURE HUMAN-AI COLLABORATION IN HEALTHCARE

The implementation of artificial intelligence (AI) in the healthcare setting has resulted in the development of collaborative systems where human knowledge and computational intelligence collaboratively assist the clinical and organizational decisions (Alowais et al., 2023). Healthcare software systems are increasingly being developed that contain AI-based features to support in diagnostics, treatment planning, clinical decision support, patient monitoring, and healthcare administration (Alowais et al., 2023). In practice, in the majority of real-world implementations, such systems are not deployed as independent systems, but as collaborative systems, which complement the functions of clinicians and other healthcare professionals (as opposed to substituting human judgment). The collaboration of human and AI in the medical field is a complicated process, as medical decisions are characterized by high stakes, health-related information is sensitive, and the work must be supervised by a person all the time (Mennella et al., 2024). Although AI systems can be used to process high volumes of data and produce predictive or prescriptive information with considerable efficiency, interpretation, validation and final decision-making are left to be carried out by human users. This mutual responsibility brings a socio-technical force where the performance of the system, the credibility of the user and security are closely connected. Any system impairment or system failure may have a direct influence on patient safety and care quality (Carayon, 2006). Security aspects are at the basis of empowering successful human-AI cooperation. The medical data is the most valuable, and the security breaches that a cyberattack can result in make healthcare information systems the leading victims of cyberattacks. The expansion of the attack surface by introducing AI technologies further increases the attack surface by including an additional number of data pipelines, additional learning models, and automated decision-making systems. A threat can be not only ordinary vectors of the cybersecurity threats, such as unauthorized access or ransom, but also AI-specific ones, such as the manipulation of the training data, exploiting the weaknesses of the model, or abusing the automated recommendations. Human factor in working in teams adds more risks to such risk; excessive reliance on the outcomes of artificial intelligence and lack of transparency in the work of algorithms (Senthilvelan, 2025).

Trust is another vital prerequisite of the successful collaboration in healthcare between human beings and AI. The clinicians are to be guaranteed safe, reliable and compatible AI systems that are aligned to the clinical objectives. Security breach, data integrity breach or inexplainable behavior of a system can bring this trust down leading to inadequate harnessing of AI tools or careless use of low-quality outputs. Consequently, to facilitate safe cooperation, along with efficient technical safety, an open system design, responsibility frameworks, and systems that would make AI-mediated choices explainable and auditable should be observed (OLAWORE et al., 2025).

As far as software engineering is concerned; to achieve secure human-AI interaction, security concerns must be integrated throughout the system lifecycle. These include that security requisite should be applied during system design, a high-quality authentication and access control system need to be adopted, data confidentiality and integrity should be maintained and continual monitoring of how the system operates should be conducted. Security-by-design and privacy-by-design are particularly useful in the healthcare context where regulatory compliance and ethics must be considered against technological innovation (Semantha et al., 2020). Along with technical precautions, organizational and governance factors are also significant determinants of the security of human-AI cooperation. The healthcare institutions should establish policies and guidelines that will determine the use of AI systems and define the role of humans and machine and provide a consistency with the relevant data protection and healthcare laws. Effective working depends on the alignment of technical controls and governance systems that help in the accountability, risk control as well as ethical control (Arjoon, 2006). It is in this part that the underlying idea of the rest of the chapter is established with the assertion of the importance of security in human-AI collaboration in healthcare software systems. Follow-up sections expound on this in line with the analysis of system architectures, cyber security threats, human aspects, governance processes, and software engineering practices that all combine to make safe and reliable AI-assisted healthcare environments.

# PRACTICAL SECURITY TOOLS AND FRAMEWORKS FOR HEALTHCARE AI SYSTEMS

The implementation of secure human–AI collaboration in healthcare requires not only conceptual governance mechanisms but also deployment of practical engineering tools that are actively used in advanced healthcare ecosystems. Modern hospitals and AI-enabled clinical platforms increasingly rely on specialized security frameworks to ensure data integrity, privacy preservation, and trustworthy AI deployment.

## FEDERATED LEARNING IN HOSPITAL NETWORKS

Federated learning allows AI models to be trained across multiple hospitals without centralizing patient data. Instead of sharing raw data, institutions share model parameters, significantly reducing privacy risks. For example, multi-hospital radiology networks in Europe and North America use federated learning to train diagnostic imaging models while complying with data protection laws. This approach reduces centralized breach risk by minimizing sensitive data transfer.

## DIFFERENTIAL PRIVACY MECHANISMS

Differential privacy techniques inject controlled noise into datasets or model outputs to prevent re-identification of patients. Frameworks such as TensorFlow Privacy enable healthcare AI developers to limit information leakage during model training. In environments where AI models are trained on large electronic health record (EHR) datasets, differential privacy reduces membership inference attack risks.

## SECURE MLOPS AND MODEL MONITORING

Healthcare AI systems require continuous monitoring to detect model drift, adversarial manipulation, and performance degradation. Secure MLOps platforms integrate:

- Automated model validation pipelines
- Drift detection algorithms
- Access logging and traceability
- Version control of trained models

These tools ensure accountability and prevent unauthorized model modification that could influence clinical decision-making.

## ZERO TRUST ARCHITECTURE (ZTA)

Zero Trust models assume that no user or system component is inherently trusted. In AI-enabled healthcare systems, Zero Trust principles include:

- Multi-factor authentication
- Continuous identity verification
- Least-privilege access control
- Micro-segmentation of AI services

This reduces risks of lateral movement attacks inside hospital networks.

## NIST AI RISK MANAGEMENT FRAMEWORK (AI RMF)

The NIST AI RMF provides structured guidance for identifying, assessing, and mitigating AI-related risks. It supports governance by aligning AI lifecycle management with risk categories such as safety, fairness, transparency, and security. Integrating AI RMF into healthcare software engineering strengthens compliance and audit readiness.

## ROLE-BASED ACCESS CONTROL (RBAC)

RBAC ensures that clinicians, administrators, and technical staff access only necessary data and AI functions. This reduces insider threat risk and improves traceability of decision support interactions.

## EXPLAINABLE AI DASHBOARDS

Explainable AI (XAI) dashboards provide visual insights into model predictions. By presenting confidence scores, feature importance metrics, and uncertainty indicators, these tools support clinician trust calibration and improve detection of anomalous AI outputs.

## AI-BASED HEALTHCARE SOFTWARE ARCHITECTURES

In the contemporary healthcare systems, human-AI cooperation is based on AI-powered healthcare software architectures. These architectures combine data collection units, computational intelligence as well as user facing applications to facilitate clinical, administrative, and operational processes. In contrast to conventional healthcare information systems AI-enabled designs should support a continuous process of learning data, updating models and interactive decision support and should be highly reliable, secure and compliant with regulations (Sharma & Kaushik, 2025).

On a basic level, AI-oriented healthcare systems are often designed in a layered or modular fashion, allowing the separation of concerns between data management, intelligence processing and user interaction. The data layers have the responsibility of gathering, archiving, and preparing heterogeneous healthcare data such as electronic health records, medical imaging, wearable device sensor information, and laboratory results. Since this information is sensitive in nature, architectural design should be built with the mechanism of secure data storage, access control and encryption to avoid unauthorized release or manipulation (Lin et al., 2017). The intelligence layer lays the foundation of machine learning systems, rule systems, or analytical engines that convert uncoded healthcare data into the actionable information. These components may be diagnostic algorithms, predictive risk models, natural language processing systems, and recommendation engines. In human-AI collaborative settings using AI, explainability and transparency should be offered in this layer to enable clinicians to interpret, evaluate, and make correct responses to AI generated products. Other architectural decisions such as modularization of the utilized models and common interfaces are also rather significant in making such monitoring easier as well as reducing the chances of opaque or untraceable system behavior (Tang et al., 2007). The interaction and application layer is employed to facilitate interaction of human and AI systems. This layer contains clinical dashboards, decision-support interfaces, alerting system, and reporting applications, which can give AI-driven insights in forms that can be easily consumed by the clinical workflow. It is also possible that improperly created interfaces can also be a threat to usability and security, i.e. their suggestions can be misunderstood, or confidential data can be accidentally disclosed. As a result, the anthropocentric values and the security issues must be put in mind in the architectural design to enable the safe and effective working (Rafsanjani and Nabizadeh, 2023; Sulman et al., 2025).The current AI architecture in healthcare is more dependent on distributed and cloud computing to enable scalability and computation. Although these types of infrastructures are flexible, efficient, and provide new security opportunities, they also create new security issues around data transmission, reliance on third-party services, and the shared computing resources. The use of such architectural measures like secure APIs, (Khan et al., 2026) containerization, and isolation of the key elements are needed to mitigate the effects of possible attacks and provide the system with resilience. In a shared setting, it is especially essential to establish a secure communication pathway between human users and AI services to guarantee trust and integrity of the system (Shneiderman, 2020).

The other feature of AI-based healthcare software architectures is interoperability. The healthcare systems need to be integrated with the already existing hospital information systems, medical devices and external sources of data. The interoperability of standards allows data to be easily exchanged and provides more attack surfaces when not well secured. Architectural structures should thus be able to provide good balance between openness and controlled access so that the interoperability would not affect confidentiality and stability of the system (Di Martino et al., 2018; Kharl, 2026; Noor et al., 2026; Waheed et al., 2026). Regarding the governance and lifecycle aspects, AI-based structures should allow maintaining constant surveillance, auditing, and renewal of system elements. The AI models can deteriorate with time, as the data patterns or clinical practices can change, and thus require retraining and validation. Secure architectural design makes it possible to make controlled updates and versioning, maintaining accountability to system behavior. This is a critical feature in the human-AI collaboration since it is necessary to make sure that clinicians are dealing with efficient and current AI systems(Naeem et al.).

## CYBERSECURITY THREATS IN HEALTHCARE AI SYSTEMS

The subject of cybersecurity threats is a severe issue to effective and safe implementation of AI-based healthcare software systems (Naeem et al., 2026). With the growing adoption of AI technologies by healthcare organizations to assist in clinical decision-making and operational systems, the complexity of these systems and their interconnection place healthcare organizations at risk of numerous security threats (Figure 1). With human-AI collaborative settings, cybersecurity events can be cascading, not only because of the potential to affect the availability of systems and data integrity but also because of the effects on the clinical trustworthiness, patient well-being, and the responsibility of an organization (Igwe-Nmaju & Anadozie, 2022).

Cyberattacks on traditional healthcare information systems are not a new occurrence because medical data is valuable, and healthcare services are vital. This threat scope is greatly enlarged with the addition of AI elements. AI systems are based on extensive data sets, ongoing models training, and logic-based automated decisions, which all result in the creation of new attack surfaces. Attackers can use weak points in the data, model, application, or infrastructure tier, and the threat analysis of the system design must be comprehensive and thorough to ensure its safety (Ten et al., 2010).

*Figure 1. Cyber security Threats using AI* **(Author's own work)**

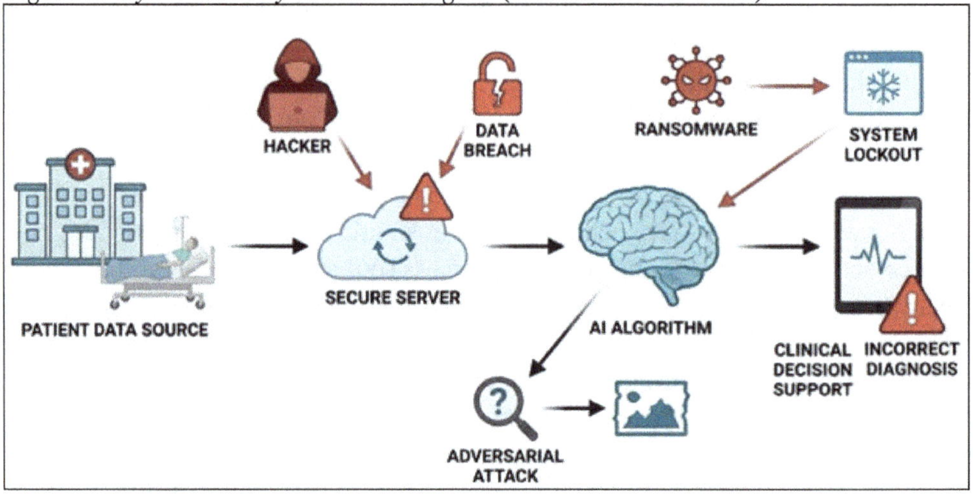


Another relevant category of threat is model-level attacks that utilize inner working of AI algorithms. Model inversion and membership inference attacks are some of the techniques that can be applied to acquire sensitive information about training data, which may expose private patients' information. Adversarial attacks can distort input data with imperceptible details that lead AI models into giving out wrong outputs even without manifestations of interference. Such attacks are especially harmful in the healthcare setting since they can be left unnoticed, and at the same time, affect clinical judgments directly (Pellino & Pellino, 2015). Communication between humans and AI creates more vulnerabilities associated with system abuse and overuse. The trust that clinicians have in AI systems can be abused by attackers, who can either manipulate outputs or interfaces and provide false or misleading recommendations. The risk of human error can be also increased due to social engineering attacks along with weakened AI systems. Poor training or insufficient skills on the shortcomings of AI systems can further increase such risks, and human users are an indirect means of attack in collaborative settings (Habbal et al., 2024).

Healthcare AI systems are also prone to danger at infrastructure level. Examples of the attacks vulnerable to distributed architecture, cloud services, and third-party integrations are denial-of-service attacks, unauthorized access, and supply chain attacks. Artificial intelligence systems that are based on external services or shared computational resources can have external vulnerabilities that are not directly controlled by healthcare institutions. At the infrastructure level, the disruption of the workflow in a human-AI partnership can disrupt clinical operations and reduce the effectiveness of the systems, casting doubt on the trust in AI-assisted care delivery (Okolo et al., 2021). The outcomes of cybersecurity attacks on healthcare AI systems are not limited to money loss or loss of operations. Data breaches and malfunctions can damage the relationships between clinicians and patients, impede the adoption of AI technologies, and result into regulatory fines. In extreme situations, undermined AI systems can add to the harm of patients by affecting clinical decisions using faulty or distorted data. These implications underline the necessity to view cybersecurity risks as not technical issues but as systemic risks that may be affecting the entire ecosystem of the human-AI cooperation (Sarker et al., 2023). The answer to the dangers of the cybersecurity risks of the healthcare AI systems should be holistic and involve technical safeguards, human consciousness, and organizational policies. The threat identification and mitigation process are to be founded on the specifics of AI technologies and the terms of collaboration in which they are used. This section outlines the threat landscape, which will be used to inform further discussions regarding the importance of human factors and governance systems and safe software engineering that should be embraced to create resilient and reliable human-AI collaborative practices in medical care (Varri, 2025).

The problem of cybersecurity in AI systems in healthcare will be revealed at several levels of data processing, model execution, and human interaction. Such threats not only affect the functionality of the system, but also have a direct impact on the clinician trust and decision-making in human-AI collaborative settings. The primary categories of cybersecurity threats and their impacts on collaboration are summarized in Table 1.

*Table 1. Cybersecurity Threats and Impacts in Healthcare AI Systems*

| Threat Category | Description | Impact on Human–AI Collaboration | Mitigation Strategy |
|---|---|---|---|
| Data Poisoning | Manipulation of training data | Incorrect AI recommendations | Data validation pipelines + anomaly detection |
| Adversarial Inputs | Crafted malicious inputs | Undetected diagnostic errors | Robust model testing + adversarial training |
| Model Inversion | Extraction of sensitive training data | Privacy breach | Differential privacy + access controls |
| Unauthorized Access | Weak authentication exploitation | Loss of clinician trust | Multi-factor authentication + RBAC |
| Ransomware | System encryption or shutdown | Clinical workflow disruption | Network segmentation + secure backups |
| Human Exploitation | Social engineering | Unsafe AI reliance | Staff cybersecurity training |

## HUMAN FACTORS AND TRUST IN AI COLLABORATION

Human components are the determining factors of the efficiency and safety of AI-based healthcare systems. Although AI technologies are associated with the new possibilities of analytical work, the effectiveness of their implementation in healthcare settings is highly contingent on how human actors interact, comprehend, and trust these systems. The perception of the clinicians and healthcare professionals in the human-AI cooperation environment as well as their behaviors and cognitive limitations are important factors of the security and reliability of the system (Asan et al., 2020). Human-AI collaboration has a fundamental component of trust. Healthcare workers should have confidence in the fact that AI systems will give correct, safe, and clinically significant results. The trust in AI, however, is not fixed and may be destroyed by the errors of the system, the absence of transparency, or security accidents. The issue of overtrust can cause overreliance, in which clinicians will follow AI suggestions without adequate scrutiny. On the other hand, lack of trust may lead to low use of AI tools thereby reducing the potential benefits. Both extremes are dangers to patient safety and effectiveness of the system, especially in the security-sensitive healthcare setting (Herath et al., 2024).

Explainability is one of the major human factors that determine trust. AI systems with the functionality of opaque or black box models may complicate the process of clinicians understanding recommendation generation. Such a lack of transparency can decrease trust in the outputs of the systems or cause unacceptable acceptance of incorrect recommendations. Explainability helps to make informed decisions, identify errors, and implement accountability in safe healthcare collaboration. Security wise, explainable systems can also be used to detect unusual behavior that can lead to cyber manipulation or system hacking (Zhang et al., 2022).

Another way human-AI interactions are structured in a healthcare environment is cognitive workload and time pressure. Clinicians usually work under a time-constrained atmosphere and decisions have to be fast. The AI systems that are created without regards to human cognitive restrictions can overload the users with hordes of alerts or complicated user interfaces. Under these conditions, there is a high chance of human error, such as the misinterpretation of AI outputs or lack of awareness of security warnings. These vulnerabilities can be used by attackers who can manipulate system outputs or interfaces to cause some wrong activity in the human-AI workflows (Chen et al., 2024). Training and user competence are the factors which are relevant in the process of ensuring secure collaboration. Medical employees may be of various levels of familiarity with AI-based technologies and cybersecurity notions. The deficiency of training can result in the abuse of AI systems, unprotected work with information, or failure to identify suspicious activity of the system. Quality collaboration assumes that the users are expected to know the possibilities and restrictions of AI systems and their input to the assurance of the security and integrity of the data (Shneiderman, 2020). Human factors are also overlapping with organizational culture and governance. The more institutions can foster the appropriate trust in AI systems is that institutions which foster transparency, accountability and life-long learning. Clear guidelines regarding human and system accountabilities help reduce the vagueness of the decision-making and incident response. When a healthcare organization operates in a team-based environment, it is possible to have clear-cut methods to escalation and audit processes so that human operators can respond to AI system anomalies or security breaches (Olatuyi, 2025). In cybersecurity terms, humans may be considered the weakest point of the defense of the system. Nevertheless, users may also provide a vital point of defense in human-AI collaboration should they be well supported. Introducing interfaces that support situational awareness, providing training that underlines the safe use of AI tools, and the governance models that foster the use of AI tools responsibly will help minimize human vulnerabilities.

Trust in AI systems must be calibrated rather than maximized. Excessive reliance may reduce clinician vigilance, whereas insufficient trust can limit adoption of beneficial AI tools. Security incidents, model drift, or unexplained predictions can destabilize trust calibration, emphasizing the importance of transparency and continuous validation mechanisms.

## GOVERNANCE AND REGULATION OF HEALTHCARE AI

Regulatory frameworks and the governance of AI-powered systems in healthcare are key to the compliance of such systems in terms of ethical, secure, and legal operation. With the use of AI technologies integrated into clinical decision-making and healthcare processes, the conventional governance paradigms of information systems will have to change to respond to the distinct risks presented by automation, data-driven inference, and human-AI interaction (Figure 2). A sound governance provides the structures, policies and accountability measures necessary to deal with these risks throughout the healthcare ecosystem (Siddiqi et al., 2009). Healthcare AI governance involves both internal and external control. On the organizational level, governance structures establish roles and responsibility of the AI system development, implementation, and utilization. The description of accountability between human users, system developers, and institutional leadership should be clear, especially in the collaborative setting in which AI systems can affect clinical decisions and yet not take over the authority of the human. In the absence of clear governance frameworks, the accountability of mistakes, security breaches, or harming patients might become unidentified, which destroys credibility and legal accountability (Wachter & Pronovost, 2009).

Recent international regulatory developments have strengthened AI governance expectations in healthcare. The WHO guidance on Ethics and Governance of AI for Health emphasizes transparency, accountability, and risk management. Similarly, emerging AI regulatory frameworks in Europe and North America introduce risk-based categorization for high-stakes AI systems, including medical decision-support tools. Healthcare institutions operating across jurisdictions must align internal governance with these evolving regulatory standards.

*Figure 2.* **Governance and Regulation of Healthcare AI (Author's own work)**

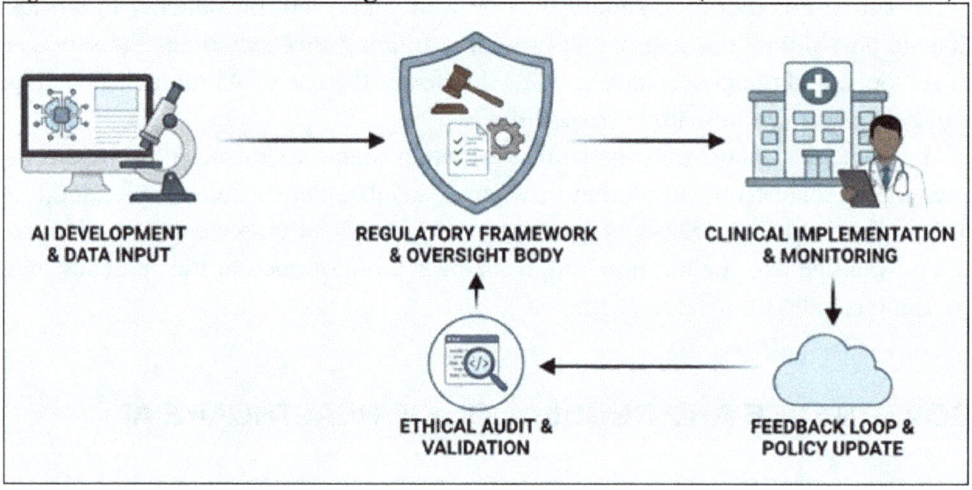


The regulation of AI systems in healthcare is also influenced by regulatory requirements. The field of healthcare is prone to severe confidentiality and data protection requirements, and the application of AI is accompanied by new factors of regulation concerning transparency, fairness, and safety. The laws protecting health information privacy, medical equipment software, and AI responsibility have limitations on the collection, processing, and sharing of data. Mechanisms governing AI should have in place that the systems adhere to these requirements across all stages of their life, such as the model training, deployment, and continuous updating (Sinha & Lee, 2024).

One of the aspects of healthcare AI governance is ethical oversight. Ethical issues associated with human-AI cooperation are prejudice, informed consent, and the correct utilization of automated suggestions. Governance frameworks should respond to such issues as the assessment of fairness and reliability of AI systems, the detection and correction of data or model biases, and the assistance of clinicians in making professional judgments. Cybersecurity is profoundly associated with ethical governance because the hacked or distorted AI systems may widen biases or offer unsafe suggestions without being identified (Kaushik et al., 2024). Governance structures have the basis of coordinated risk management and incident response, as far as security is concerned. The control policies on access, data sharing and monitoring of the system assist in minimizing the chances of unauthorized usage or malicious use of AI systems. Well-established governance processes can ensure speed in responding, investigating, and removing a security incident in the event of a security incident. Such processes are vital in a human-AI cooperative setting so that the technical teams and clinical staff are aware of their roles in case of cybersecurity incidents (Sarker et al., 2023).

The regulation styles also differ internationally, and therefore, governance of healthcare AI is more complicated. The healthcare organizations that conduct cross-jurisdictional business are compelled to address incomparable legal requirements, dealing with the protection of data, AI responsibility, and patient rights. The structures of governance are then supposed to be flexible to enable adherence to different sets of regulations (Organization, 2024). The fact that the internal governance practices are of a higher quality and consistency with the generally accepted standards and best practices in the field of healthcare information security and AI ethics promotes the importance of this issue. Human-AI cooperation, transparency and trust are also encouraged by appropriate governance. The stakeholders can consider the use of the AI systems, decision-making processes, and risk management with the help of documentation, auditing, and reporting systems. Regulatory compliance made easier is not the only outcome of such processes, which contribute to making clinicians and patients feel confident and accepting of AI-enabled healthcare services (Williamson & Prybutok, 2024). Table 2 depicts the interaction between technical safeguards and governance mechanisms in relation to the fact that socio-technical controls must be coordinated within healthcare AI systems.

*Table 2. Governance Mechanisms and Technical Controls in Healthcare AI*

| Governance Dimension | Governance Mechanism | Supporting Technical Controls |
|---|---|---|
| Accountability | Defined human oversight roles | Audit logs and decision traceability |
| Regulatory Compliance | Data protection policies | Encryption and access control |
| Ethical Oversight | Bias and fairness review | Model validation and monitoring |
| Risk Management | Security and privacy assessments | Continuous threat monitoring |
| Transparency | Documentation requirements | Explainable AI interfaces |

## SECURE SOFTWARE ENGINEERING FOR HEALTHCARE AI

Secure software engineering is a key facilitator of credible human-AI interdisciplinary collaboration in healthcare systems. As AI technologies become integrated into the healthcare software, the conventional software engineering practices need to be expanded to deal with the specific security, safety, and reliability issues that are posed by data-based and adaptable components (Preston, 2024). Security, in the context of healthcare, is an issue that should be addressed as a core design issue and not as a secondary consideration, since the failure of a system or security breach can lead to dire consequences (Kwon & Johnson, 2018).

Healthcare AI systems must have security requirements that are to be discovered at the beginning of software development. The requirements engineering should consider data confidentiality, integrity, availability, and healthcare regulations (Ansari et al., 2020). Clarity of boundaries between human use and AI elements in human-AI collaborative systems, where human control is required and where AI outputs must be verified before affecting clinical decision making, should also be defined by requirements (Figure 3). Clear security requirements can be used to minimize ambiguity, and assist in the consistent implementation of system parts (Lindgren, 2025; Wen, 2024).

During the implementation of healthcare AI systems, the role of architectural design is primary in maintaining security. Modular architectures allow isolating key architectures like the data storage, model training and decision-support services (Almadani et al., 2025). This isolation minimizes the effects of possible tradeoffs and helps in managing restricted access to confidential information and algorithms. Role-based access control, component-level authentication, and secure communication patterns are among the secure architectural patterns that need to be implemented to secure human users and the AI services in the collaborative settings (Dhinakaran et al., 2025).

*Figure 3.* **Secure Software Engineering for Healthcare AI (Author's own work)**

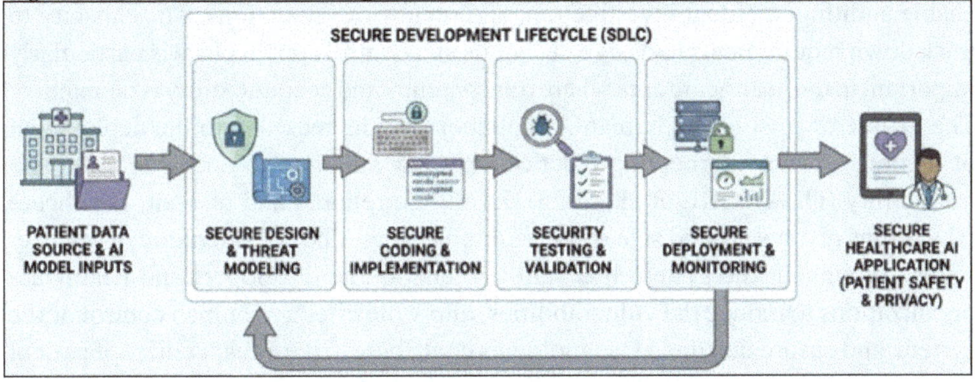


The implementation practices should also follow the principles of secure code, to avoid the common vulnerabilities that include injection attacks, inappropriate authentication and insecure data processing. In the case of AI-enabled systems, computer pipelines of machine learning, such as data preprocessing, model training, and deployment, need to be secured as well. Integrity of the training data and model artifacts is of special importance, since the models that have been compromised may give inappropriate results that can influence human decision-making. Safe version control and validation is used to ensure accountability and traceability during the development process (Meng et al., 2018).

The necessary aspects of secure healthcare AI software engineering are testing and validation. In addition to the functional testing, systems are also expected to be tested regarding security so as to find vulnerabilities in the traditional software components and the AI-based components. The testing should test how the systems react to abnormal input, system fault as well as the potential misuse conditions. The deployment and maintenance are also factors that bring about other security considerations that need to be usability tested to ensure that security controls unwind to add to the cognitive load, or encourage unsafe workarounds in the use of such systems (Baqar and Khanda, 2025). The AI systems commonly used in healthcare are often developed to operate in highly dynamic environments where the data distribution, practice patterns, and regulatory requirements vary over time. Secure deployment practices are controlled configuration administration, safe update systems and system behavior tracking (Ellahham et al., 2020). Security threats and reviews must be regularly done to combat the new threats and remain within the strategies. The maintenance activities within the collaborative settings will be forced to ensure that the users are made to know changes that might affect the system in supporting the decision support or workflows (Bala et al., 2024). The security and governance objectives are made facilitative and recorded. The behavior of AI models, security controls, and system design are to be well documented in order to enable auditing, incident investigation, and review of regulations. The capacity to track down requirements to design decisions and controls put in place is particularly important in the healthcare area where transparency and accountability is demanded. The degree of trust of the human-AI collaboration increases with the deployment of secure software engineering practices that pay attention to documentation and traceability (OLAWORE et al., 2025). In all, the reliable and resilient healthcare AI systems revolve around safe software engineering. The consideration of security issues throughout the system lifecycle will enable the developers and healthcare organizations to reduce the vulnerabilities, allow the effective human control of the system, and ensure that the AI technologies contribute to the enhancement of patient care rather than threaten it. The specified method of engineering assumes analyzing the privacy protection and safety mitigation initiatives in AI-based healthcare (Williamson and Prybutok, 2024).

The implementation of security in the software design lifecycle is the key to the reliability and resilience of the AI-assisted healthcare systems. Secure software engineering practices should answer not only the traditional software vulnerabilities but also the AI-related risks as well as facilitate regulatory compliance and human control. Table 3 presents key security practices mapped to the lifecycle phases of healthcare AI systems (Amugongo et al., 2025).

*Table 3. Secure Software Engineering Practices Across the AI System Lifecycle*

| Lifecycle Phase | Key Security Practices | Relevance to Healthcare AI |
|---|---|---|
| Requirements Engineering | Security and privacy requirements definition | Ensures compliance with healthcare regulations |
| System Design | Modular and layered architectures | Limits impact of component-level breaches |
| Implementation | Secure coding and data validation | Prevents exploitation of software and AI pipelines |
| Testing and Validation | Security and robustness testing | Identifies vulnerabilities before deployment |
| Deployment | Secure configuration and access control | Protects systems in operational environments |
| Maintenance | Continuous monitoring and secure updates | Addresses evolving threats and model drift |

## PRIVACY AND RISK MITIGATION IN AI SYSTEMS

The key issues surrounding the implementation of AI-based healthcare systems are privacy protection and the reduction of risks, especially in the human-AI co-operative setting. Health data is a very sensitive information that is prone to strict legal, ethical and professional requirements. The use of AI technologies increases the threat of privacy because of the volume of the data processing, the application of complex analysis, and the possibility of unintentional inference. Operational risk mitigation strategies should consequently focus on technical and organizational aspects of privacy and security (Snigdha et al., 2025).

*Table 4. Traditional IT Security vs AI-Specific Security Risks*

| Dimension | Traditional Healthcare IT | AI-Enabled Healthcare Systems |
|---|---|---|
| Data Risk | Data theft | Data theft + model manipulation |
| Integrity Risk | Database corruption | Model poisoning + drift |
| Attack Surface | Servers, endpoints | Data pipelines + models + APIs |
| Human Risk | Phishing | Phishing + AI overreliance |
| Governance | IT compliance | AI lifecycle + ethics + compliance |

Healthcare AI systems are based on vast amounts of personal and clinical data to produce valid information. This dependence adds to the threat of unauthorized access, information leakage, and re-identification of the persons even under the conditions of applying the traditional methods of anonymization (Ahmadi & RabieNezhad Ganji, 2023; Thesmar et al., 2019). The threat of privacy is further increased in collaborative environments where there could be a number of users, systems, and organizations that engage with shared information and AI services. The risk mitigation should consider the whole lifecycle of data, such as its collection, storage, processing, sharing, and disposal (Bala et al., 2024). The use of technical mechanisms is essential in ensuring privacy in healthcare AI systems. Data minimization strategies constrain the gathering and utilization of data to the extent that is necessary to run the systems. At rest and in transit, the encryption of data assists in protecting sensitive information against the unauthorized disclosure (Williamson & Prybutok, 2024). Access control mechanisms are used to grant access to authorized users and system components only to the protected data. These controls are relevant in the aspect of accountability in human-AI collaboration as they are used to establish accountability by clearly specifying who can access data and within what circumstances (Ardagna et al., 2008). Increased use of advanced privacy-enhancing methods is used to reduce AI-related risks. Differentiating privacy, secure multi-party computation and federated learning methods have a goal of minimizing exposure of sensitive data, but allow model training and inference. The methods enable healthcare organizations to take advantage of AI abilities without the need to centralize raw patient data, which will mitigate the effects of possible breaches. Their viability, however, is conditional upon a meticulous implementation and compliance with clinical and operation needs (Székely, 2022).

The monitoring and evaluation of system behavior is also a risk mitigation measure. There is a possibility that AI models can change with time through updates or changes in the data patterns that would present new privacy or security hazards (Chehri et al., 2021; Radanliev et al., 2024). Periodic audits and performance reviews assist in determining whether someone is not behaving as expected and seeking indications of misuse and compromise. Monitoring mechanisms used in the human-AI collaborative environment would need to support transparency and give actionable feedback to both technical teams and clinical users (Abikoye et al., 2024).

Technical controls are supplemented by organizational measures in dealing with privacy and risk. The data governance, consent management, and incident response policies offer a systematic risk mitigation strategy (Emma & Harri, 2023). Human user training and awareness programs contribute to making sure that human users are aware of their role in the management of sensitive data and safe interaction with AI systems. There should be explicit reporting and response procedures on privacy incidents to ensure the reduction of harms and trust (Pemmasani & Abd Nasaruddin, 2022). There is an ongoing issue in healthcare AI of balancing innovation and privacy protection. An over-protective control can reduce the utility of a system, and a lack of strong protection can put patients and organizations at a level of risk that is intolerable. Proper risk mitigation plans aim to establish this balance through incorporating privacy in the system design, the governance models, and the day-to-day operational behaviors (Akmal et al., 2024).

Overall, safe human-AI working in healthcare involves privacy and risk reduction. Entering into a unity of technical protection, organizational measures and constant monitoring, healthcare organizations will be able to minimize vulnerabilities and secure sensitive information and also use AI technologies responsibly. This discussion sets the stage of the future of the challenges and directions of research in the secure healthcare AI systems (Varri, 2025).

## FUTURE CHALLENGES IN SECURE HEALTHCARE AI

The future of safe human-AI cooperation is characterized by various new challenges emerging due to the further development of AIs technologies in the healthcare sector. Although existing systems show much promise to enhance the clinical care and operational efficiency, the pace of technology evolution, the complexity of systems, and the changing threat environment present ambiguities that need to be resolved through research, policy, and engineering creativity (Wen, 2024). The complexity of AI systems is one of the problems that are hard to handle. Contrary to conventional programs, AI models can evolve throughout time as they can be retrained or updated according to new data and clinical practice (Richardson et al., 2023). These modifications may create security vulnerability that has not been anticipated or compromise the performance of the system in rather unpredictable ways. The ongoing security, reliability, and fairness of adaptive AI systems is a research problem to which no definitive solution has been provided, especially in healthcare environments that demand continuous human supervision, which can only be achieved through safety concerns (Stoica et al., 2017).

Security management is becoming a challenging issue as the number of interdependent and distributed healthcare ecosystems increases. Presumably, next-generation healthcare AI systems will be more institutionally but less geographically dispersed, like remote care, wearable technologies. Even though the interoperability will promote the provision of more detailed and personalized care, it will result in an expanded attack surface and dependence on external services. These synergized systems will require advanced architectural and governance measures in the assurance of the protection of these systems and data privacy and system resiliency (Bala et al., 2024). The other question is the AI governance to technological innovation compatibility. Regulatory systems are usually lagging behind the technologies that they are established to regulate. As AI functionality grows, the existing regulations will be either inadequate or unclear and healthcare institutions and developers will be uncertain. One of the most significant issues still is the creation of dynamic governance frameworks capable of keeping pace with the technological shift and not losing accountability and compliance (Scherer, 2015). One of the factors that will also decide whether healthcare AI systems are secure or not is the role of the human factor. Having the AI tools improved, clinicians will be more inclined to use automated advice. In order to mitigate the human based vulnerability as well as to ensure that the overreliance does not take place, appropriate systems must be established to help in establishing the proper trust as well as promote a proper examination and effective communication of the uncertainty. The future research ought to focus on how human-AI interfaces and training systems can be created to minimize safe and effective collaboration (Asan and Choudhury, 2021). New cyber threats to the AI technologies are also being created. Resistance will develop more advanced ways of attack and it will make use of invisibility and complexity of AI systems. The necessity to reduce such threats will imply the use of more efficient detection software, increased verification of AI models, and the integration of cybersecurity intelligence in the system of AI programs monitoring. It would also be possible to predict and take action against new attack vectors, which would also become a key indicator of the long-term safety of healthcare AI systems (Azhar, 2016; Whyte, 2020).

Finally, the future of safe healthcare AI will also be affected by ethical and social considerations in a larger part. Such issues as bias, transparency, and patient autonomy will grow more acute as AI systems occupy bigger roles in healthcare provision. The answer to such problems is the use of interdisciplinary measures that incorporate the participation of technologists, clinicians, policymakers and ethicists. The establishment of secure human-AI cooperation should therefore not only be seen as a technical concern, but rather a more general socio-technical project (Goktas and Grzybowski, 2025).

## CONCLUSION

Safe human-ai collaboration in healthcare software systems is a very sensitive intersection of technologically creative, cybersecurity, governance and human-centered software development. Only in case of the combination of technical performance with the security, transparency, and reliability of the systems that they operate, the integration of AI technologies in healthcare processes can be of benefit and even acceptable. The chapter has discussed the ways of influencing the resilience of AI-enabled healthcare environments by the risks of cybersecurity, governance frameworks, and secure software engineering practice. As it is discussed, cybersecurity risks of the healthcare AI systems have extended beyond the traditional information system risks, such as manipulation of the data, use of models, and threat of human-AI interactions. The solution to these threats is hard to find alone, yet a multifaceted method of dealing with them including technical actions, organization administration, and the human aspect should be considered. Secure software engineering practices provide a foundation on which vulnerabilities are addressed and on which explainability, accountability and regulatory compliance are enabled when applied during the lifecycle of the system. Regulatory control and governance also promote safe co-operation that ensures that there are better responsibilities, ethical protection and compliance structure. At the same time, human factor and trust are also to be considered seriously to ensure that AI systems do not influence clinical decision-making negatively. Privacy protection and risk reduction efforts should be the primary concern because the healthcare AI systems are continuing to grow and expand in the distributed and interoperable environments. In general, the secure human-AI collaboration within healthcare can be viewed as the socio-technical issue that needs the coordination of activities across disciplines. By combining cybersecurity, governance, and software engineering, healthcare organizations will have a chance to build AI-powered systems, which are safe and dependable and can deliver patients with valuable benefits in patient care. The additional research and collaboration among stakeholders will become the key to the resolving of new issues and the maximum of AI in healthcare.

## REFERENCES


Abikoye, B. E., Akinwunmi, T., Adelaja, A. O., Umeorah, S. C., & Ogunsuji, Y. M. (2024). Real-time financial monitoring systems: Enhancing risk management through continuous oversight. *GSC Advanced Research and Reviews*, *20*(1), 465–476. DOI: 10.30574/gscarr.2024.20.1.0287

Ahmadi, A., & RabieNezhad Ganji, N. (2023). AI-driven medical innovations: Transforming healthcare through data intelligence. [IJBLS]. *International Journal of BioLife Sciences*, *2*(2), 132–142.

Akmal, I., Khan, H., Khushnood, A., Zulfiqar, F., & Shahbaz, E. (2024). An efficient artificial intelligence (Al) and blockchain-based security strategies for enhancing the protection of low-power loT devices in 5G networks. *Spectrum of engineering sciences, 2*(3), 528-586.

Almadani, B., Kaisar, H., Thoker, I. R., & Aliyu, F. (2025). A systematic survey of distributed decision support systems in healthcare. *Systems*, *13*(3), 157. DOI: 10.3390/systems13030157

Alowais, S. A., Alghamdi, S. S., Alsuhebany, N., Alqahtani, T., Alshaya, A. I., Almohareb, S. N., Aldairem, A., Alrashed, M., Bin Saleh, K., Badreldin, H. A., Al Yami, M. S., Al Harbi, S., & Albekairy, A. M. (2023). Revolutionizing healthcare: The role of artificial intelligence in clinical practice. *BMC Medical Education*, *23*(1), 689. DOI: 10.1186/s12909-023-04698-z

Amugongo, L. M., Kriebitz, A., Boch, A., & Lütge, C. (2025). Operationalising AI ethics through the agile software development lifecycle: A case study of AI-enabled mobile health applications. *AI and Ethics*, *5*(1), 227–244. DOI: 10.1007/s43681-023-00331-3

Ansari, M. T. J., Al-Zahrani, F. A., Pandey, D., & Agrawal, A. (2020). A fuzzy TOPSIS based analysis toward selection of effective security requirements engineering approach for trustworthy healthcare software development. *BMC Medical Informatics and Decision Making*, *20*(1), 236. DOI: 10.1186/s12911-020-01209-8

Ardagna, C. A., Cremonini, M., De Capitani di Vimercati, S., & Samarati, P. (2008). A privacy-aware access control system. *Journal of Computer Security*, *16*(4), 369–397. DOI: 10.3233/JCS-2008-0328

Asan, O., Bayrak, A. E., & Choudhury, A. (2020). Artificial intelligence and human trust in healthcare: Focus on clinicians. *Journal of Medical Internet Research*, *22*(6), e15154. DOI: 10.2196/15154

Bala, I., Pindoo, I., Mijwil, M. M., Abotaleb, M., & Yundong, W. (2024). Ensuring security and privacy in Healthcare Systems: A Review Exploring challenges, solutions, Future trends, and the practical applications of Artificial Intelligence. *Jordan Medical Journal*, *58*(3).

Carayon, P. (2006). Human factors of complex sociotechnical systems. *Applied Ergonomics*, *37*(4), 525–535. DOI: 10.1016/j.apergo.2006.04.011

Chehri, A., Fofana, I., & Yang, X. (2021). Security risk modeling in smart grid critical infrastructures in the era of big data and artificial intelligence. *Sustainability (Basel)*, *13*(6), 3196. DOI: 10.3390/su13063196

Chen, C., Gong, X., Liu, Z., Jiang, W., Goh, S. Q., & Lam, K.-Y. (2024). Trustworthy, responsible, and safe ai: A comprehensive architectural framework for ai safety with challenges and mitigations. *arXiv preprint arXiv:2408.12935*.

Dhinakaran, D., Kumar, N. J., & Ponnuviji, N. (2025). Safeguarding confidentiality and privacy in cloud-enabled healthcare systems with spectrasafe encryption and dynamic k-anonymity algorithm. *Expert Systems with Applications*, *279*, 127584. DOI: 10.1016/j.eswa.2025.127584

Di Martino, B., Rak, M., Ficco, M., Esposito, A., Maisto, S. A., & Nacchia, S. (2018). Internet of things reference architectures, security and interoperability: A survey. *Internet of Things : Engineering Cyber Physical Human Systems*, *1*, 99–112. DOI: 10.1016/j.iot.2018.08.008

Emma, O., & Harri, F. (2023). Integrating Cybersecurity Measures into Data Governance Policies for Content Management.

Habbal, A., Ali, M. K., & Abuzaraida, M. A. (2024). Artificial Intelligence Trust, risk and security management (AI trism): Frameworks, applications, challenges and future research directions. *Expert Systems with Applications*, *240*, 122442. DOI: 10.1016/j.eswa.2023.122442

Herath, H., Herath, H., Madhusanka, B., & Guruge, L. (2024). Data protection challenges in the processing of sensitive data. In *Data Protection: The Wake of AI and Machine Learning* (pp. 155–179). Springer. DOI: 10.1007/978-3-031-76473-8_8

Igwe-Nmaju, C., & Anadozie, C. (2022). Commanding digital trust in high-stakes sectors: Communication strategies for sustaining stakeholder confidence amid technological risk. *World Journal of Advanced Research and Reviews*, *15*(3), 609–630. DOI: 10.30574/wjarr.2022.15.3.0920

Kaushik, K., Khan, A., Kumari, A., Sharma, I., & Dubey, R. (2024). Ethical considerations in AI-based cybersecurity. In *Next-generation cybersecurity: AI, ML, and Blockchain* (pp. 437-470). Springer. DOI: 10.1007/978-981-97-1249-6_19

Khan, M. Z., Naeem, M. S., Khalid, S., Gill, Z., Ali, H., Iqbal, S., Shahid, S., Sulman, A., Awan, A., & Kharl, H. A. A. (2026). AI-GUIDED QSAR, MOLECULAR DYNAMICS, AND PHARMACOPHORE MODELING. *PharmA AI: Revolutionizing Drug Discovery and Healthcare with Artificial Intelligence.*

Kharl, H. A. A. (2026). *PharmA AI: Revolutionizing Drug Discovery and Healthcare with Artificial Intelligence.* IBH Publisher.

Kwon, J., & Johnson, M. E. (2018). Meaningful healthcare security. *Management Information Systems Quarterly, 42*(4), 1043–A1047. DOI: 10.25300/MISQ/2018/13580

Lin, J., Yu, W., Zhang, N., Yang, X., Zhang, H., & Zhao, W. (2017). A survey on internet of things: Architecture, enabling technologies, security and privacy, and applications. *IEEE Internet of Things Journal, 4*(5), 1125–1142. DOI: 10.1109/JIOT.2017.2683200

Lindgren, H. (2025). Emerging roles and relationships among humans and interactive AI systems. *International Journal of Human-Computer Interaction, 41*(17), 10595–10617. DOI: 10.1080/10447318.2024.2435693

Meng, N., Nagy, S., Yao, D., Zhuang, W., & Argoty, G. A. (2018). Secure coding practices in java: Challenges and vulnerabilities. Proceedings of the 40th International Conference on Software Engineering, Mennella, C., Maniscalco, U., De Pietro, G., & Esposito, M. (2024). Ethical and regulatory challenges of AI technologies in healthcare: A narrative review. *Heliyon, 10*(4). Naeem, M. S., Ahmed, S., Sulman, A., Usman, S., Farooq, M. A., Talha, M., Awan, A., Afzal, Z., Khan, M. Z., & Hanif, A. Role of Medicinal Plants in the Management of Metabolic Disorders: Mechanisms, Efficacy, and Therapeutic Prospects.

Naeem, M. S., Naeem, M., Mehmood, M., Sulman, A. A., & Kharl, H. A. A. (2026). MACHINE LEARNING IN FORMULATION OPTIMIZATION AND PROCESS CONTROL. *PharmA AI: Revolutionizing Drug Discovery and Healthcare with Artificial Intelligence.*

Noor, I., Mahmood, S., Aslam, M., Iqbal, S., Naeem, M. S., Shafaqat, M., Sulman, A., Awan, A., Aamir, H., & Kharl, A. (2026). AI ALGORITHMS AND TOOLS FOR PHARMACEUTICAL APPLICATIONS. *PharmA AI: Revolutionizing Drug Discovery and Healthcare with Artificial Intelligence.*

Okolo, C. T., Kamath, S., Dell, N., & Vashistha, A. (2021). "It cannot do all of my work": Community health worker perceptions of AI-enabled mobile health applications in rural India. Proceedings of the 2021 CHI conference on human factors in computing systems, Pellino, I. M., & Pellino, G. (2015). Consequences of defensive medicine, second victims, and clinical-judicial syndrome on surgeons' medical practice and on health service. *Updates in Surgery*, *67*(4), 331–337.

Pemmasani, P. K., & Abd Nasaruddin, M. A. (2022). Strengthening public sector data governance: Risk management strategies for government organizations. *International Journal of Modern Computing*, *5*(1), 108–118.

Preston, K. (2024). Bridging the gap: how human factors can support the development of AI technology in healthcare.

Radanliev, P., De Roure, D., Maple, C., Nurse, J. R., Nicolescu, R., & Ani, U. (2024). AI security and cyber risk in IoT systems. *Frontiers in Big Data*, *7*, 1402745. DOI: 10.3389/fdata.2024.1402745

Richardson, N., Kothapalli, S., Onteddu, A. R., Kundavaram, R., & Talla, R. R. (2023). AI-Driven Optimization Techniques for Evolving Software Architecture in Complex Systems. *ABC Journal of Advanced Research*, *12*(2), 71–84. DOI: 10.18034/abcjar.v12i2.783

Sarker, I. H., Janicke, H., Mohammad, N., Watters, P., & Nepal, S. (2023). AI potentiality and awareness: a position paper from the perspective of human-AI teaming in cybersecurity. International Conference on Intelligent Computing & Optimization, Sharma, N., & Kaushik, P. (2025). Integration of AI in healthcare systems—A discussion of the challenges and opportunities of integrating AI in healthcare systems for disease detection and diagnosis. *AI in Disease Detection: Advancements and Applications*, 239-263.

Shneiderman, B. (2020). Bridging the gap between ethics and practice: Guidelines for reliable, safe, and trustworthy human-centered AI systems. [TiiS]. *ACM Transactions on Interactive Intelligent Systems*, *10*(4), 1–31. DOI: 10.1145/3419764

Siddiqi, S., Masud, T. I., Nishtar, S., Peters, D. H., Sabri, B., Bile, K. M., & Jama, M. A. (2009). Framework for assessing governance of the health system in developing countries: Gateway to good governance. *Health Policy (Amsterdam)*, *90*(1), 13–25. DOI: 10.1016/j.healthpol.2008.08.005

Sinha, S., & Lee, Y. M. (2024). Challenges with developing and deploying AI models and applications in industrial systems. *Discover Artificial Intelligence*, *4*(1), 55. DOI: 10.1007/s44163-024-00151-2

Snigdha, E. Z., Jalil, M. S., Dahwal, F. M., Saeed, M., Mehedy, M. T. J., & Hasan, S. K. (2025). Cybersecurity in Healthcare IT Systems: Business Risk Management and Data Privacy Strategies. *The American Journal of Engineering and Technology, 7*(03), 163–184. DOI: 10.37547/tajet/Volume07Issue03-15

Stoica, I., Song, D., Popa, R. A., Patterson, D., Mahoney, M. W., Katz, R., Joseph, A. D., Jordan, M., Hellerstein, J. M., & Gonzalez, J. E. (2017). A berkeley view of systems challenges for ai. *arXiv preprint arXiv:1712.05855.*

Székely, B. (2022). Mitigating the privacy risks of AI through privacy-enhancing technologies. *Acta Universitatis Sapientiae. Legal Studies, 11*(2), 35–64.

Ten, C.-W., Manimaran, G., & Liu, C.-C. (2010). Cybersecurity for critical infrastructures: Attack and defense modeling. *IEEE Transactions on Systems, Man, and Cybernetics. Part A, Systems and Humans, 40*(4), 853–865. DOI: 10.1109/TSMCA.2010.2048028

Thesmar, D., Sraer, D., Pinheiro, L., Dadson, N., Veliche, R., & Greenberg, P. (2019). Combining the power of artificial intelligence with the richness of healthcare claims data: Opportunities and challenges. *PharmacoEconomics, 37*(6), 745–752. DOI: 10.1007/s40273-019-00777-6

Varri, D. B. S. V. (2025). Human-AI collaboration in healthcare security.

Wachter, R. M., & Pronovost, P. J. (2009). Balancing "no blame" with accountability in patient safety. *The New England Journal of Medicine, 361*(14), 1401–1406. DOI: 10.1056/NEJMsb0903885

Waheed, H., Waheed, F., Ashiq, E., Afzal, A., Sarosh, A., Maqbool, W., Sulman, A., Awan, A., & Kharl, H. A. A. (2026). INTRODUCTION TO ARTIFICIAL INTELLIGENCE AND MACHINE LEARNING IN PHARMACY. *PharmA AI: Revolutionizing Drug Discovery and Healthcare with Artificial Intelligence.*

Wen, H. (2024). Human-AI collaboration for enhanced safety. In *Methods in Chemical Process Safety* (Vol. 8, pp. 51–80). Elsevier.

Williamson, S. M., & Prybutok, V. (2024). Balancing privacy and progress: A review of privacy challenges, systemic oversight, and patient perceptions in AI-driven healthcare. *Applied Sciences (Basel, Switzerland), 14*(2), 675. DOI: 10.3390/app14020675

Zhang, Z., Al Hamadi, H., Damiani, E., Yeun, C. Y., & Taher, F. (2022). Explainable artificial intelligence applications in cyber security: State-of-the-art in research. *IEEE Access : Practical Innovations, Open Solutions, 10*, 93104–93139. DOI: 10.1109/ACCESS.2022.3204051

# Chapter 2
# Designing Human-AI Collaborative Workflows in Healthcare:
## Roles, Trust, and Clinical Decision Support

**Andi Asrifan**
http://orcid.org/0000-0002-9934-6129
*Universitas Negeri Makassar, Indonesia*

**Nurhajar Patinrosi**
http://orcid.org/0009-0005-2453-3201
*UIN Palopo, Indonesia*

**Sahabuddin Sahabuddin**
http://orcid.org/0000-0002-9074-3822
*Universitas Negeri Makassar, Indonesia*

## ABSTRACT

*Artificial intelligence (AI) is progressively revolutionizing healthcare systems by facilitating more data-driven, efficient, and precise clinical decision-making. This study examines the design and execution of human–AI collaborative workflows in healthcare, emphasizing roles, trust, and clinical decision support systems. It analyzes the integration of AI technologies into clinical settings via efficient workflow design, user-centric system development, and organizational preparedness. The discourse underscores the synergistic functions of physicians and AI systems, accentuating the significance of clinical acumen, elucidative algorithms, and transparent decision-support mechanisms. The study examines the ethical, technical, and organizational*

DOI: 10.4018/979-8-3373-9119-9.ch002

*problems related to AI use in healthcare environments. The results indicate that effective human–AI collaboration necessitates robust governance structures, workforce training, and ongoing system assessment to guarantee dependable, safe, and patient-centered healthcare provision.*

## 1. FOUNDATIONS OF HUMAN–AI COLLABORATION IN HEALTHCARE

### 1.1 Evolution of Artificial Intelligence in Healthcare Systems

AI is one of the most groundbreaking healthcare technologies. In recent decades, AI has evolved from rule-based systems to complicated machine learning and deep learning models that can analyze medical data. This trend indicates computational advances and the rising accessibility of large health datasets from electronic health records, medical imaging systems, genetic databases, and wearable health devices. AI has become essential to improving diagnostic precision, clinical efficacy, and tailored patient care as healthcare systems increasingly use digital infrastructures.

AI was first used in healthcare in the 1970s and 1980s using expert systems. These systems mostly used rule-based reasoning to help clinicians diagnose and treat diseases using "if–then" principles. The MYCIN system was an early example of using patient symptoms and test results to recommend bacterial infection treatments (Papadopoulos et al., 2022, p. 715). Early expert systems showed the potential of computational support in clinical decision-making, but they were limited by rigid rule frameworks, knowledge base upgrades, and inability to handle large amounts of complex data.

Machine learning in the late 1990s and early 2000s revolutionized healthcare AI applications. Machine learning algorithms may find patterns in large datasets without writing decision rules, unlike rule-based systems. These algorithms can identify medical characteristics, predict illness, and analyze clinical data. Patient data are analyzed using machine learning algorithms to predict hospital readmissions, identify early sickness indications, and optimize therapeutic recommendations based on patient characteristics.

Recent advances in deep learning and neural network topologies have greatly improved healthcare AI systems. Radiographic pictures, pathology slides, and genomic sequences are ideal for deep learning models. AI algorithms can help doctors detect malignancies, fractures, and cardiovascular disorders in medical imaging (Fatima et al., 2023, p. 1). These computers analyze images using convolutional neural networks to find patterns humans may miss. Thus, AI is improving radiology, oncology, cardiology, and ophthalmology diagnostics.

AI has improved healthcare prediction analytics and diagnostics. Physicians can identify high-risk patients and intervene earlier in disease management using predictive models. Predictive algorithms can predict hospitalized patients' sepsis risk, ICU decline, and predisposition to chronic diseases including diabetes and cardiovascular disease. These traits help move from reactive to preventative treatment.

Integrating intelligent clinical decision support tools into hospital information infrastructures is a major success in AI-enabled healthcare. Healthcare facilities increasingly use electronic health record systems that store large volumes of patient data. AI algorithms can analyze these statistics in real time and provide clinicians with relevant patient care information (Fahim et al., 2025). These technologies let doctors diagnose, offer evidence-based treatments, detect drug interactions, and track patient states. Despite these advances, AI is meant to help physicians.

Medical decisions sometimes involve complex contextual factors, ethical considerations, and patient relationships—human factors. Thus, AI in healthcare has prioritized collaborative approaches where human expertise and AI improve therapeutic outcomes. Human–AI collaborative workflows that combine technical intelligence with clinical acumen are becoming more popular due to this transformation.

## 1.2 Conceptualizing Human–AI Collaborative Workflows

Healthcare professionals and artificial intelligence technologies work together to improve medical decision-making and patient care. Without replacing human expertise with AI, this perspective emphasizes the complementary strengths of humans and technology. AI technologies give computing efficiency, vast data analysis, and pattern recognition, but humans have contextual comprehension, moral reasoning, empathy, and experience insight. These synergistic characteristics can improve diagnosis, therapy, and clinical procedures when properly integrated.

Collaborative intelligence highlights that AI works best with human expertise. Healthcare workers sometimes make complex decisions that include interpreting various data sources, assessing ambiguous data, and considering patient preferences (Cuéllar et al., 2024, p. 12). AI systems can analyse enormous amounts of medical data, find hidden patterns, and make evidence-based suggestions. Clinicians can then evaluate these outputs based on patient history, clinical expertise, and ethics.

In hybrid decision-making workflows, AI-generated insights inform human judgment but do not replace it. Radiological images can be analyzed by an AI system to detect abnormal tissue proliferation. After reviewing these findings, the radiologist can verify the AI's interpretation and use additional clinical data to make a diagnosis (Alanazi et al., 2024, p. 742). This collaborative approach ensures that AI is an auxiliary tool while human oversight and responsibility are maintained in medical decisions.

Human–AI collaboration requires transparency and interpretability. Clinicians trust AI systems more when they understand their recommendations. Explainable AI systems explain algorithmic decisions to help healthcare experts evaluate the system's rationality and therapeutic relevance (Adeniran et al., 2024). Clinical settings require transparency since decisions affect patient safety and treatment outcomes.

Successful human-AI collaboration requires careful workflow design. AI technologies should improve therapeutic methods, not hinder them. Poorly designed systems can increase cognitive strain, workload, and decision-making ambiguity for doctors. Thus, human–AI workflows are designed with usability, dependability, and therapeutic relevance in mind.

Additionally, collaborative healthcare systems must address responsibility and accountability. While AI systems may suggest treatments, clinicians make the final decision. AI output interpretation and clinical application require explicit recommendations (Ueda et al., 2023, p. 7). Healthcare businesses may create secure and efficient collaboration systems by separating human and AI roles.

## 1.3 The Role of Clinical Decision Support Systems (CDSS)

Clinical Decision Support Systems (CDSS) constitute a crucial technical interface facilitating human–AI collaboration within healthcare settings. Clinical Decision Support Systems (CDSS) are computer-based platforms intended to aid healthcare professionals in clinical decision-making by analyzing patient data and offering pertinent recommendations. These systems amalgamate medical knowledge, patient data, and algorithmic analysis to facilitate diagnostic processes, treatment planning, and risk evaluation.

Historically, initial Clinical Decision Support Systems (CDSS) were intimately associated with rule-based expert systems that offered recommendations grounded in established clinical guidelines. Contemporary Clinical Decision Support Systems increasingly integrate machine learning and artificial intelligence methodologies, facilitating more advanced analysis of patient data (Siddiq, 2021, p. 1581). These sophisticated computers can analyze extensive datasets, derive knowledge from historical medical records, and produce predicted insights that facilitate evidence-based clinical decision-making.

A main role of CDSS is to offer diagnostic support. AI-driven diagnostic instruments may evaluate patient symptoms, laboratory findings, and imaging data to ascertain potential medical disorders (Lysaght et al., 2019, p. 302). For instance, CDSS may propose possible diagnoses based on symptomatology or emphasize anomalies identified in radiological scans. These tips assist doctors in contemplating alternate diagnoses and mitigating the risk of diagnostic inaccuracies.

A fundamental aspect of CDSS is the facilitation of treatment planning. Through the examination of clinical guidelines and patient-specific data, CDSS can propose suitable treatment alternatives customized to the unique requirements of each patient. The system may provide ideal prescription regimens considering patient allergies, medical history, and current health issues. These guidelines aid doctors in choosing evidence-based therapies that conform to recognized medical standards.

Clinical Decision Support Systems (CDSS) also play a crucial role in medication management and patient safety. Drug interaction notifications are a prevalent component of most healthcare information systems. When clinicians prescribe pharmaceuticals, Clinical Decision Support Systems (CDSS) can automatically assess potential drug interactions, dose inaccuracies, or contraindications based on patient characteristics (Sutton et al., 2020). These notifications assist in averting adverse medication events and improving patient safety.

Predictive risk modeling constitutes a significant capability of contemporary Clinical Decision Support Systems (CDSS). AI-driven predictive models can evaluate patient data to assess the probability of future health issues. Predictive tools can identify individuals at elevated risk for hospital readmission, infection, or cardiovascular incidents. By recognizing these hazards promptly, healthcare providers can execute preventive measures that enhance patient outcomes and diminish healthcare expenses.

Although CDSS offer substantial advantages, their efficacy is contingent upon their incorporation into clinical workflows and the endorsement by healthcare practitioners. Systems that produce an overabundance of alerts or inconsequential recommendations can result in alert fatigue, causing doctors to disregard system cautions (Kusumadewi & Miladiyah, 2023, p. 1754). Consequently, the design of CDSS must emphasize relevance, accuracy, and usability to guarantee that recommendations effectively assist clinical practice.

## 2. ROLES AND RESPONSIBILITIES IN HUMAN–AI CLINICAL COLLABORATION

### 2.1 Defining the Role of Clinicians in AI-Augmented Healthcare

The use of artificial intelligence into healthcare systems has created new prospects for enhancing diagnostic precision, clinical efficiency, and patient outcomes. The effective use of AI technology is contingent upon the active involvement of healthcare professionals who analyze, validate, and utilize AI-generated insights in clinical practice (Park & Langlotz, 2025). Healthcare professionals, including physicians and nurses, are pivotal in ensuring that AI-assisted decision-making matches with patient requirements, medical ethics, and the specific realities of clinical contexts. As healthcare systems progressively integrate AI tools, physicians must modify their professional responsibilities to properly interact with intelligent technologies while retaining accountability for patient care.

Clinicians continue to be the principal decision-makers in healthcare settings, notwithstanding the analytical assistance offered by AI systems. Medical decisions frequently necessitate intricate assessments that demand a profound comprehension of patient history, social environment, psychological circumstances, and ethical issues (Jia & Zhao, 2025, p. 5414). AI systems can produce suggestions derived from data patterns; yet they are incapable of fully encompassing the intricate elements that affect therapeutic decisions (Vitacca et al., 2022, p. 4). Treatment recommendations proposed by an AI model may inadequately incorporate patient preferences, comorbidities, cultural factors, or economical limitations. Consequently, doctors must rigorously assess AI-generated outputs and incorporate them with their professional skills prior to implementation in patient care.

Another crucial duty of clinicians in AI-enhanced healthcare is to validate and verify AI recommendations. AI systems, especially those utilizing machine learning, are not infallible and may generate errors stemming from biased training data, inadequate datasets, or constraints in algorithm design (Almotairi et al., 2022, p. 3). Healthcare personnel must meticulously assess AI outputs to ascertain the clinical appropriateness and safety of the suggestions for the patient. This human monitoring functions as an essential safeguard that mitigates the risk of erroneous diagnoses or unsuitable therapies stemming from algorithmic inaccuracies.

Alongside clinical judgment, healthcare workers contribute vital human attributes to patient care that AI systems are incapable of emulating. Empathy, compassion, and interpersonal communication are fundamental elements of efficient healthcare provision. Patients frequently depend on professionals for both medical care and emotional assistance amid challenging health circumstances (Ferguson, 2025). AI technologies can aid in diagnostic analysis or treatment planning; but they cannot supplant the human connection that fosters confidence between patients and healthcare providers. Consequently, doctors are accountable for conveying medical knowledge to patients, elucidating treatment alternatives, and assisting them in healthcare decision-making.

Moreover, healthcare professionals must acquire new skills pertaining to digital health technologies and artificial intelligence literacy. As AI systems gain prominence in healthcare settings, healthcare personnel must comprehend their operational mechanisms, inherent constraints, and the interpretation of their outputs (Malerbi et al., 2023, p. 1). AI literacy empowers doctors to critically evaluate algorithmic suggestions and identify instances when AI-generated insights may be incorrect or unsuitable. Training programs and ongoing professional development initiatives are thus becoming increasingly essential for equipping healthcare workers to utilize AI technologies successfully.

Clinicians in AI-enhanced healthcare engage in transdisciplinary collaboration. Healthcare AI systems are typically created through collaborations among medical professionals, data scientists, engineers, and technology experts. Clinicians provide domain expertise that guarantees AI technologies are clinically pertinent, morally robust, and consistent with actual healthcare procedures (Reuben et al., 2024, p. 6). Clinicians influence the design, assessment, and execution of AI technologies, thereby fostering systems that genuinely enhance patient-centered care.

Ultimately, delineating the role of doctors in AI-enhanced healthcare necessitates acknowledging that AI serves as a tool intended to assist—not supplant—medical professionals. Human judgment, ethical accountability, and patient-centered communication are fundamental components of healthcare delivery. Integrating AI insights with clinical experience enables healthcare workers to improve the quality and efficacy of medical decision-making.

## 2.2 The Role of AI Systems in Clinical Workflows

Artificial intelligence systems are becoming increasingly vital in facilitating clinical operations inside contemporary healthcare settings. These systems are engineered to examine extensive medical data, discern patterns that may elude human detection, and offer insights that facilitate clinical decision-making. AI technologies enhance human analytical abilities, assisting healthcare workers in managing intricate information, increasing diagnostic precision, and refining treatment strategies.

A significant application of AI in clinical operations is the processing of medical data. Healthcare systems produce vast amounts of data from sources including electronic health records, laboratory results, imaging systems, and wearable health monitoring devices. AI algorithms can process and analyze datasets at speeds much surpassing human capability, enabling healthcare professionals to discern significant patterns and trends (Chatterjee et al., 2024, p. 14). AI models can analyze patient records to discover early signs of chronic disease, ascertain risk factors linked to hospital readmission, or monitor health trends at the population level.

Medical imaging exemplifies a domain in which AI systems have exhibited considerable potential. Deep learning algorithms excel in the analysis of radiological images, including X-rays, CT scans, MRI scans, and ultrasound pictures. AI algorithms trained on extensive datasets of medical images can accurately identify abnormalities, including cancers, fractures, and organ irregularities. These technologies aid radiologists by emphasizing questionable regions in pictures and offering preliminary evaluations that facilitate diagnostic procedures. AI technologies enhance efficiency by diminishing the time needed for the analysis of intricate images, enabling physicians to concentrate on more sophisticated interpretative responsibilities.

AI systems additionally enhance predictive analytics in clinical operations. Predictive models utilize historical patient data to assess the probability of forthcoming medical occurrences. AI algorithms can foresee the likelihood of patient deterioration in intensive care units, identify patients at elevated risk for cardiovascular disease, or predict the possibility of postoperative complications (Abut et al., 2023, p. 2). These predictive insights empower healthcare providers to implement preventative measures and intervene earlier in the disease trajectory, potentially enhancing patient outcomes and decreasing healthcare expenditures.

A significant role of AI in clinical operations is to assist with therapy suggestions. AI-driven decision support systems can evaluate clinical guidelines, patient attributes, and treatment results to provide suitable therapeutic approaches. Oncology decision support systems can evaluate genomic data and clinical records to propose individualized cancer therapy strategies. Likewise, AI algorithms can aid clinicians in determining suitable pharmaceuticals by considering patient allergies, drug interactions, and treatment history.

Notwithstanding these capabilities, AI systems are primarily regarded as decision-support instruments rather than independent decision-makers. AI technologies are proficient in analyzing extensive datasets and recognizing statistical patterns; yet, they are deficient in contextual comprehension, ethical reasoning, and experiential judgment, which are attributes of human physicians (Saadeh et al., 2025, p. 2). The fundamental role of AI in clinical workflows is to deliver analytical insights that aid healthcare workers in making educated decisions.

Moreover, AI technologies can facilitate the optimization of administrative functions within healthcare institutions. Automated documentation, scheduling support, and data management technologies can alleviate the administrative load on clinicians (Samajdar et al., 2025). By automating repetitive processes, AI technologies enable healthcare personnel to allocate more time to direct patient care and clinical problem-solving.

The primary function of AI systems in clinical workflows is to augment the analytical and operational capabilities of healthcare systems. When correctly integrated, AI technology can enhance productivity, minimize errors, and facilitate more tailored patient care approaches. These systems are most effective when utilized in conjunction with human clinicians who understand and implement AI-generated insights within the whole framework of medical practice.

## 2.3 Collaborative Decision-Making Between Humans and AI

Collaborative decision-making between humans and artificial intelligence constitutes a crucial element of AI-integrated healthcare systems. Instead of substituting clinicians, AI technologies serve as analytical collaborators that offer data-driven insights to enhance medical decision-making. Successful collaboration between humans and AI necessitates meticulously crafted interaction models that enable physicians to assess, evaluate, and authenticate algorithmic recommendations prior to their implementation in clinical practice.

A prevalent form of human–AI interaction has AI systems delivering initial analyses, with physicians retaining ultimate decision-making authority. In diagnostic imaging, AI systems may examine scans to detect probable anomalies. The clinician thereafter examines the AI-generated findings, assesses their pertinence in relation to patient data, and decides if additional diagnostic tests or treatments are warranted (Spear et al., 2023, p. 2). This collaborative process enables AI to improve the efficiency and precision of data processing while maintaining human supervision.

Another significant approach entails AI systems operating as real-time decision support instruments in clinical practice. In this context, AI algorithms perpetually assess patient data and offer recommendations during consultations or treatment planning sessions. A clinical decision support system may notify a clinician of possible drug interactions during medication prescriptions or provide alternative therapies in accordance with clinical guidelines. These real-time advice aid clinicians in making informed judgments while diminishing the probability of medical errors.

Trust and openness are essential components in collaborative decision-making between humans and artificial intelligence. Clinicians must comprehend and assess the rationale underlying AI-generated suggestions. Explainable AI systems seek to elucidate the processes by which algorithms reach their findings, enabling doctors to evaluate the alignment of the system's suggestions with clinical expertise. Clinicians are more inclined to believe and utilize recommendations from AI systems that exhibit transparency and reliability.

Human–AI collaboration necessitates systems enabling doctors to veto AI outputs when deemed essential. AI systems may sporadically produce erroneous or deceptive suggestions due to data constraints or algorithmic biases (Yoon et al., 2024, p. 17). In such instances, therapists must possess the capacity to interrogate, amend, or dismiss AI-generated ideas. Adopting this human-in-the-loop methodology guarantees that healthcare practitioners maintain paramount accountability for patient care determinations.

Besides technological issues, collaborative decision-making include organizational and cultural factors within healthcare organizations. Healthcare practitioners must cultivate confidence in AI systems by training, experience, and demonstrable system reliability. Organizations must formulate explicit policies concerning the interpretation of AI suggestions and the allocation of responsibility between clinicians and AI technologies.

The efficacy of human–AI collaborative decision-making relies on the creation of workflows that utilize the advantages of both humans and machines. AI systems offer sophisticated analytical capabilities and swift data processing, but physicians deliver contextual insight, ethical judgment, and empathetic patient care (Sokol et al., 2025). By integrating these synergistic capabilities, healthcare systems can attain enhanced diagnostic accuracy, improved treatment outcomes, and more efficient healthcare delivery.

## 3. DESIGNING EFFECTIVE HUMAN–AI COLLABORATIVE WORKFLOWS

### 3.1 Workflow Integration in Clinical Environments

The effective deployment of artificial intelligence in healthcare relies not only on the complexity of the algorithms but also on the efficiency of their integration into current clinical workflows. Healthcare settings are intricate systems defined by rapid decision-making, interdisciplinary cooperation, and stringent regulatory mandates. If AI solutions disturb existing clinical processes or elevate the cognitive burden on healthcare personnel, their adoption is improbable, irrespective of their technical proficiency. Consequently, the design of efficient human–AI collaborative processes necessitates meticulous alignment between technology systems and clinical procedures.

A crucial factor in process integration is interoperability with electronic health record (EHR) systems. EHR platforms function as the primary repository for patient information, encompassing medical history, laboratory results, medication records, imaging reports, and physician notes. AI systems must effortlessly access and evaluate these datasets to yield useful insights (Devi, 2024, p. 4). Interoperability guarantees that AI applications may interact with current healthcare information systems without necessitating manual data entry or supplementary administrative procedures. When AI systems are completely linked with EHR platforms, doctors can obtain AI-generated suggestions immediately within their current digital workflow environments.

Effortless data interchange between AI tools and EHR systems mitigates the likelihood of errors linked to disjointed information systems. In numerous healthcare facilities, professionals depend on various digital platforms to obtain patient information, resulting in inefficiencies and incomplete data interpretation. AI systems that directly interact with EHR infrastructures can evaluate extensive patient datasets in real time, facilitating more precise clinical insights and diminishing the necessity for physicians to manually aggregate information from various sources.

System usability is a crucial element in the integration of AI technologies within clinical settings. Healthcare personnel face considerable time restrictions, and any added complexity from digital tools may provoke resistance to their implementation. AI systems must be engineered with intuitive interfaces that enable physicians to swiftly obtain pertinent insights without traversing convoluted menus or deciphering ambiguous representations (Wu et al., 2024, p. 15). An intuitive design alleviates the cognitive load on physicians and guarantees that AI technologies facilitate, rather than obstruct, clinical decision-making.

Another crucial element of process integration entails synchronizing AI tools with current clinical practices. Hospitals and healthcare institutions adhere to standardized protocols for disease diagnosis, treatment administration, and patient information documentation. AI technology ought to enhance these traditional processes instead than compelling clinicians to embrace totally new workflows. AI diagnostic technologies ought to be integrated into current imaging review systems utilized by radiologists, rather than necessitating doctors to upload images to distinct platforms. Likewise, AI-generated therapy recommendations ought to be integrated into prescription management systems utilized by clinicians during standard patient appointments.

Successful workflow integration necessitates collaboration between healthcare professionals and technology developers throughout the design and implementation stages. Clinicians provide significant insights into the functioning of medical workflows, encompassing the issues related to time constraints, patient complexity, and interdisciplinary cooperation (Ndabu et al., 2021, p. 11). Engaging healthcare professionals in system design guarantees that AI solutions are customized to address actual clinical requirements and can be implemented without interrupting patient care.

Ultimately, the incorporation of AI into healthcare operations necessitates a harmonious approach that merges scientific advancement with practical applicability. AI systems must be integrally included into healthcare infrastructures, compatible with digital health data, and consistent with current medical practices. When these criteria are satisfied, AI technologies can augment clinical efficiency, boost diagnostic precision, and facilitate more informed decision-making while maintaining the continuity of patient care.

## 3.2 Human-Centered Design for AI-Assisted Clinical Systems

Human-centered design is essential for ensuring that AI-assisted clinical systems are successful, user-friendly, and aligned with the requirements of healthcare professionals. In contrast to several other technical environments, healthcare settings necessitate solutions that facilitate swift decision-making, ensure patient safety, and operate dependably under high-pressure circumstances. AI tools that neglect the practical realities of clinical practice may induce confusion, elevate cognitive burden, or foster distrust among healthcare personnel. Consequently, the design of AI-assisted healthcare technology necessitates a robust emphasis on usability, transparency, and physician involvement.

A fundamental tenet of human-centered design is the emphasis on user experience. Healthcare personnel must swiftly and accurately understand AI-generated insights during patient care operations. Interfaces must provide information clearly and succinctly, emphasizing essential recommendations while reducing superfluous complexity (Nasarian et al., 2023, p. 38). AI systems that aid in medical imaging analysis may employ visual overlays to emphasize regions of concern within radiological images. These visual indicators allow clinicians to swiftly recognize any anomalies while retaining authority over the diagnostic interpretation process.

Explainable artificial intelligence is an essential element of human-centered AI design in healthcare. Numerous AI systems, especially those utilizing deep learning models, function as intricate "black box" algorithms, rendering their decision-making processes challenging to elucidate. In clinical settings, healthcare workers must comprehend the rationale behind an AI system's specific recommendations (Salahuddin et al., 2021). Explainable AI strategies seek to deliver interpretable insights into algorithmic thinking, including the identification of data elements that influenced predictions and the elucidation of patterns that contributed to diagnoses. When clinicians get the rationale behind AI advice, they are more inclined to trust and efficiently employ the technology.

The visualization of AI-generated insights is crucial in human-centered system design. Healthcare practitioners routinely analyze intricate datasets, encompassing imaging scans, laboratory findings, and patient histories. Effective AI systems convey these findings via intuitive visual formats, such dashboards, heat maps, risk assessments, or trend graphs. These visual instruments assist physicians in interpreting AI outputs more effectively, enabling the integration of algorithmic insights into their decision-making processes.

An additional critical factor in the design of AI-assisted clinical systems is facilitating decision-making under time constraints. Healthcare personnel frequently operate in settings that necessitate swift decision-making to manage critical medical circumstances. AI systems must consequently provide timely and pertinent insights without inundating therapists with superfluous information. Alert systems must prioritize essential warnings and reduce superfluous alerts that may lead to alert fatigue. By delivering solely the most pertinent insights, AI systems assist doctors in prioritizing patient care.

Clinician involvement is crucial for effective human-centered design. Healthcare professionals must engage in the creation and assessment of AI systems to guarantee that the technologies correspond with actual clinical requirements (Wang et al., 2023, p. 14). Participatory design methodologies enable clinicians to offer input on system functionality, interface design, and workflow integration. This collaborative procedure enhances system usability and bolsters clinician acceptance and confidence in AI technologies.

## 3.3 Building Trust in Human–AI Clinical Collaboration

Trust is a key component affecting the successful implementation of artificial intelligence in healthcare settings. Even the most sophisticated AI systems may not produce significant outcomes if clinicians lack trust in the accuracy, reliability, or safety of their suggestions. Healthcare professionals bear responsibility for patient outcomes and must ensure that AI-supported insights enhance clinical decision-making. Establishing confidence in human–AI collaboration necessitates transparency, algorithmic explainability, performance dependability, and stringent validation procedures.

Transparency is fundamental in fostering confidence between clinicians and AI systems. Healthcare personnel must comprehend the objectives, functionalities, and constraints of AI systems employed in clinical environments. Clinicians may be reluctant to trust the suggestions of AI systems when they function as opaque "black boxes" (Choudhury, 2022, p. 5). Transparent systems explicitly convey the methodology behind forecasts, the data sources utilized, and the potential uncertainties inherent in the model. This transparency enables doctors to critically assess AI recommendations and integrate them into therapeutic reasoning with increased confidence.

Algorithmic explainability is intrinsically linked to transparency. Explainable AI methodologies seek to render algorithmic judgments comprehensible to human users. An AI system forecasting cardiovascular disease risk may identify particular patient attributes—such as blood pressure, cholesterol levels, or lifestyle factors—that influenced the prognosis. Offering these elucidations enables physicians to evaluate whether the AI's rationale corresponds with recognized medical knowledge. Clinicians are more inclined to believe and incorporate algorithmic insights into clinical practice when they can comprehend the rationale behind the forecasts.

Performance reliability constitutes a crucial element of confidence in AI-assisted healthcare systems. Clinicians must ensure that AI models reliably yield accurate and trustworthy outcomes across diverse patient groups and therapeutic settings (Asan et al., 2020, p. 3). This reliability necessitates thorough testing of AI algorithms with multiple datasets that encompass various demographic groupings and medical situations. Inadequate validation of AI systems may yield biased or wrong predictions, eroding trust and potentially jeopardizing patient safety.

Validation techniques are essential for verifying that AI technologies comply with clinical standards prior to their implementation in healthcare settings. Clinical validation entails the assessment of AI systems through the utilization of authentic medical data and the evaluation of their efficacy in comparison to recognized diagnostic or therapeutic standards. Regulatory authorities in numerous nations mandate such validation to guarantee that AI tools comply with safety and efficacy criteria prior to their deployment in healthcare facilities. Ongoing assessment of AI performance post-deployment is essential to guarantee that models retain accuracy as clinical conditions and patient demographics change.

The level of trust in human–AI collaboration is affected by the extent of control clinicians exert over AI-assisted judgments. Healthcare personnel must possess the authority to evaluate, interrogate, and supersede AI-generated suggestions when deemed essential (Almotairi et al., 2022, p. 3). Preserving a human-in-the-loop architecture guarantees that clinicians maintain final accountability for patient care decisions. This perspective emphasizes that AI operates as an auxiliary instrument rather than an independent decision-maker.

Training and education are crucial in fostering clinician trust in AI systems. Healthcare practitioners who comprehend the operational mechanics of AI systems are more inclined to utilize them efficiently and ethically. Educational programs that impart AI principles, data analysis abilities, and ethical issues enable clinicians to cultivate the confidence required for collaboration with intelligent technologies.

# 4. IMPLEMENTATION STRATEGIES FOR HUMAN–AI CLINICAL SYSTEMS

## 4.1 Organizational Readiness for AI Integration in Healthcare

The integration of artificial intelligence in healthcare systems necessitates not just technology advancement but also thorough organizational preparedness. Healthcare organizations must implement the requisite structures, resources, and governance frameworks to facilitate the integration of AI technologies inside clinical settings. In the absence of sufficient institutional preparation, even advanced AI tools may not realize their intended effects. Organizational readiness includes assessing leadership commitment, digital infrastructure capabilities, workforce preparedness, and regulatory compliance in healthcare businesses.

Leadership support is a pivotal factor affecting the successful application of AI. Healthcare leaders are crucial in defining strategic priorities, distributing resources, and cultivating a culture that promotes technological innovation. When organizational leaders actively endorse digital transformation projects, they foster a climate conducive to the adoption of AI-based solutions by physicians and staff (Rahimi et al., 2024, p. 25). Leadership engagement guarantees that AI efforts are congruent with overarching institutional objectives, including the enhancement of patient outcomes, the optimization of operational efficiency, and the preservation of superior healthcare quality standards. Strategic leadership is crucial for directing long-term investments in digital technologies and for instituting governance frameworks that ensure the ethical and responsible utilization of AI.

Digital infrastructure constitutes a critical element of organizational preparedness. AI systems depend significantly on extensive quantities of high-quality data to operate efficiently. Healthcare businesses must maintain resilient digital infrastructures that can securely store, process, and transmit patient data. Electronic health record systems, medical imaging platforms, laboratory information systems, and other digital health technologies must exhibit interoperability to facilitate seamless data sharing. Moreover, healthcare organizations require dependable computing resources, secure cloud infrastructures, and robust data processing skills that enable AI algorithms to assess clinical information instantaneously.

Data quality and governance are crucial for equipping healthcare companies for AI integration. Inconsistent or missing patient data might markedly diminish the precision of AI predictions and clinical recommendations. Healthcare organizations must implement robust data management practices to assure the accuracy, completeness, and uniformity of health records (Mandl et al., 2024). Data governance policies are essential for safeguarding patient privacy and ensuring adherence to national and international data protection standards. These regulations delineate the protocols for the collection, storage, analysis, and dissemination of patient data within AI-integrated healthcare settings.

Workforce readiness constitutes a vital component of corporate preparation. Healthcare personnel must possess the requisite knowledge and abilities to engage effectively with AI technologies. This encompasses clinicians, administrative people, health informatics experts, and information technology staff who underpin the digital framework of healthcare organizations. Training programs and professional development initiatives are crucial for enabling healthcare staff to comprehend the functionality of AI tools, analyze their outputs, and integrate these systems into clinical workflows.

Regulatory compliance is a crucial factor in the deployment of AI systems in healthcare. Medical technology must comply with stringent regulatory criteria intended to safeguard patient safety and guarantee the dependability of clinical instruments. Healthcare organizations must assess whether AI applications comply with national regulations concerning medical devices, patient data protection, and clinical decision support technology (Vardas et al., 2025). Adherence to these standards fosters public confidence and guarantees that AI systems function within defined legal and ethical parameters.

## 4.2 Training Healthcare Professionals for AI Collaboration

As artificial intelligence becomes more incorporated into healthcare systems, the competencies demanded of healthcare personnel are changing. Successful collaboration between clinicians and AI technologies necessitates that healthcare professionals acquire new competencies to analyze, assess, and implement AI-generated insights in clinical practice (Mendes, 2025). It is imperative to train healthcare workers for collaboration with AI to ensure that technical advancements result in significant enhancements in patient care.

A crucial competency for clinicians utilizing AI technologies is AI literacy. AI literacy denotes a fundamental comprehension of the operational mechanisms of AI technologies, encompassing the essential principles of machine learning, data processing, and predictive modeling. Healthcare personnel should not become AI engineers; however, they must comprehend the capabilities and limitations of AI technologies to utilize them properly. AI literacy enables doctors to analyze algorithmic outputs, identify potential biases or mistakes, and ascertain when AI recommendations warrant scrutiny or validation through further clinical evaluation.

Data interpretation abilities are an essential competency for healthcare providers in AI-enhanced settings. AI systems frequently produce intricate outputs, including prediction risk scores, probability assessments, or visual representations of patterns in medical pictures. Clinicians must appropriately understand these outputs and integrate them into their clinical reasoning processes (Giordano et al., 2021, p. 6). A predictive model may suggest that a patient is at elevated risk for complications post-surgery. Clinicians must assess this prognosis in conjunction with other clinical indicators, patient history, and professional judgment to ascertain the most suitable course of action.

Digital competencies are becoming progressively vital in contemporary healthcare systems. Healthcare professionals must be proficient in engaging with digital health technology, such as electronic health records, telemedicine platforms, and AI-driven diagnostic instruments. Digital competency enables healthcare providers to adeptly navigate technology interfaces, retrieve pertinent patient information, and employ AI-assisted advice during consultations. As digital health technologies advance, continuous training programs will be essential to ensure healthcare personnel remain informed about new tools and optimal practices.

Interdisciplinary collaboration constitutes a crucial aspect of AI training within healthcare settings. The creation and execution of AI systems generally entail teams consisting of clinicians, data scientists, software engineers, and healthcare administrators. Efficient cooperation among these entities is crucial for guaranteeing that AI technologies are both technically sound and clinically pertinent. Clinicians offer domain experience that informs the creation of AI models, whilst data scientists and engineers supply technical knowledge pertinent to algorithm development and system integration.

Educational institutions and healthcare organizations are essential in equipping healthcare workers for collaboration with AI. Medical schools, nursing programs, and continuing education efforts are progressively integrating digital health and AI-related subjects into their curricula (Issa et al., 2024, p. 10). These educational programs seek to prepare future healthcare workers with the requisite expertise to operate within technologically sophisticated clinical settings.

Simulation-based training can serve as an effective method for equipping clinicians to engage with AI systems. Clinical simulations enable healthcare workers to utilize AI-assisted decision-making tools in realistic circumstances, ensuring patient safety is not compromised. These activities enable doctors to acquire practical expertise in reading AI-generated recommendations, addressing potential errors, and incorporating algorithmic insights into patient care.

Ultimately, preparing healthcare workers for AI collaboration necessitates the cultivation of technical expertise, digital competencies, and interdisciplinary communication skills. When doctors comprehend the functionality of AI technologies and their appropriate use in clinical practice, they are more adept at utilizing these tools efficiently. This training guarantees that human expertise is vital in healthcare delivery, while AI technology augment the analytical proficiency of medical experts.

## 4.3 Monitoring and Evaluating AI-Supported Clinical Workflows

The effective deployment of AI technologies in healthcare necessitates ongoing monitoring and assessment to guarantee that these systems function safely, efficiently, and in accordance with therapeutic objectives. Monitoring and evaluation frameworks assist healthcare companies in assessing the efficacy of human–AI collaborative workflows and pinpointing areas requiring enhancement. Through the rigorous assessment of AI-enhanced clinical systems, healthcare organizations can ascertain that technological advancements lead to improved patient outcomes and enhanced healthcare efficiency.

Diagnostic accuracy is a crucial metric for assessing AI-enhanced clinical procedures. AI systems intended for diagnostic assistance must exhibit elevated accuracy in disease identification and patient state prediction (Varnosfaderani & Forouzanfar, 2024). Evaluation generally entails juxtaposing AI-generated predictions with validated clinical diagnoses or expert evaluations. Elevated diagnostic precision signifies that AI systems can dependably assist physicians in recognizing medical disorders and suggesting suitable remedies.

Patient outcomes serve as a vital metric for assessing the efficacy of AI-integrated healthcare systems. The primary objective of incorporating AI technologies into healthcare is to enhance patient health and well-being. Evaluation frameworks assess whether AI-assisted therapies result in enhanced clinical outcomes, like decreased mortality rates, reduced hospital readmissions, or earlier disease identification. Through the analysis of patient outcomes, healthcare companies can ascertain the efficacy of AI technology in providing measurable advantages for patients.

Workflow efficiency is a crucial parameter for evaluating the influence of AI technologies in healthcare settings. AI solutions are frequently implemented with the anticipation that they will enhance clinical efficiency and alleviate administrative constraints (Bajpai, 2023, p. 7). Assessing workflow efficiency entails analyzing elements such as the duration of diagnostic evaluations, the rapidity of clinical decision-making, and the overall productivity of healthcare teams. Enhancements in workflow efficiency demonstrate that AI technologies are effectively improving the operational performance of healthcare organizations.

Clinician satisfaction is a crucial factor in assessing AI-enhanced clinical workflows. Healthcare personnel are more inclined to accept and routinely utilize AI solutions when they regard them as beneficial and trustworthy. Surveys, interviews, and observational studies can evaluate physicians' experiences with AI systems, encompassing their impressions of usability, trustworthiness, and use in clinical practice. Comprehending physician viewpoints aids healthcare organizations in recognizing possible obstacles to adoption and enhancing system design accordingly.

System dependability and safety are critical elements of evaluation frameworks. AI technologies must function reliably and sustain stable performance across many therapeutic settings Morley et al. (2021, p. 9). Evaluating system dependability entails analyzing parameters such as operational uptime, error rates, and the incidence of erroneous predictions or recommendations. Moreover, safety assessments guarantee that AI systems do not pose unforeseen hazards to patients or healthcare professionals.

Ongoing monitoring is crucial due to the potential evolution of AI systems as new data emerges, or healthcare situations fluctuate. Machine learning models developed using historical data may necessitate regular retraining to preserve their accuracy and relevance. Continuous assessment enables healthcare companies to determine when models require revision and guarantees that AI solutions maintain efficacy in practical clinical settings.

# 5. CHALLENGES, ETHICAL CONSIDERATIONS, AND FUTURE DIRECTIONS

## 5.1 Ethical and Regulatory Challenges in AI-Supported Healthcare

The use of artificial intelligence into healthcare systems offers substantial prospects for enhancing clinical decision-making and patient outcomes. Nevertheless, technology also presents intricate ethical and regulatory dilemmas that must be resolved to guarantee responsible and secure deployment. Given that healthcare decisions significantly impact human welfare, AI technologies employed in clinical settings must comply with rigorous ethical norms and regulatory frameworks that safeguard patient rights, promote openness, and uphold responsibility in medical practice.

A significant ethical concern related to AI-assisted healthcare is patient privacy. AI systems depend significantly on extensive datasets that encompass sensitive medical information, such as personal identities, medical histories, genetic data, and diagnostic records (Zeb et al., 2024, p. 123). The collecting, storage, and analysis of such data pose problems about confidentiality and data security. Unauthorized access to health data or incorrect data exchange may jeopardize patient privacy and potentially result in discrimination or misuse of personal health information. Healthcare firms must develop robust data security rules and encryption technology to secure patient information while allowing AI systems to evaluate medical data efficiently.

Another ethical dilemma pertains to algorithmic bias in AI systems. Machine learning models are developed with historical information, and if these datasets exhibit biases pertaining to gender, race, socioeconomic position, or geographic location, the resultant algorithms may yield inequitable or discriminating results. An AI system trained predominantly on data from a certain population may exhibit diminished accuracy when utilized with patients from diverse demographic groupings. Such gaps may result in misdiagnoses, inequitable treatment recommendations, or inequalities in healthcare access. Mitigating algorithmic bias necessitates meticulous data selection, broad training datasets, and ongoing monitoring to guarantee that AI systems yield fair and equitable results across various patient demographics.

Transparency constitutes a vital ethical consideration in AI-assisted healthcare. Numerous sophisticated AI systems, especially deep learning models, function through intricate computer processes that are challenging for humans to comprehend. The absence of transparency may provide difficulties for physicians in comprehending the rationale behind an AI system's specific advice (Weiner et al., 2024, p. 6). In healthcare settings, decisions frequently require justification to patients, regulatory authorities, and professional colleagues. Consequently, it is imperative to develop explainable AI systems that offer interpretable insights into algorithmic reasoning to uphold confidence and responsibility in clinical decision-making.

Accountability poses a considerable ethical dilemma when AI technology are utilized in healthcare decision-making. When an AI system is implicated in a medical blunder or erroneous advice, the attribution of responsibility for the outcome may be ambiguous. Healthcare workers retain accountability for patient care decisions; nevertheless, the impact of algorithmic recommendations may obfuscate liability issues. Consequently, explicit rules must be formulated to delineate the duties and responsibilities of clinicians, healthcare institutions, and technology developers in the utilization of AI-assisted decision-making tools.

Regulatory frameworks are crucial in tackling ethical concerns and guaranteeing the safe implementation of AI technologies in healthcare systems. Numerous nations have instituted regulatory frameworks for medical technology that encompass mandates for clinical validation, risk evaluation, and continuous oversight of AI-driven systems (Gill et al., 2023, p. 1647). Regulatory bodies frequently mandate that developers prove AI technologies comply with safety, accuracy, and dependability standards prior to their use in clinical environments.

Alongside national rules, international organizations and professional medical associations are progressively formulating recommendations for the ethical application of AI in healthcare. These frameworks underscore themes such patient autonomy, equity, transparency, and accountability. Ethical guidelines advocate for developers and healthcare organizations to emphasize patient safety, reduce bias, and guarantee that AI technologies augment rather than supplant human clinical judgment.

## 5.2 Technical and Organizational Barriers to Implementation

Despite the increasing promise of artificial intelligence in healthcare, certain technical and organizational obstacles persist, impeding its extensive adoption. Effectively integrating AI technologies into healthcare systems necessitates addressing issues associated with data quality, system interoperability, corporate culture, and financial limitations. Comprehending these obstacles is crucial for formulating methods that facilitate the efficient incorporation of AI tools into therapeutic settings.

Data quality issues constitute a major technological hurdle in AI-enhanced healthcare systems. Artificial intelligence systems depend on extensive datasets to discern patterns and produce predictive insights. Medical data are frequently insufficient, inconsistent, or fragmented across many information systems (Zeb et al., 2024, p. 123). Patient records may exhibit incomplete information, erroneous entries, or inconsistencies in data formatting among various healthcare organizations. Subpar data quality can markedly diminish the precision and dependability of AI models, resulting in erroneous predictions or deceptive clinical recommendations.

Healthcare firms must thus engage in enhanced data management methods, standardized data formats, and quality assurance processes to guarantee the effective operation of AI systems.

Interoperability constraints are a significant obstacle to the application of AI in healthcare settings. Healthcare organizations frequently employ various digital systems to oversee patient information, encompassing electronic health records, laboratory systems, imaging databases, and pharmaceutical administration platforms. If these systems are not engineered for effective intercommunication, the integration of AI tools becomes increasingly challenging. The absence of interoperability may necessitate manual data transfers or intricate system upgrades, so elevating costs and diminishing efficiency. Establishing standardized data sharing protocols and interoperable health information systems is essential for facilitating seamless AI integration.

Organizational opposition to technological change constitutes an additional obstacle to AI adoption. Healthcare personnel may exhibit reluctance to embrace AI technologies due to apprehensions about job displacement, augmented workload, or uncertainty surrounding the dependability of algorithmic recommendations. Certain clinicians may regard AI systems as intrusive technology that disrupt conventional healthcare practices (Adibi et al., 2025, p. 17). Addressing this opposition necessitates the implementation of effective change management strategies that highlight the supportive function of AI technology in augmenting, rather than supplanting, clinical competence. Involving healthcare experts in the design and deployment of AI systems can foster confidence and enhance acceptability.

Financial limitations may hinder the implementation of AI technologies in healthcare organizations. Creating, executing, and sustaining AI systems frequently necessitates significant expenditures in digital infrastructure, data management systems, and specific technical proficiency. Smaller healthcare facilities or organizations with constrained finances may struggle to dedicate resources for sophisticated AI systems. Furthermore, continuous maintenance, software updates, and cybersecurity protocols augment the long-term expenses related to AI installation.

The incorporation of AI tools into intricate healthcare systems introduces further operational difficulties. Healthcare settings encompass complex workflows that require interactions among physicians, nurses, laboratory technicians, administrative personnel, and other professions (Sarker, 2023, p. 347). AI technology must be meticulously incorporated into these procedures without compromising patient care or exacerbating administrative costs. Inadequately built technologies can introduce superfluous stages in clinical workflows or produce an abundance of alerts that inundate healthcare workers.

Overcoming these technical and organizational obstacles necessitates collaborative efforts among healthcare institutions, technology developers, legislators, and regulatory bodies. Investments in digital infrastructure, standardized data systems, workforce training, and collaborative design methodologies can mitigate numerous problems related to AI adoption. By proactively addressing these obstacles, healthcare organizations can cultivate settings in which AI technologies augment clinical practice and boost healthcare outcomes.

## 5.3 Future Directions of Human–AI Collaboration in Healthcare

Human knowledge and artificial intelligence are shaping healthcare's future. As AI systems improve and healthcare data grows, human–AI collaboration may improve. These innovations are expected to transform how doctors diagnose, treat, and customize treatments.

Explainable AI is a major advancement in AI-assisted healthcare. Clinicians must understand algorithmic predictions as AI models get increasingly complex. Advanced explainability techniques will likely be used in future AI systems to clarify model data interpretation and recommendation creation (Alkan et al., 2025, p. 13). These advances will increase clinician trust and help them use AI data more confidently.

AI is expected to impact personalized medicine. Traditional medical treatments often use uniform clinical guidelines that may not account for patient differences. AI-driven predictive analytics can analyze genetic, lifestyle, and clinical data to determine patient-specific therapy alternatives. These data can help healthcare practitioners create more personalised treatment strategies, which may improve efficacy and reduce negative effects.

Healthcare innovation is growing with autonomous clinical support systems. Due to ethical and regulatory issues, complete autonomy in medical decision-making is unlikely, although AI systems will provide increasingly advanced therapeutic treatment (Goh et al., 2025). AI-driven monitoring systems can continuously analyze patient data from wearable sensors and hospital devices and inform clinicians of early health worsening. These systems could improve healthcare prevention.

Intelligent healthcare ecosystems that integrate AI technologies across healthcare delivery are a major future achievement. These environments allow AI systems to analyze data from electronic health records, diagnostic imaging platforms, genomic databases, and remote monitoring devices. These integrated systems can provide holistic patient health perspectives and improve clinical decision-making by combining data from multiple sources.

Natural language processing should improve clinician-digital health system communication. AI systems that evaluate clinical notes, medical literature, and patient communications may help healthcare workers find relevant information. AI-driven solutions may condense patient data, highlight key clinical markers, or offer relevant research to support therapy recommendations.

Despite technological advances, healthcare will depend on strong human–AI cooperation. AI systems cannot replicate empathy, ethical judgment, and contextual understanding, therefore healthcare staff will remain crucial in patient care (Akinnagbe, 2024, p. 409). AI will increasingly collaborate with doctors to improve their analytical skills.

## CONCLUSION

The incorporation of artificial intelligence into healthcare systems signifies a fundamental change in the design and execution of clinical decision-making, patient management, and medical processes. The increasing accessibility of extensive health data, along with advancements in machine learning and predictive analytics, has generated novel prospects for augmenting diagnostic precision, refining treatment strategies, and optimizing healthcare delivery. The efficacy of these technologies relies not solely on their technical capabilities but also on healthcare organizations' capacity to create collaborative environments in which human expertise and artificial intelligence operate synergistically.

The collaboration between humans and AI in healthcare underscores the necessity of harmonizing technology advancement with clinical expertise. AI systems are proficient at analyzing intricate datasets and recognizing patterns that may elude human perception; however, doctors offer contextual insight, ethical judgment, and patient-focused communication that are vital to medical practice. Creating efficient collaborative workflows necessitates the careful incorporation of AI technologies into clinical procedures, underpinned by human-centered system design, transparent algorithms, and dependable decision-support systems.

The successful implementation relies on organizational preparedness, employee training, and ongoing assessment of AI-supported systems. Healthcare organizations must guarantee that professionals have the requisite digital capabilities to evaluate AI-generated insights while retaining accountability for patient care decisions. Simultaneously, robust governance frameworks are essential to tackle ethical issues of data privacy, algorithmic bias, and regulatory adherence.

Future advancements in explainable AI, predictive analytics, and intelligent healthcare ecosystems are anticipated to enhance the significance of human–AI collaboration in medical practice. These advancements will facilitate more individualized and proactive healthcare strategies while assisting doctors with progressively advanced analytical instruments. The future of healthcare will hinge on establishing lasting collaborations between human knowledge and intelligent technologies, ensuring that innovation improves clinical practice while upholding the core values of safety, trust, and patient-centered care.

## REFERENCES


Abut, S., Okut, H., Zackula, R., & Kallail, K. J. (2023). Deep neural networks and applications in medical research. In *Artificial intelligence*. IntechOpen., DOI: 10.5772/intechopen.112371

Adeniran, A. A., Onebunne, A. P., & William, P. (2024). Explainable AI (XAI) in healthcare: Enhancing trust and transparency in critical decision-making. *World Journal of Advanced Research and Reviews*, *23*(3), 2447–2658. DOI: 10.30574/wjarr.2024.23.3.2936

Adibi, A., Xu, C., Ji, Z., Kaur, J., Chen, W., Healey, E., Nuwagira, B., Ye, W., Woollard, G., Xu, M., Cui, H. T., Xi, J., Chang, T., Bikia, V., Zhang, N., Noori, A., Yuan, X., Hossain, M. B., Frank, H. A., . . . Jabbour, S. (2025). Recent advances, applications and open challenges in machine learning for health: Reflections from research roundtables at ML4H 2024 symposium. *arXiv*. https://doi.org//arxiv.2502.06693DOI: 10.48550

Akinnagbe, O. B. (2024). Human-AI collaboration: Enhancing productivity and decision-making. *International Journal of Education Management and Technology*, *2*(3), 387–417. DOI: 10.58578/ijemt.v2i3.4209

Alanazi, M. M. F., Almutairi, S., Alarjani, N., Alghaylan, M. Y. A., Aljawhari, M. S. M., & Alkhulaifi, A. A. S. (2024). Advancements in AI-driven diagnostic radiology: Enhancing accuracy and efficiency. *International Journal of Health Sciences*, *8*(S1), 737–749. DOI: 10.53730/ijhs.v8nS1.14928

Alkan, M. F., Zakariyya, I., Leighton, S., Sivangi, K. B., Anagnostopoulos, C., & Deligianni, F. (2025). Artificial intelligence-driven clinical decision support systems. *arXiv*. https://doi.org//arxiv.2501.09628DOI: 10.48550

Almotairi, A. H., Alswegi, F. H., Almutairi, M., Almotiry, F. S. F., Rakhimi, M. N. H. A., Aljamily, A. H. M., Aldosari, N. M. M., & Alaoufi, R. Y. (2022). A review in the application of artificial intelligence in many medical sectors. *Journal of Population Therapeutics and Clinical Pharmacology = Journal de la Thérapeutique des Populations et de la Pharmacologie Clinique*. Advance online publication. DOI: 10.53555//jptcp.v29i04.5772

Asan, O., Bayrak, A. E., & Choudhury, A. (2020). Artificial intelligence and human trust in healthcare: Focus on clinicians. *Journal of Medical Internet Research*, *22*(6), e15154. Advance online publication. DOI: 10.2196/15154 PMID: 32558657

Bajpai, A. (2023). Advancing healthcare through artificial intelligence: Innovations at the intersection of AI and medicine. *Journal of Propulsion Technology*, *44*(2). Advance online publication. DOI: 10.52783/tjjpt.v44.i2.131

Chatterjee, I., Das, K. C., & Mukherjee, K. (2024). Revolutionizing innovations and impact of artificial intelligence in healthcare. *International Journal for Multidisciplinary Research*, *6*(3), 19333. Advance online publication. DOI: 10.36948/ijfmr.2024.v06i03.19333

Choudhury, A. (2022). Toward an ecologically valid conceptual framework for the use of artificial intelligence in clinical settings. *JMIR Human Factors*, *9*(2), e35421. Advance online publication. DOI: 10.2196/35421 PMID: 35727615

Cuéllar, M.-F., Dean, J., Doshi-Velez, F., Hennessy, J. L., Konwinski, A., Koyejo, S., Moiloa, P., Pierson, E., & Patterson, D. (2024). Shaping AI's impact on billions of lives. *arXiv*. https://doi.org//arxiv.2412.02730DOI: 10.48550

Devi, M.M Syamala Devi. (2024). Artificial intelligence in medicine. *International Journal for Multidisciplinary Research*, *6*(1), 12490. Advance online publication. DOI: 10.36948/ijfmr.2024.v06i01.12490

Fahim, Y. A., Hasani, I. W., Kabba, S., & Ragab, W. M. (2025). Artificial intelligence in healthcare and medicine: Clinical applications, therapeutic advances, and future perspectives. *European Journal of Medical Research*, *30*(1), 848. DOI: 10.1186/s40001-025-03196-w PMID: 40988064

Fatima, I., Grover, V., Khan, I. R., Ahmad, N., & Yadav, A. (2023). Artificial intelligence in medical field. *EAI Endorsed Transactions on Pervasive Health and Technology*, *9*. Advance online publication. DOI: 10.4108/eetpht.9.4713

Ferguson, J. (2025). The human element: Ethical guardrails for AI in modern medicine. *The American Journal of Cosmetic Surgery*, *42*(3), 149–154. DOI: 10.1177/07488068251359686

Gill, A. Y., Saeed, A., Rasool, S., Husnain, A., & Hussain, H. K. (2023). Revolutionizing healthcare: How machine learning is transforming patient diagnoses. *Journal of Wood Science*, *2*(10), 1638–1652. DOI: 10.58344/jws.v2i10.449

Giordano, C., Brennan, M., Mohamed, B., Rashidi, P., Modave, F., & Tighe, P. (2021). Accessing artificial intelligence for clinical decision-making. *Frontiers in Digital Health*, *3*, 645232. Advance online publication. DOI: 10.3389/fdgth.2021.645232 PMID: 34713115

Goh, E., Bunning, B., Khoong, E. C., Gallo, R. J., Milstein, A., Centola, D., & Chen, J. H. (2025). Physician clinical decision modification and bias assessment in a randomized controlled trial of AI assistance. *Communications Medicine*, *5*(1), 59. DOI: 10.1038/s43856-025-00781-2 PMID: 40038550

Issa, W. B., Shorbagi, A., Alshorman, A., Rababa, M., Majed, K. A., Radwan, H., Raffat, F. A., Al-Yateem, N., Mottershead, R., Abdelrahim, D. N., Hijazi, H., Khasawneh, W., Ibrahim, A., Abbas, N., & Fakhry, R. (2024). Shaping the future: Perspectives on the integration of artificial intelligence in health profession education. *Research Square*. https://doi.org/DOI: 10.21203/rs.3.rs-4396289/v1

Jia, J., & Zhao, S. (2025). Ethical and legal governance of generative AI in Chinese healthcare. *Journal of Multidisciplinary Healthcare*, *5405*, 5405–5419. Advance online publication. DOI: 10.2147/JMDH.S541271 PMID: 40917542

Kusumadewi, S., & Miladiyah, I. (2023). Do clinical decision support systems improve patient safety? *Indonesian Journal of Electrical Engineering and Computer Science*, *30*(3), 1748. DOI: 10.11591/ijeecs.v30.i3.pp1748-1761

Lysaght, T., Lim, H. Y., Xafis, V., & Ngiam, K. Y. (2019). AI-assisted decision-making in healthcare. *Asian Bioethics Review*, *11*(3), 299–314. DOI: 10.1007/s41649-019-00096-0 PMID: 33717318

Malerbi, F. K., Nakayama, L. F., Dychiao, R. G., Ribeiro, L. Z., Villanueva, C., Celi, L. A., & Regatieri, C. V. (2023). Digital education for the deployment of artificial intelligence in health care. *Journal of Medical Internet Research*, *25*, e43333. Advance online publication. DOI: 10.2196/43333 PMID: 37347537

Mandl, K. D., Gottlieb, D., & Mandel, J. C. (2024). Integration of AI in healthcare requires an interoperable digital data ecosystem. *Nature Medicine*, *30*(3), 631–634. DOI: 10.1038/s41591-023-02783-w PMID: 38291298

Mendes, J. M. (2025). Reimagining healthcare education through nurturing AI-driven innovation. *BMC Medical Education*, *25*(1), 1644. DOI: 10.1186/s12909-025-08254-9 PMID: 41291684

Morley, J., Morton, C. E., Karpathakis, K., Taddeo, M., & Floridi, L. (2021). Towards a framework for evaluating AI systems for health. SSRN *Electronic Journal*. https://doi.org/DOI: 10.2139/ssrn.3826358

Ndabu, T., Mulgund, P., Sharman, R., & Singh, R. (2021). Perceptual gaps between clinicians and technologists on health IT errors. *JMIR Human Factors*, *8*(1). Advance online publication. DOI: 10.2196/21884 PMID: 33544089

Papadopoulos, P., Soflano, M., Chaudy, Y., Adejo, W., & Connolly, T. (2022). A systematic review of rule-based clinical decision support systems. *Health Technology (Hong Kong)*, *12*(4), 713. DOI: 10.1007/s12553-022-00672-9

Park, S. H., & Langlotz, C. P. (2025). Crucial role of understanding in human-AI interaction for clinical adoption. *Korean Journal of Radiology*, *26*(4), 287. DOI: 10.3348/kjr.2025.0071 PMID: 40015562

Rahimi, A. K., Pienaar, O., Ghadimi, M., Canfell, O. J., Pole, J. D., Shrapnel, S., van der Vegt, A., & Sullivan, C. (2024). Implementing AI in hospitals to achieve a learning health system. *Journal of Medical Internet Research*, *26*, e49655. Advance online publication. DOI: 10.2196/49655 PMID: 39094106

Reuben, J. S., Meiri, H., & Arien-Zakay, H. (2024). AI's pivotal impact on redefining stakeholder roles in healthcare. *Frontiers in Digital Health*, *6*. Advance online publication. DOI: 10.3389/fdgth.2024.1458811 PMID: 39564581

Saadeh, M., Janhonen, J., de Beer, E. S., Castelyn, C., & Hoffman, D. N. (2025). Automation complacency in medical decision-making. *AI and Ethics*, *5*(6), 5783–5793. Advance online publication. DOI: 10.1007/s43681-025-00825-2

Salahuddin, Z., Woodruff, H. C., Chatterjee, A., & Lambin, P. (2021). Transparency of deep neural networks for medical image analysis. *Computers in Biology and Medicine*, *140*, 105111. DOI: 10.1016/j.compbiomed.2021.105111 PMID: 34891095

Samajdar, S. S., Chatterjee, R., Mukherjee, S., Dey, A. K., Saboo, B., Pal, J., Joshi, S., & Chatterjee, N. (2025). Artificial intelligence in healthcare: Current trends and future directions. *Current Medical Issues*, *23*(1), 53–60. DOI: 10.4103/cmi.cmi_93_24

Sarker, M. (2023). Assessing the integration of AI technologies in enhancing patient care delivery. *Journal of Knowledge Learning and Science Technology*, *2*(2), 338–351. DOI: 10.60087/jklst.vol2.n2.p351

Siddiq, M. (2021). Integration of machine learning in clinical decision support systems. *Eduvest*, *1*(12), 1579–1591. DOI: 10.59188/eduvest.v1i12.809

Sokol, K., Fackler, J. C., & Vogt, J. E. (2025). Artificial intelligence should support clinical reasoning. *npj. Digital Medicine*, *8*(1), 345. DOI: 10.1038/s41746-025-01725-9 PMID: 40494886

Spear, J., Ehrenfeld, J. M., & Miller, B. J. (2023). Applications of artificial intelligence in health care delivery. *Journal of Medical Systems*, *47*(1), 121. Advance online publication. DOI: 10.1007/s10916-023-02018-y PMID: 37975946

Sutton, R. T., Pincock, D., Baumgart, D. C., Sadowski, D., Fedorak, R. N., & Kroeker, K. I. (2020). Overview of clinical decision support systems. *npj. Digital Medicine*, *3*(1), 17. DOI: 10.1038/s41746-020-0221-y PMID: 32047862

Ueda, D., Kakinuma, T., Fujita, S., Kamagata, K., Fushimi, Y., Ito, R., Matsui, Y., Nozaki, T., Nakaura, T., Fujima, N., Tatsugami, F., Yanagawa, M., Hirata, K., Yamada, A., Tsuboyama, T., Kawamura, M., Fujioka, T., & Naganawa, S. (2023). Fairness of artificial intelligence in healthcare. *Japanese Journal of Radiology*, *42*(1), 3–15. DOI: 10.1007/s11604-023-01474-3 PMID: 37540463

Vardas, E. P., Marketou, M., & Vardas, P. (2025). Medicine, healthcare and the AI act. *European Heart Journal. Digital Health*, *6*(4), 833–839. DOI: 10.1093/ehjdh/ztaf041 PMID: 40703136

Varnosfaderani, S. M., & Forouzanfar, M. (2024). The role of AI in hospitals and clinics. *Bioengineering (Basel, Switzerland)*, *11*(4), 337. DOI: 10.3390/bioengineering11040337 PMID: 38671759

Vitacca, M., Giardini, A., Gazzi, L., & Vitacca, M. (2022). Hidden biases in clinical decision-making. *Monaldi Archives for Chest Disease*. Advance online publication. DOI: 10.4081/monaldi.2022.2339 PMID: 36069639

Wang, L., Zhang, Z., Wang, D., Cao, W., Zhou, X., Zhang, P., Liu, J., Fan, X., & Tian, F. (2023). Human-centered design of AI clinical decision systems. *Frontiers of Computer Science*, *5*. Advance online publication. DOI: 10.3389/fcomp.2023.1187299

Weiner, E., Dankwa-Mullan, I., Nelson, W. A., & Hassanpour, S. (2024). Ethical challenges in AI clinical integration. *arXiv*. https://doi.org//arxiv.2412.03576DOI: 10.48550

Wu, S., Cao, W., Fu, S., Yao, B., Yang, Z., Yin, C., Mishra, V., Addison, D., Zhang, P., & Wang, D. (2024). CardioAI system for cardiotoxicity detection. *arXiv*. https://doi.org//arxiv.2410.04592DOI: 10.48550

Yoon, S., Goh, H., Lee, P. C., Tan, H. C., Teh, M. M., Lim, D. S. T., Kwee, A., Chandran, S., Carmody, D., Swee, D. S., Tan, S. Y. T., Wong, A. J.-W., Choo, C. H., Wee, Z., & Bee, Y. M. (2024). AI-enabled prescription advisory tool study. *JMIR Human Factors*, *11*. Advance online publication. DOI: 10.2196/50939 PMID: 38869934

Zeb, S., Abbasi, N., & Fahad, M. (2024). AI in healthcare: Revolutionizing diagnosis and therapy. *International Journal of Multidisciplinary Sciences and Arts*, *3*(3), 118–128. DOI: 10.47709/ijmdsa.v3i3.4546

## ADDITIONAL READING


Abbas, Q., Khan, M. T., & Alharbi, S. M. (2025). Explainable AI in clinical decision support systems: A systematic review of transparency, trust, and implementation challenges. *Journal of Medical Systems*, *49*(1), 112. DOI: 10.1007/s10916-025-02145-7 PMID: 40932673

Elechi, U., Roberts, J., & Mensah, P. (2025). Artificial intelligence in healthcare: A narrative review of clinical applications and organizational readiness. *Journal of Healthcare Leadership*, *17*, 45–63. DOI: 10.2147/JHL.S553748 PMID: 41488817

Jung, I.-C., Schuler, K., Zerlik, M., Grummt, S., Sedlmayr, M., & Sedlmayr, B. (2025). Overview of basic design recommendations for user-centered explanation interfaces for AI-based clinical decision support systems: A scoping review. *Digital Health*, *11*, 1–18. DOI: 10.1177/20552076241308298 PMID: 39866885

Jung, J., Park, H., & Kim, S. (2025). Evaluating the impact of explainable AI on clinicians' acceptance of machine learning–based clinical decision support systems. *International Journal of Medical Informatics*, *198*, 105894. DOI: 10.1016/j.ijmedinf.2025.105894

Liu, S., Wright, A., McCoy, A. B., & Sittig, D. F. (2024). Leveraging explainable artificial intelligence to optimize clinical decision support alert criteria. *Journal of the American Medical Informatics Association : JAMIA*, *31*(4), 968–977. DOI: 10.1093/jamia/ocae019 PMID: 38383050

Oei, S. P., van der Velde, M., & Vos, M. (2025). Artificial intelligence in clinical decision support and the prediction of adverse events: Challenges and future pathways. *Frontiers in Digital Health*, *7*, 1403047. Advance online publication. DOI: 10.3389/fdgth.2025.1403047 PMID: 40520218

Rezaeian, O., Smith, J., & Patel, N. (2025). The impact of AI explanations on clinicians' trust and diagnostic accuracy in breast cancer. *Applied Ergonomics*, *129*, 104577. DOI: 10.1016/j.apergo.2025.104577 PMID: 40577970

Shawi, R. E., & Jamel, L. (2025). Leveraging ChatGPT and explainable AI for enhancing clinical decision support. *Scientific Reports*, *15*(1), 38786. DOI: 10.1038/s41598-025-22784-8 PMID: 41193683

Tun, H. M., Rahman, F., & Lee, A. (2025). Trust in artificial intelligence–based clinical decision support systems: A systematic review. *Journal of Medical Internet Research*, *27*, e69678. DOI: 10.2196/69678 PMID: 40772775 van Leersum, C. M., van der Zande, I., & Habli, I. (2025). Human centred explainable AI decision-making in healthcare. *Healthcare Analytics*, *5*, 100312. DOI: 10.1016/j.health.2025.100312

## KEY TERMS AND DEFINITIONS

**Algorithmic Bias:** A systematic bias in AI-generated results resulting from imbalanced training data, erroneous model assumptions, or inequitable data representation, resulting in unjust treatment recommendations for specific patient populations.

**Artificial Intelligence:** A computational skill that allows machines to emulate human thinking, learning, prediction, and pattern recognition to facilitate healthcare analysis and decision-making.

**Clinical Decision Support System:** A digital system that evaluates patient data and medical expertise to furnish clinicians with evidence-based suggestions for diagnosis, therapy, and risk management.

**Explainable Artificial Intelligence:** A design methodology for artificial intelligence that renders algorithmic thinking transparent and interpretable, enabling healthcare professionals to comprehend the generation of forecasts or suggestions.

**Human–AI Collaboration:** A clinical workflow approach wherein healthcare professionals and AI systems collaborate by integrating human judgment, ethical reasoning, and empathy with machine-driven data analysis.

**Interoperability:** The capacity of various healthcare technologies, databases, and digital platforms to interchange, understand, and utilize data seamlessly across clinical systems.

**Predictive Analytics:** An analytical technique grounded in data that utilizes historical and real-time patient information to predict health risks, illness development, or treatment outcomes.

**System Reliability:** The extent to which an AI-assisted healthcare system reliably operates with precision, safety, and consistency across various clinical scenarios and patient demographics.

**Transparency:** The clarity of an AI system that enables users to comprehend its objectives, data origins, reasoning, and constraints in clinical decision support.

**Workflow Integration:** The integration of AI tools into established clinical practices and hospital information systems to enhance efficiency, usability, and continuous patient care.

# Chapter 3
# Explainability-as-a-Defense (XaaD) for Secure Healthcare AI

**Shaik Johny Basha**
http://orcid.org/0000-0003-1000-6564
*Jawaharlal Nehru Technological University, Kakinada, India*

**Veeraiah Duggineni**
http://orcid.org/0000-0002-4230-4606
*Lakireddy Bali Reddy College of Engineering, India*

**Sumalatha Lingamgunta**
*Jawaharlal Nehru Technological University, Kakinada, India*

## ABSTRACT

*The rapid adoption of AI in healthcare has made the clinical functionality more convenient at the expense of exposing multifaceted cybersecurity risks which are difficult to detect using the traditional perimeter-based approach to security. Although explainable AI is fully deployed with intent to achieve transparency and regulation compliance, the prospects of explainable AI as a native security control have not been pursued. The chapter is a presentation of Explainability-as-a-Defense (XaaD) a framework which transforms the results of AI explanations into continuous behavioral fingerprints to perform proactive cybersecurity monitoring. A XaaD architecture that takes advantage of a layered architecture with explainability generation, drift detection, and human-in-the-loop validation is proposed, which is shown in the example of a clinical decision support, medical chatbots, IoMT analytics, and federated learning. XaaD re-imagines explainability as a post-hoc interpretability condition into an active form of defensive health care AI performance of trust.*

DOI: 10.4018/979-8-3373-9119-9.ch003

# 1. INTRODUCTION

## 1.1 The Rise of AI-Enabled Healthcare Systems

The integration of artificial intelligence into healthcare represents one of the most consequential technology transitions in the history of medicine. Over the past decade, machine learning algorithms, deep neural networks, and large language models have migrated from research laboratories into active clinical environments, reshaping workflows across diagnostics, therapeutics, patient monitoring, and healthcare administrative operations globally (Topol, 2019). Radiology departments now deploy convolutional neural networks capable of detecting pulmonary nodules, diabetic retinopathy, and intracranial hemorrhages with sensitivity rates rivaling experienced clinicians across diverse healthcare settings from teaching hospitals in North America and Europe to district health facilities in lower-and-middle-income countries (Topol, 2019; Noor et al., 2025).

The global healthcare AI market is projected to reach over $110 billion by 2030, growing at a compound annual rate exceeding 38% (MarketsandMarkets, 2025). This growth is not confined to well-resourced institutional settings; AI is penetrating rural telehealth platforms, mobile diagnostic units, and home-based monitoring ecosystems, extending advanced clinical intelligence to previously underserved populations. Critically, these systems are deeply embedded within complex, interconnected digital infrastructures that interface with hospital information systems, laboratory platforms, pharmacy dispensing systems, and insurance claims networks.

## 1.2 Cybersecurity Challenges in Clinical AI Pipelines

The cybersecurity landscape confronting healthcare organizations has grown dramatically more hostile in parallel with the sector's digital transformation. Healthcare consistently ranks among the most targeted industries globally (American Hospital Association, 2025). In 2024 alone, healthcare data breaches exposed over 276 million patient records, with average breach costs reaching $10.93 million per incident, the highest of any industry (IBM Security, 2023; HIPAA Journal, 2025). The introduction of AI into clinical pipelines has not merely inherited these existing vulnerabilities; it has generated an entirely new and qualitatively distinct category of cybersecurity challenges operating at the reasoning layer of deployed models.

Adversarial input attacks exploit the mathematical brittleness of neural networks by introducing carefully crafted perturbations that are imperceptible to human observers, causing AI to produce dangerously incorrect predictions with high confidence (Kaviani et al., 2022). Model poisoning attacks corrupt the training pipeline, embedding hidden behaviors that lie dormant until triggered. Backdoor attacks insert

Trojan triggers into pre-trained foundation models, a particularly insidious threat given the increasing reliance on publicly available pre-trained models fine-tuned for clinical tasks (He et al., 2024). What makes these threats uniquely dangerous is their technical subtlety: an adversarial perturbation that causes a chest X-ray AI to miss a malignancy generates no network intrusion alert, no security log entry, and leaves no forensic trace detectable by conventional tools.

## 1.3 Limitations of Traditional AI Security Mechanisms

The cybersecurity frameworks governing healthcare AI were largely developed before the clinical AI era. Standards such as the NIST Cybersecurity Framework and the HIPAA Security Rule operate at the infrastructure layer, addressing threats to systems and data rather than threats to algorithmic reasoning. The NIST AI Risk Management Framework (NIST, 2023) introduced AI-specific governance guidance yet stops short of prescribing real-time architectural mechanisms for continuous model security verification.

Adversarial robustness techniques including adversarial training and certified defenses are fundamentally reactive: they defend against attack types anticipated at training time and provide no protection against novel attack vectors, model substitution, or supply chain compromise (Vadillo et al., 2025). Regulatory frameworks including the FDA's AI/ML-based SaMD pathway (FDA, 2021) and the EU AI Act (European Parliament, 2024) impose robustness and transparency requirements but stop short of prescribing operational mechanisms for continuous reasoning-layer security verification.

## 1.4 Explainability Beyond Trust: A Security Opportunity

Explainable AI (XAI) has emerged as a critical domain motivated by the imperative to make opaque models interpretable to the humans who depend upon their outputs. Techniques such as SHAP (Lundberg and Lee, 2017) and LIME (Ribeiro et al., 2016), alongside Grad-CAM and attention visualization, have been developed for post-hoc interpretability across diverse architectures. In healthcare, XAI has been positioned primarily as serving trust-building and regulatory compliance, which are legitimate but incomplete objectives (Noor et al., 2025).

A SHAP explanation for a diagnostic decision encodes the model's internal attribution of decision weight across all input features at a specific inference, functioning as a fingerprint of the model's reasoning process at that moment. Under normal operation, explanation fingerprints for clinically similar cases exhibit statistically consistent attribution patterns. This consistency is disrupted by adversarial interference: adversarial inputs force the model to assign weight to irrelevant or manipulated features, producing explanation signatures that diverge detectably from established baselines. Existing work has demonstrated that adversarial attacks on post-hoc explanation methods produce measurable distortions in feature attribution outputs (Slack et al., 2020), confirming that explanation anomalies are empirically observable security signals, not merely theoretical constructs. It is important to note, however, that explanation methods themselves carry known limitations regarding faithfulness and stability, which are addressed directly in Sections 2.3 and 10.1, and which constitute a central design challenge for the XaaD framework.

## 1.5 Research Problem, Propositions, and Chapter Objectives

The central research problem addressed in this chapter is as follows: given that healthcare AI systems face adversarial attacks that operate at the model reasoning layer and are undetectable by conventional security tools, and given that explainability outputs already generated for transparency and governance purposes encode behavioral fingerprints of model reasoning, can those explanation outputs be formally operationalized as real-time cybersecurity signals to detect attacks that evade all existing monitoring mechanisms?

This problem matters because the current state of healthcare AI security exhibits a critical gap: model reasoning is simultaneously the primary target of the most dangerous adversarial attacks and the component entirely unobserved by all existing security tooling. The gap between these states defines the scope of this chapter.

As this chapter presents a conceptual framework and theory-building, its claims are structured as formal propositions:

- Proposition 1: Adversarial attacks that alter healthcare AI model behavior necessarily produce measurable changes in explanation output distributions, independently of whether prediction accuracy metrics degrade.
- Proposition 2: Explanation drift, defined as statistically significant deviation from a validated baseline explanation distribution, can serve as an early-warning signal for selected adversarial machine learning attack classes in healthcare AI systems.
- Proposition 3: A layered XAI-based monitoring architecture can complement infrastructure-layer and robustness-layer security to provide detection coverage at the AI reasoning layer, which is currently unaddressed by any existing security framework.

These propositions are theoretically motivated by prior literature (Slack et al., 2020; Baniecki and Biecek, 2024; Vadillo et al., 2025) and are offered as a research agenda for empirical validation in future work, as discussed in Section 10. The chapter pursues five specific objectives: to formally establish the theoretical basis for treating explanation outputs as security observable; to propose the XaaD five-layer architecture as an implementable security framework; to introduce explanation drift as a measurable indicator of adversarial interference; to demonstrate how explanation monitoring complements traditional cybersecurity tools; and to analyze practical implementation scenarios across clinical AI domains.

The remainder of this chapter is organized as follows. Section 2 provides background healthcare AI applications, cybersecurity threats, and XAI techniques, including a critical examination of XAI limitations. Section 3 introduces the XaaD paradigm and its theoretical principles. Section 4 formalizes explanation drift and the detection algorithm. Section 5 presents the five-layer system architecture. Section 6 examines human-AI collaboration dimensions. Section 7 presents application scenarios. Section 8 addresses security, privacy, and ethical implications. Section 9 discusses implementation challenges and limitations. Section 10 outlines future research directions, and Section 11 concludes the chapter.

## 2. BACKGROUND AND CONCEPTUAL FOUNDATIONS

This section establishes foundational knowledge for a multidisciplinary audience by surveying healthcare AI applications, the cybersecurity threat landscape, and explainable AI techniques.

### 2.1 Overview of Healthcare AI Applications

Clinical Decision Support Systems (CDSSs) integrate patient data from electronic health records, laboratory results, and physiological monitoring streams to generate real-time recommendations, risk scores, and treatment guidance (Elhaddad et al., 2024). AI-powered CDSSs have demonstrated measurable clinical impact across sepsis management, cardiac risk stratification, oncological risk scoring, and drug-interaction detection (Ouanes and Farhah, 2024). A notable example is the deployment of sepsis prediction models in large academic medical centers, where AI-generated early warnings have reduced sepsis mortality but have also revealed the security risk: any successful data poisoning attack against the EHR inputs underpinning such systems could produce systematically incorrect high-stakes recommendations before clinical staff detect any performance anomaly.

Deep learning models, predominantly convolutional neural networks, have demonstrated diagnostic performance rivaling specialists across radiology, pathology, and ophthalmology (Topol, 2019). From a security perspective, medical images are particularly vulnerable to adversarial perturbations: pixel-level noise imperceptible to radiologists can cause diagnostic networks to misclassify malignant lesions as benign (Kaviani et al., 2022). The 2020 demonstration by Finlayson et al. that adversarial attacks could manipulate AI-assisted diagnosis at negligible cost provided an early empirical signal that deployment-time security for medical imaging AI is a real and present challenge. Spatial explanation methods such as Grad-CAM produce heatmaps whose anomalous activation patterns under adversarial attack may be detectable before incorrect predictions cause clinical harm, which is a core mechanism proposed by XaaD.

LLM-based medical chatbots handle patient triage, symptom assessment, and clinical queries across hospital portals and telehealth platforms (Sezgin, 2024). Their natural language interface creates unique security exposure: prompt injection attacks can override safety guardrails, generate dangerous medical advice, or facilitate social engineering (Chen and Esmaeilzadeh, 2024). It must be noted, however, that the interpretability of attention maps in transformer models as genuine explanations of reasoning remains contested in the literature, a point addressed in Section 2.3.

## 2.2 Cybersecurity Threat Landscape in Healthcare AI

Healthcare ranked as the most cyberattacked industry globally in 2024, with over 276 million patient records exposed (HIPAA Journal, 2025; AHA, 2024). Average breach costs reached $10.93 million per incident, the highest of any sector (IBM Security, 2023). Beyond immediate operational disruption, ransomware incursions with extended dwell times can silently corrupt AI training pipelines, constituting inadvertent data poisoning whose clinical consequences emerge only after model retraining. The 2020 Universal Health Services ransomware attack affecting 400 US hospitals and the 2021 Ireland Health Service Executive incident illustrate both the scale and the AI-specific risks of prolonged infrastructure compromise.

Adversarial machine learning (AML) encompasses attacks that exploit the mathematical properties of models rather than network perimeters and are therefore invisible to conventional security controls. Table 1 summarizes the primary attack types, their target stage, healthcare examples, and detectability by standard security tooling. The consistent finding across this taxonomy is that conventional IDS and SIEM systems cannot detect most training-time attacks and many inference-time attacks, which defines the security gap that XaaD is designed to address (Kaviani et al., 2022; He et al., 2024; Vadillo et al., 2025).

*Table 1. Adversarial machine learning attack taxonomy for healthcare AI systems*

| Attack Type | Target Stage | Healthcare Example | Detectable by IDS / SIEM | Theoretical XaaD detection capability |
|---|---|---|---|---|
| Data Poisoning | Training | Corrupting EHR data for sepsis predictor | No | Gradual SHAP drift over weeks |
| Backdoor/Trojan | Training | Hidden trigger misclassifies tumors in radiology AI | No | Sudden attribution spike to trigger features |
| Adversarial Input | Inference | Perturbed X-ray causes missed cancer diagnosis | No | Abrupt Grad-CAM spatial shift |
| Prompt Injection | Inference | Malicious query overrides LLM chatbot guardrails | No | Attention weight shift to injected tokens |
| Model Substitution | Deployment | Attackers replace production AI with malicious clone | No | Wholesale explanation fingerprint mismatch |
| Model Inversion | Inference | Reconstructing patient records from model outputs | Rarely | Atypical attribution concentration on ID fields |
| Model Extraction | Inference | Cloning CDSS via repeated API queries | Partially | Unusual query volume; explanation instability |

Insiders including MLOps engineers, data scientists, and privileged administrators can directly modify model weights, corrupt training pipelines, or insert backdoors without generating any network intrusion alert (Riggi, 2024). Because these attacks originate from authenticated, authorized users, access-log-based security controls offer no reliable detection.

## 2.3 Explainable AI (XAI): Concepts, Techniques, and Known Limitations

Feature attribution methods quantify each input feature's contribution to a specific model prediction. SHAP, grounded in cooperative game theory, assigns each feature a Shapley value representing its marginal contribution averaged across all feature subsets (Lundberg and Lee, 2017). LIME constructs locally faithful linear approximations of model behavior around individual instances (Ribeiro et al., 2016), while Grad-CAM produces spatial heatmaps for image-based models.

However, a critical body of literature documents significant limitations in these methods that directly affect their reliability as security signals. SHAP and LIME explanations exhibit inherent statistical variability across runs on identical inputs, a property documented extensively by Alvarez-Melis and Jaakkola (2018), who showed that explanation outputs can be sensitive to minor implementation choices. Slack et al. (2020) demonstrated that post-hoc explanation methods including SHAP and LIME can themselves be adversarially manipulated to produce deceptive explanations that conceal model bias while appearing faithful. Adebayo et al. (2018) showed that certain saliency methods fail basic sanity checks, producing visually similar maps even when model weights are fully randomized. These findings are not peripheral critiques; they represent central challenges to the XaaD proposal that any deployment must be addressed through multi-method monitoring, statistical stability testing, and conservative threshold calibration.

The interpretability of attention maps in transformer models is particularly contested. While attention weights indicate which tokens influence downstream computations, Jain and Wallace (2019) argued that attention weights do not reliably reflect feature importance and cannot be treated as faithful explanations of model decisions. This challenge is specifically relevant to XaaD's chatbot monitoring scenario and is explicitly acknowledged in Section 10. Notwithstanding these limitations, the empirical observation from Slack et al. (2020) remains: adversarial attacks produce detectable changes in explanation distributions even when those explanations are imperfect, suggesting that explanation anomaly detection may be robust to some faithfulness limitations even when individual explanation values are not fully faithful.

Model-agnostic methods including SHAP and LIME are immediately deployable as security overlays across heterogeneous clinical AI ecosystems (Noor et al., 2025). Model-specific methods including Grad-CAM and attention visualization exploit internal architectural information to produce richer signals. For explanation outputs to serve as security observables, they must be validated as clinically coherent under normal operation: a SHAP explanation attributing dominant weight to troponin and patient age in a cardiac risk model is clinically coherent; one attributing dominant weight to encounter identifiers is clinically incoherent and constitutes a security signal regardless of whether the prediction appears normal (Elhaddad et al., 2024).

## 2.4 Adjacent Approaches: How XaaD Relates to Existing Defense Methods

XaaD is not the only proposed mechanism for monitoring deployed AI model integrity. Several adjacent approaches exist, and situating XaaD relative to them is essential for accurately characterizing its contribution. Out-of-distribution (OOD) detection methods identify inputs that fall outside the training distribution, which may indicate adversarial perturbation or distributional shift (Yang et al., 2024). While valuable, OOD detection operates at the input layer and does not observe model reasoning; an adversarial input crafted to remain in-distribution while altering model attribution patterns would evade OOD detection.

Uncertainty quantification methods including Bayesian neural networks and conformal prediction provide calibrated confidence estimates that may signal anomalous inference conditions. Conformal risk control offers statistical guarantees on model error rates under distribution shift but does not provide attribution-level explanation of what features drove a specific anomalous prediction. Runtime monitoring frameworks in safety-critical machine learning, such as those proposed in the ML assurance literature, track performance metrics including accuracy, calibration, and drift in output distributions. XaaD's proposed contribution is to complement rather than replace these approaches, adding a reasoning-layer monitoring signal that the existing set of defenses does not provide. The integration of explanation-based monitoring with OOD detection and uncertainty quantification as a composite AI assurance layer represents a productive direction for future empirical research.

## 2.5 Gap Analysis: Why Explainability Is Not Used as Defense

Despite the theoretical and empirical case for treating XAI outputs as security observables, explainability has not been operationalized as a defense mechanism. Table 2 maps the five identified gaps to their root causes and XaaD's proposed responses. The gap analysis distinguishes what is currently known, what remains uncertain, what is actively contested, and what XaaD is uniquely positioned to address.

*Table 2. Gap analysis mapping research gaps to XaaD responses*

| # | Gap | Status | Root Cause | XaaD Response |
|---|---|---|---|---|
| 1 | Disciplinary separation between security and XAI communities | Known; unaddressed | Parallel research traditions with no cross-pollination | XaaD aims to bridge XAI and cybersecurity through a unified framework |
| 2 | XAI tools designed for human consumption, not automated monitoring | Known; unaddressed | Tool architecture assumes terminal human output | XaaD's monitoring layer intercepts outputs for automated anomaly comparison before display |
| 3 | No explanation baseline standards exist | Known; unaddressed | Regulatory frameworks require performance metrics but not explanation distribution baselines | XaaD's Baseline Engine establishes stratified explanation fingerprint libraries per clinical context |
| 4 | Computational overhead of real-time XAI | Known; partially addressed | SHAP/LIME expensive at inference time | XaaD's tiered monitoring applies full analysis only upon lightweight anomaly trigger |
| 5 | No unifying framework for XAI-as-defense | Known; contested (XAI faithfulness limits remain unresolved) | Neither community has formalized this paradigm, and XAI reliability for this purpose is uncertain | XaaD proposes the first five-layer conceptual architecture; empirical validation is identified as future work |

## 3. FROM TRANSPARENCY TO SECURITY: THE XaaD PARADIGM

This section formally introduces the XaaD paradigm, establishing the theoretical and conceptual basis upon which the framework's architecture, detection mechanisms, and clinical application scenarios are built.

### 3.1 Rethinking Explainability as a Security Primitive

In conventional security engineering, a security primitive denotes a building block with mathematically characterized guarantees sufficient for composition into larger defense architecture (Stallings and Brown, 2018). Cryptographic hash functions and digital signatures are canonical examples, possessing provable resistance properties under defined threat models. This chapter uses the term more loosely: XaaD proposes that explanation outputs constitute a security observable in the sense that they provide a measurable, continuously available signal whose statistical properties under normal operation are sufficiently stable to support baseline-referenced anomaly detection. This is a weaker claim than a cryptographic primitive, and it is important to acknowledge that this claim inherits all the faithfulness and stability limitations of the underlying XAI methods, as detailed in Section 2.3.

Three observable properties motivate this repositioning. First, adversarial attacks that manipulate model behavior necessarily alter internal feature attribution patterns, producing statistically detectable shifts in explanation outputs even when the prediction appears plausible (Slack et al., 2020; Baniecki and Biecek, 2024). This is theoretically motivated but not yet empirically benchmarked in clinical deployment settings. Second, explanation outputs are generated as a byproduct of legitimate clinical AI operation, requiring no separate data collection infrastructure. Third, explanation patterns for a stable clinical model exhibit sufficient statistical regularity to support baseline-referenced anomaly detection.

### 3.2 Core Principles of Explainability-as-a-Defense

A clinically validated AI model should produce explanations consistent with its learned decision logic across similar inputs. Reasoning Consistency holds that, for a given patient cohort and clinical context, the relative importance of features driving predictions should remain stable within statistically defined bounds. Violations, manifested as sudden changes in which features dominate attribution, may constitute a detection signal for acute adversarial attacks such as backdoor activation and adversarial input manipulation (Vadillo et al., 2025). The qualification 'may constitute' is deliberate: whether such violations reliably indicate adversarial interference rather than benign model instability under clinical heterogeneity is an empirical question that requires validation.

Explainability Stability requires that small, clinically insignificant variations in input data produce proportionally small variations in explanation outputs. A model under adversarial perturbation will violate explanation stability in characteristic ways: minor input modifications produce disproportionately large attribution changes. Monitoring explanation stability provides a continuous integrity check that operates independently of prediction accuracy metrics, potentially detecting attack classes that preserve accuracy while corrupting reasoning (Alvarez-Melis and Jaakkola, 2018). It is noted, however, that explanation instability is also a property of normal SHAP and LIME behavior on high-dimensional data, requiring careful threshold calibration to distinguish adversarial from benign instability.

XaaD preserves Human Interpretability of security alerts by ensuring that detected explanation anomalies are communicated in medically meaningful terms. A security alert stating that dominant attribution has shifted from troponin and ejection fraction to patient encounter ID is actionable for a cardiologist in a way that a raw statistical anomaly score is not. This principle ensures XaaD integrates into clinical governance workflows, establishing shared accountability between technical and clinical stakeholders (Noor et al., 2025).

## 3.3 Threat Assumptions and Trust Boundaries

XaaD operates under a defined threat model. It assumes a deployed clinical AI system whose model weights, training pipeline, and inference infrastructure may be subject to compromise. The trust boundary encompasses the explanation generation layer: XaaD assumes that the XAI monitoring module itself remains uncompromised, and that its baseline fingerprint library was generated from a validated pre-deployment model. This is analogous to the trust assumption in intrusion detection systems, which assume that the monitoring infrastructure itself operates with integrity (Sommer and Paxson, 2010). Importantly, this assumption is potentially fragile: Baniecki and Biecek (2024) demonstrate that explanation methods themselves can be adversarially targeted to produce deceptive outputs. XaaD does not resolve this attack surface; it acknowledges it as a recognized limitation addressed in Section 10.3, and proposes multi-method monitoring across SHAP, LIME, and attention maps as a partial mitigation.

## 3.4 Comparison with Existing Security Approaches

Table 3 positions XaaD against the three primary existing approaches to clinical AI security: network-layer security, adversarial robustness training, and model performance monitoring. The comparison demonstrates that XaaD aims to occupy the intersection of real-time operation, AI reasoning-layer coverage, and attack-type generality, a combination not achievable by any single existing approach.

*Table 3. Comparison of XaaD with existing healthcare AI security approaches*

| Approach | Operates At | Real-Time? | May Detect Previously Unseen Reasoning Anomalies? | Clinical Reasoning Coverage? |
|---|---|---|---|---|
| Network-Layer Security (IDS/SIEM) | Infrastructure | Yes | No | No |
| Adversarial Robustness Training | Model Training | No | Limited | Partial |
| Model Performance Monitoring | Output Metrics | Yes | Limited | No |
| XaaD | AI Reasoning Layer | Potentially | Under defined assumptions | Partial-to-strong (context-dependent) |

Network-layer security tools detect infrastructure breaches but are entirely blind to attacks on AI reasoning. Adversarial robustness training strengthens models against anticipated attack patterns but provides no real-time detection capability and offers no protection against novel attacks unseen during training. Model performance monitoring detects output degradation but cannot distinguish adversarial manipulation from benign performance drift and is specifically evaded by attacks designed to preserve accuracy metrics. XaaD aims to address by monitoring the behavioral fingerprint of the model's reasoning process in real time, representing a fundamentally different and complementary security posture (Baniecki & Biecek, 2024; Vadillo et al., 2025).

## 4. EXPLANATION DRIFT AS A CYBERSECURITY SIGNAL

This section introduces explanation drift which is the chapter's primary original contribution as a formally defined, measurable, and clinically interpretable cybersecurity signal for healthcare AI systems.

### 4.1 Definition of Explanation Drift

Concept drift in machine learning refers to changes in the statistical relationship between input features and model outputs over time (Hinder et al., 2024). Explanation drift is a distinct and more specific phenomenon occurring at the reasoning layer rather than the output layer. To build intuition before the formal definition: in a cardiac risk CDSS operating normally, SHAP values would consistently assign high importance to troponin levels and ejection fraction. This shift may be imperceptible from accuracy metrics alone because the model may still produce plausible-looking predictions.

## Explanation Drift

Let $M$ denote a deployed clinical AI model with explanation function $\varphi: X \rightarrow \mathbb{R}^d$, where $X$ is the input space and $d$ is the number of features. For input $x_t \in X$ at time $t$, let $E(x_t) = \varphi(M, x_t)$ be the explanation vector.

Let $B = \{E(x_i): i \in \mathcal{V}\}$ denote the baseline explanation distribution, where $\mathcal{V}$ is the validated pre-deployment inference set. The baseline distribution is characterized by mean $\mu\_B$ and covariance $\Sigma\_B$.

***Explanation drift*** is said to occur at time $t$ if the divergence measure $D(E(x_t) \parallel B)$ exceeds a statistically defined threshold $\delta > 0$:

$$D(E(x_t) \parallel B) > \delta$$

where $D$ is the Jensen-Shannon divergence (for distributional comparison) or Mahalanobis distance (for instance-level comparison.

The **XaaD Security Score (XSS)** at time $t$ is defined as:

$$XSS(t) = \alpha \cdot FeatureDrift(t) + \beta \cdot CoherenceScore(t) + \gamma \cdot TemporalConsistency(t)$$

where $FeatureDrift(t)$ = KL divergence between current and baseline SHAP distributions; $CoherenceScore(t)$ = clinical validity rating of the explanation [0,1]; $TemporalConsistency(t)$ = stability of explanations across similar inputs over time; and α, β, γ are domain-tuned weights with $\alpha + \beta + \gamma = 1$. $XSS(t) > \delta$ triggers a security intervention.

FeatureDrift(t) is the KL divergence between the current and baseline SHAP distributions, normalized to [0,1] by dividing by a domain-calibrated maximum divergence value; higher values indicate greater drift and higher security concern. CoherenceScore(t) is the inverse clinical validity rating: it is set to 0 when the explanation is fully clinically coherent and increases toward 1 as clinical incoherence grows; this ensures all three components increase monotonically with security concern. TemporalConsistency(t) is the inverse temporal stability score, set to 0 when explanations are fully stable across consecutive similar inputs and increasing toward 1 as instability grows. The threshold δ is calibrated per deployment using held-out baseline inferences: a starting value of 0.35 is recommended, but δ should be set to achieve a false positive rate acceptable for the clinical context, which requires empirical calibration prior to deployment.

The choice of Jensen-Shannon divergence for distributional comparison is motivated by its symmetry and boundedness (0 to 1 in bit units), which simplifies threshold setting relative to the unbounded KL divergence. Mahalanobis distance is preferred for instance-level comparison because it accounts for feature correlations in the explanation baseline, reducing false positives in high-dimensional clinical data. This choice requires that the baseline covariance matrix Σ_B is well-conditioned, which may not hold for sparse clinical datasets; regularization of Σ_B is recommended in such cases.

This formal definition distinguishes explanation drift from benign performance degradation. It degrades without necessarily altering feature-attribution structure by enabling XaaD to detect attack classes specifically engineered to evade performance monitoring (Vadillo et al., 2025; Salih et al., 2024).

## 4.2 Three Types of Explanation Drift and Their Attack Signatures

Sudden drift manifests as an abrupt, large magnitude shift in feature attribution across a small number of inference events. This is the characteristic signature of inference-time attacks including adversarial input manipulation and backdoor activation (Slack et al., 2020). In the cardiac risk scenario, sudden drift appears as a single-step transfer of attribution weight from troponin and ejection fraction to encounter ID, detectable within milliseconds.

Gradual drift unfolds over extended horizons as the explanation distribution incrementally departs from its baseline. This is the proposed signature of slow data poisoning, in which adversarially crafted training examples progressively shift decision boundaries (Abdul Razak et al., 2023). Contextual drift occurs when explanation patterns deviate from sub-context expectations without deviating from the global baseline. This may indicate workflow manipulation attacks targeting specific patient subgroups. It requires stratified baseline modeling: maintaining separate explanation fingerprints per clinical context, patient cohort, and demographic subgroup. It is important to note that explanation baselines constructed without demographic stratification risk encoding existing clinical disparities as the expected norm, potentially normalizing inequitable reasoning patterns. Baseline construction must therefore account for subgroup representativeness.

## 4.3 Distinguishing Legitimate Clinical Change from Malicious Drift

A critical operational challenge is differentiating security-motivated drift from legitimate explanation changes caused by seasonal disease prevalence shifts, protocol updates, or demographic changes in the patient population (Sahiner et al., 2023). XaaD addresses this through three mechanisms: a Clinical Change Log that registers documented clinical events and suspends drift alerts during expected explanation transitions; drift pattern analysis that distinguishes clinically coherent gradual transitions from adversarially abrupt or feature-incoherent shifts; and the Clinical Coherence Validator, which cross-checks drifting attribution patterns against a structured medical knowledge base. The false positive rate under benign clinical change is an open empirical question; conservative threshold calibration and mandatory human review at medium severity levels are essential safeguards during initial deployment.

## 4.4 Explanation Drift Detection Pipeline

Algorithm 1 presents the detection pipeline. The two-stage design reflects the computational constraint that full SHAP analysis at every inference is impractical for high-throughput clinical systems. The lightweight Mahalanobis pre-screening in Stage 2 uses the pre-computed baseline mean and covariance to filter normal inferences rapidly, incurring negligible latency. Only inferences flagged by Stage 2 proceed to full statistical analysis in Stage 3. Latency analysis for specific deployment environments is identified as a future work priority.

### Algorithm 1: XaaD Explanation Drift Detection Pipeline

```
Input: Clinical AI model M, XAI method φ, inference input xₜ,
   Baseline distribution B = (μ_B, Σ_B), threshold δ,
   Clinical Change Log CCL, Medical Knowledge Base MKB
Output: XaaD Security Score XSS(t), Alert level, Response action
```

---

```
Stage 1 - Explanation Generation:
   E(xₜ) ← φ(M, xₜ) // Generate explanation vector
Stage 2 - Lightweight Divergence Check:
   d_fast ← MahalanobisDistance(E(xₜ), μ_B, Σ_B)
   if d_fast < δ_low then return XSS = LOW, no alert // Fast exit
```

```
Stage 3 - Full Statistical Analysis:
   FeatureDrift(t) ← KLDivergence(E(xₜ), B)
   CoherenceScore(t) ← ValidateAgainstMKB(E(xₜ))
   TemporalConsistency(t)← CorrelateWithHistory(E(xₜ), E_history)
   XSS(t) ← α·FeatureDrift(t) + β·CoherenceScore(t) + γ·Tempo-
ralConsistency(t)
Stage 4 - Drift Classification:
   if XSS(t) > δ then:
      Check CCL for registered clinical events    // Suppress
false positives
      if not in CCL then:
         DriftType ← Classify(rate, magnitude, coherence)
         // DriftType ∈ {SUDDEN, GRADUAL, CONTEXTUAL}
         ThreatClass ← MapToAttackTaxonomy(DriftType)
Stage 5 - Graduated Response:
   if XSS(t) ∈ (δ, 0.5]: Log alert, notify security team
   if XSS(t) ∈ (0.5, 0.75]: Flag output for mandatory clinical review
   if XSS(t) ∈ (0.75, 0.90]: Suspend AI output, activate human fallback
   if XSS(t) > 0.90: Trigger AI Circuit Breaker, isolate model,
freeze recent outputs for forensic audit
```

The two-stage divergence check in Stages 2–3 is a deliberate design choice to address computational overhead: the lightweight Mahalanobis distance computation provides a rapid filter that exits without full SHAP analysis for most normal inferences, reserving the computationally intensive full statistical analysis only for flagged candidates (Salih et al., 2024). This tiered architecture ensures that XaaD's real-time operation imposes minimal latency on clinical workflows under normal conditions.

## 4.5 Clinical Interpretability of Drift Events

XaaD generates dual-format drift alerts: a technical summary specifying divergence magnitude, affected features, drift type, and candidate threat class; and a clinical narrative in medically interpretable language. For a sudden attack in a cardiac CDSS, the clinical narrative reads: 'The model's cardiac risk decision is now predominantly weighted toward administrative metadata rather than cardiac biomarkers. This pattern is clinically incoherent and warrants immediate suspension of AI-assisted decisions pending review.' This dual-format communication supports shared accountability between security teams and clinical staff, developed further in Section 6.

### 4.6 Illustrative Clinical Example of Explanation Drift

Consider a cardiac risk prediction model where baseline SHAP explanations consistently assign high importance to troponin levels and ejection fraction. Under normal operation, these features dominate attribution across similar patients. Although the model may still output plausible risk scores, the explanation vector deviates significantly from the baseline distribution.

For example:

- Baseline explanation: [Troponin: 0.42, Ejection Fraction: 0.35, Age: 0.18, Others: 0.05]
- Under attack: [Troponin: 0.12, Ejection Fraction: 0.10, Encounter ID: 0.48, Others: 0.30]

This shift results in a high Mahalanobis distance and elevated XSS, triggering a drift alert. This example illustrates how explanation drift can expose anomalies that remain invisible to output-based monitoring.

## 5. XaaD SYSTEM ARCHITECTURE FOR HEALTHCARE AI

This section presents the XaaD reference architecture, a five-layer system design that operationalizes the theoretical principles and detection mechanisms introduced in Sections 3 and 4 into a deployable, clinically integrated security infrastructure. The architecture is designed as a non-invasive security overlay: it complements rather than replaces existing clinical AI infrastructure and can be implemented across heterogeneous healthcare AI deployments without requiring modification of production models (Oke et al., 2025; Qureshi et al., 2024).

### 5.1 Layered Architecture Overview

Figure 1 presents the XaaD five-layer architecture designed as a non-invasive security overlay that complements rather than replaces existing clinical AI infrastructure. The architecture can, in principle, be implemented across heterogeneous healthcare AI deployments without requiring modification of production models, although the practical feasibility of this depends significantly on vendor cooperation, API accessibility, and infrastructure maturity, as discussed in Section 10. A circuit breaker feedback path from Layer 5 to Layer 1 enables automated suspension of AI-assisted decisions when critical drift thresholds are breached.

*Figure 1. XaaD Five-Layer Security Architecture*

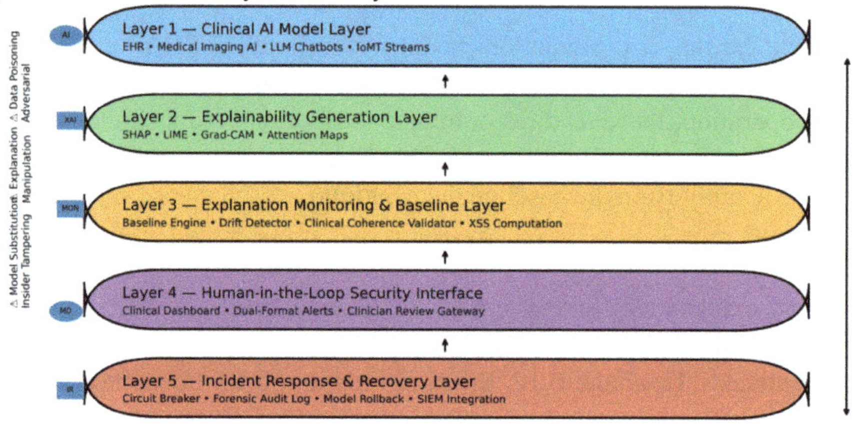


## 5.2 Layer 1: Clinical AI Model Layer

This layer encompasses all deployed AI systems: structured data models on EHR inputs, medical imaging AI processing DICOM data, LLM-based chatbots, and IoMT-driven predictive models. The layer is monitored but not modified by XaaD. The read-only posture is a deliberate design choice that ensures XaaD integration does not introduce new attack surfaces into the clinical AI pipeline itself (Oke et al., 2025). It must be acknowledged that the maturity of XaaD's monitoring capability differs significantly across these model classes: SHAP-based monitoring on tabular CDSS models is the most technically mature context and stability caveats documented in Section 2.3.

## 5.3 Layer 2: Explainability Generation Layer

This layer intercepts each model inference and concurrently generates an explanation vector using the XAI method appropriate to the model architecture: SHAP for structured data models, LIME for model-agnostic approximations, Grad-CAM for convolutional imaging networks, and attention map extraction for transformer-based models. The layer implements the two-stage computational strategy from Algorithm 1, using lightweight Mahalanobis pre-screening followed by full SHAP analysis only for flagged inferences, to minimize added latency. Explanation vectors are simultaneously forwarded to Layer 3 for security monitoring and to clinical interfaces for transparency display, ensuring the security overlay does not compromise the transparency function for which XAI was originally deployed.

## 5.4 Layer 3: Explanation Monitoring and Baseline Layer

Layer 3 is the core security engine. The Explanation Baseline Engine maintains stratified explanation fingerprints per clinical context, patient cohort, and diagnostic category, generated from pre-deployment model validation runs. The Drift Detector computes XSS in real time. The Clinical Coherence Validator cross-checks detected anomalies against a structured medical knowledge base. The Clinical Change Log suppresses false-positive alerts during documented clinical transitions. Critically, baseline construction requires careful attention to subgroup representativeness: baselines drawn from demographically unrepresentative validation sets may encode clinical bias as a normal pattern, with both equity and security implications (Sahiner et al., 2023).

## 5.5 Layer 4: Human-in-the-Loop Security Interface

This layer translates Layer 3 outputs into clinically actionable alerts delivered through a unified dashboard. A Clinician Review Gateway routes AI outputs flagged at medium-severity XSS levels to mandatory human review before clinical action. The operational burden imposed on clinical staff by alert review has not been empirically quantified; estimated alert review throughput, escalation workflows, and the cost of unnecessary AI suspension at high-false-positive rates must be assessed in pilot deployments before full clinical rollout (Naiseh et al., 2023).

## 5.6 Layer 5: Incident Response and Recovery Layer

Layer 5 operationalizes the graduated response actions. The AI Circuit Breaker suspends model inference at XSS $> 0.90$ and activates human-only clinical fallback protocols. The Model Rollback Manager coordinates reversion to a previously validated model version. The SIEM Integration Module forwards structured security event data to the organization's existing security operations infrastructure. The medico-legal governance questions raised by automated circuit breaker activation in clinical care contexts, including liability for decisions made after AI suspension, require institutional policy frameworks and legal guidance before deployment.

## 5.7 Deployment Equity Considerations

A significant concern with XaaD's five-layer architecture is its implementation burden. The framework requires explainability infrastructure, a dedicated monitoring engine, a clinical knowledge base, a human review workflow, and SIEM integration, all of which presuppose organizational maturity, technical resources, and vendor cooperation that large academic medical centers are more likely to possess than rural, community, or resource-constrained institutions. There is a real risk that XaaD could become a capability available primarily to well-resourced hospitals, creating a new dimension of healthcare cybersecurity inequity. Addressing this requires open-source reference implementations, cloud-hosted baseline sharing services, and regulatory incentives encouraging healthcare AI vendors to provide XaaD-compatible explanation export interfaces as a standard product feature rather than a custom integration. Table 4 provides a consolidated summary of each layer's primary function, key components, and the attack classes it addresses.

*Table 4. XaaD five-layer architecture summary*

| Layer | Name | Key Components | Primary Function | Attacks Addressed |
|---|---|---|---|---|
| 1 | Clinical AI Model | EHR models, imaging AI, LLM chatbots, IoMT | Inference & prediction | All (monitored, not modified) |
| 2 | Explainability Generation | SHAP, LIME, Grad-CAM, Attention maps | Explanation vector generation | Adversarial input, backdoor (detection trigger) |
| 3 | Monitoring & Baseline | Baseline Engine, Drift Detector, Clinical Coherence Validator, CCL | Real-time drift detection & XSS | All AML attack types, insider tampering |
| 4 | Human-in-the-Loop Interface | Clinical dashboard, dual-format alerts, clinician review gateway | Clinical oversight & alert delivery | Reduces impact of undetected drift |
| 5 | Incident Response | Circuit Breaker, Forensic Log, Rollback, SIEM | Containment, recovery & audit | Post-detection response to all attack classes |

Together, these five layers form a continuous monitoring and response loop that enables healthcare organizations to detect, interpret, and mitigate adversarial interference at the level of AI reasoning rather than merely at the infrastructure level.

## 6. HUMAN-AI COLLABORATION IN XaaD

XaaD is fundamentally a socio-technical framework. Its security effectiveness depends not only on technical detection mechanisms but equally on the quality of collaboration between AI systems and the clinicians, security professionals, and administrators who interpret, validate, and act upon its outputs.

## 6.1 Clinicians as Security Stakeholders

XaaD repositions clinicians as security stakeholders whose domain expertise is operationally essential to the framework's effective functioning. Clinicians contribute to the Clinical Coherence Validator by validating expected explanation patterns for their patient cohorts; they interpret dual-format drift alerts that require medical judgment to contextualize; and they exercise the authority to override circuit breaker decisions based on clinical urgency. This repositioning reflects broader findings in human-AI teaming research that effective collaboration in critical care requires active clinician involvement in AI governance (Bienefeld et al., 2024).

## 6.2 Cognitive Task Allocation

Algorithm 1 handles high-frequency statistical divergence computation, tasks for which automated systems are faster and more consistent than human operators. Human reviewers are engaged only for tasks requiring clinical contextualization: assessing whether a flagged anomaly reflects a clinically plausible emerging condition, a known protocol change, or a genuine security threat. This division exploits the complementary strengths of human and AI cognition, consistent with established principles of effective human-AI decision support in high-stakes clinical environments (Gomez et al., 2024; Bienefeld et al., 2024).

## 6.3 Trust Calibration and Shared Accountability

XaaD addresses trust calibration by making the AI model's security status explicitly visible through the XSS displayed on the clinical dashboard. A clinician viewing a recommendation alongside an XSS of 0.08 has grounds for appropriate confidence; one viewing a recommendation alongside an XSS of 0.72 has grounds for heightened scrutiny without requiring technical security knowledge to interpret the signal. Accountability is shared: the XSS at the time of each clinical decision is preserved in the Forensic Audit Log, creating an accountable record of the security context within which every human-AI decision was made (Dzindolet et al., 2024).

## 6.4 Avoiding Automation Bias

Three design features mitigate automation bias within XaaD. The Clinical Change Log requires human registration of expected clinical events. Medium-severity alerts mandate clinician review rather than automated response. The circuit breaker override capability preserves clinician authority to maintain AI-assisted care in exceptional circumstances where full suspension would cause immediate patient harm (Gomez et al., 2024).

### 6.5 Training and Awareness

Effective XaaD deployment requires training for three stakeholder groups: clinical staff on XSS interpretation and drift alert response; security operations staff on the healthcare AI threat taxonomy and drift type classification; and AI developers on Baseline Engine configuration and forensic audit standards. Interdisciplinary training programs bringing these groups together are essential for the shared vocabulary and mutual accountability that XaaD's sociotechnical design presupposes (Bienefeld et al., 2024; Naiseh et al., 2023).

## 7. ILLUSTRATIVE PROOF-OF-CONCEPT DESIGN

This section presents an illustrative proof-of-concept design to demonstrate how explanation drift could be evaluated empirically. A representative healthcare dataset (e.g., MIMIC-III or a tabular clinical dataset) may be used to train a baseline model such as XGBoost or Random Forest. Explanation vectors can be generated using SHAP under normal conditions and compared with those generated under simulated adversarial perturbations, such as feature manipulation or poisoning-like shifts. Drift can be quantified using Mahalanobis distance for instance-level detection and Jensen-Shannon divergence for distribution-level comparison. The evaluation would measure detection rate, false positive rate under benign clinical variation, and latency overhead introduced by explanation monitoring. This proof-of-concept is intended to illustrate the feasibility of XaaD rather than provide full clinical validation. Comprehensive empirical validation across diverse model classes and deployment environments remains a priority for future work.

## 8. USE CASES AND APPLICATION SCENARIOS

This section presents five application scenarios illustrating how XaaD's detection mechanisms may address security challenges across healthcare AI deployment contexts. These are conceptual scenarios intended to demonstrate plausibility and design coherence. The scenarios are drawn on the adversarial attack taxonomy in Table 1 and the detection mechanisms in Section 4.

## 8.1 AI-Enhanced Clinical Decision Support Systems

In CDSS deployments, XaaD operates as a continuous integrity monitor for models generating risk scores from EHR data. The Clinician Review Gateway would escalate flagged predictions to attending physicians before corrupted recommendations reach clinical action (Elhaddad et al., 2024; Gambetti et al., 2025). SHAP-based monitoring on tabular EHR models is the most technically mature XaaD deployment context and closest to current proof-of-concept feasibility.

## 8.2 Medical Chatbots and Virtual Assistants

For LLM-based chatbots, XaaD monitors attention-map distributions at each inference step. A prompt injection attack would produce a characteristic attention anomaly: abrupt attribution shift toward injected instruction tokens rather than clinical content (Chen and Esmaeilzadeh, 2024). XaaD's monitoring may detect this shift within the same inference cycle. The important caveat from Section 2.3 applies: attention maps in transformers are contested as faithful explanations; this scenario therefore has higher uncertainty than the CDSS scenario and requires dedicated empirical validation of attention anomaly detection performance for prompt injection specifically.

## 8.3 IoMT and Wearable-Driven AI Systems

IoMT environments present distinctive challenges due to constrained edge resources. XaaD implements lightweight Mahalanobis pre-screening locally on the IoMT device, forwarding only flagged inferences to a connected edge server for full SHAP analysis. A spoofing attack injecting fabricated physiological readings into a wearable arrhythmia detector would alter feature attribution toward artificial signal regularities, producing contextual explanation drift detectable at the edge server (Abbas et al., 2024; Feki et al., 2023).

## 8.4 Federated Learning Across Healthcare Institutions

In federated learning settings, XaaD provides explanation-level monitoring at each institution's local inference environment. Each institution maintains its own explanation baseline calibrated to its local patient population. A compromised global model update would produce explanation fingerprint divergence from the locally established baseline, triggering an institution-level drift alert before the corrupted model enters clinical use (Abbas et al., 2024; Pfitzner et al., 2021).

## 8.5 Cross-Hospital Threat Intelligence Sharing

When a hospital detects and classifies a specific explanation drift pattern, the anonymized drift signature can be shared with partner institutions through a federated threat intelligence network, enabling proactive baseline updates before the same attack pattern reaches their drift threshold. This collective defense mechanism is conceptually compelling but raises significant implementation challenges including data governance for shared drift signatures, the risk of adversaries using shared signatures to engineer mimicry attacks, and the absence of established standards for explanation signature representation and exchange (AHA, 2024).

*Table 5. XaaD use-case scenarios, explanation signals, and response actions*

| Scenario | Attack Type | Explanation Signal | XaaD Response |
|---|---|---|---|
| CDSS | Data poisoning | SHAP drift | Clinician review |
| Chatbot | Prompt injection | Attention anomaly | Circuit breaker |
| IoMT | Sensor spoofing | Feature attribution shift | Edge alert |
| Federated Learning | Model poisoning | Baseline divergence | Update rejection |
| Cross-hospital | Sector attack | Drift taxonomy | Shared intelligence |

Together, these scenarios illustrate how XaaD extends explanation-based security monitoring across diverse healthcare AI environments, from centralized hospital CDSS deployments to distributed federated learning networks and IoMT ecosystems.

# 9. SECURITY, PRIVACY, AND ETHICAL IMPLICATIONS

XaaD's operation introduces important considerations spanning privacy, ethics, regulatory compliance, and accountability that must be addressed for responsible deployment.

## 9.1 Privacy Risks in Explainability Outputs

SHAP explanation vectors encode feature attribution patterns derived from patient data and may indirectly reveal sensitive clinical information. If stored without adequate access controls, explanation logs could constitute protected health information subject to HIPAA and GDPR requirements (Thiyagarajan et al., 2025; Konnoth, 2024). XaaD addresses this through explanation-level de-identification: Shapley values are stored as normalized statistical aggregates rather than patient-linked records, and access to raw explanation logs is restricted to security personnel with appropriate authorization.

## 9.2 Ethical Risks of Misinterpreted Explanations

Explanation anomalies detected by XaaD could, if misinterpreted, lead to unjustified suspension of beneficial AI tools or generate unwarranted clinical alarm. The dual-format alert system mitigates this risk by requiring clinical context before security action is taken at medium severity levels. A particularly important ethical risk is that explanation baselines constructed from historically collected clinical data may encode existing disparities in care as the expected norm: if clinically similar patients receive systematically different attribution patterns across demographic groups due to historical inequity in EHR data quality, XaaD's baseline may normalize inequitable reasoning. Baseline construction must explicitly assess and address subgroup representativeness (Gerke et al., 2025).

## 9.3 Regulatory Alignment and Operational Requirements

XaaD's Forensic Audit Log directly supports HIPAA Security Rule requirements for audit controls and information system activity reviews. Under HIPAA, covered entities are required to implement hardware, software, and procedural mechanisms that record and examine activity in information systems containing protected health information; XaaD's explanation event log satisfies this requirement at the AI model layer. The Clinical Coherence Validator and explanation baseline documentation provide evidence of ongoing model monitoring consistent with FDA post-market surveillance expectations for AI/ML-based SaMD (FDA, 2021). The EU AI Act's requirements for robustness, logging, and human oversight of high-risk AI systems map to Layers 3, 4, and 5 of the XaaD architecture (European Parliament, 2024). Beyond regulatory compliance, operational questions remain: how would XaaD's baseline and drift threshold documentation be evaluated in a regulatory audit? What constitutes sufficient evidence of baseline validity for FDA purposes? These operational details require guidance from regulatory authorities and are recommended as a priority for future standards development.

## 9.4 Explainability Logs as Potential Forensic Evidence

XaaD's immutable forensic audit log preserves a timestamped record of every explanation vector, XSS score, drift classification, and clinical action taken during a security event. This record may constitute structured evidence relevant to regulatory investigations, clinical negligence proceedings, and insurance liability assessments, depending on jurisdiction and applicable evidentiary standards. Whether explanation logs would be admissible as forensic evidence in specific legal contexts is a legal question beyond the scope of this chapter and requires assessment by qualified legal counsel in each jurisdiction (Gerke et al., 2025; Konnoth, 2024).

### 9.5 Accountability in Human-AI Security Decisions

Because the XSS at the time of each human-AI decision is preserved in the audit log, post-incident analysis can determine whether harm arose despite a low XSS (indicating acceptable security status at decision time) or in the presence of an elevated XSS that was not appropriately escalated. This structured accountability aligns with the consensus that explainability must be integrated with documentation and audit trails rather than deployed as a standalone transparency measure (Gerke et al., 2025). Unresolved governance questions include the liability implications of automated circuit breaker activation and the responsibilities of clinical staff who override a high-XSS alert to continue AI-assisted care.

## 10. IMPLEMENTATION CHALLENGES AND LIMITATIONS

The limitations of XaaD must be stated directly and prominently, not confined to a late section. The most important limitation is that the XaaD framework as presented is a conceptual architecture; none of its detection claims have been empirically validated. This is not a minor qualification: the framework's core proposition that explanation drift reliably indicates adversarial interference rather than benign instability, demographic shift, or model recalibration effects remains an open empirical question. The following subsections detail the specific challenges that any future empirical evaluation and deployment must address.

### 10.1 The Fundamental Tension: XAI Instability and XaaD Reliability

The most significant theoretical challenge is the fundamental tension between XaaD's reliance on explanation outputs as security signals and the documented instability and limited faithfulness of those outputs under normal operation (Alvarez-Melis and Jaakkola, 2018; Slack et al., 2020; Adebayo et al., 2018). If SHAP values are noisy across runs on identical inputs, then distinguishing adversarial explanation drift from normal explanation variance requires careful statistical characterization of the baseline noise distribution, conservative threshold calibration, and sustained divergence requirements across multiple consecutive inferences rather than single-inference alerts. This tension is a central design challenge for XaaD, not a peripheral implementation detail, and it must be addressed empirically before the framework can be deployed in safety-critical clinical settings.

## 10.2 Unknown False Positive and False Negative Rates

The false positive rate of XaaD's drift detection under benign clinical change has not been quantified. In dynamic clinical environments with seasonal disease prevalence shifts, protocol updates, and demographic changes, the expected rate of false-positive drift alerts may be substantial if threshold calibration is insufficiently conservative. Equally, the false negative rate for specific attack classes that are designed to minimize explanation change (adversarial explanation mimicry, discussed in Section 10.3) is unknown. Before deployment, a rigorous evaluation on held-out clinical data under both clean and adversarially perturbed conditions is essential.

## 10.3 Adversarial Explanation Mimicry

A sophisticated adversary with knowledge of XaaD's baseline fingerprints could craft attacks that manipulate model behavior while preserving surface-level explanation patterns, effectively mimicking normal explanation outputs (Baniecki and Biecek, 2024). This represents XaaD's most significant theoretical vulnerability, as it would allow an attacker who knows the monitoring system to engineer attacks that evade detection entirely. Mitigation strategies including periodic undisclosed baseline rotation and multi-method monitoring across SHAP, LIME, and attention maps are proposed but have not been evaluated. This limitation is directly analogous to the evasion problem in network intrusion detection, where adversaries engineer traffic to resemble benign patterns (Sommer and Paxson, 2010).

## 10.4 Scalability and Latency in High-Throughput Environments

Full SHAP computation at every clinical inference is computationally expensive for high-throughput systems processing thousands of predictions per hour. The two-stage architecture mitigates but does not eliminate this overhead. Deployment in large-scale EHR-integrated systems will require hardware acceleration, inference batching, and asynchronous explanation generation strategies. For imaging AI processing high-resolution DICOM data with Grad-CAM, the computational overhead is substantially larger than for tabular CDSS models. Latency benchmarks have not been established.

## 10.5 Integration with Legacy Hospital IT and Vendor-Locked Systems

Many healthcare organizations operate clinical AI systems on legacy infrastructure with limited API accessibility. XaaD's Layer 2 explanation-generation interception requires programmatic access to model inference pipelines that may not be available in vendor-locked deployments. Adoption depends on healthcare AI vendors providing XaaD-compatible explanation export interfaces as standard product features, which in turn requires either regulatory mandates or market incentives that do not currently exist.

## 10.6 Uncertain Transferability Across Model Classes

XaaD's design is most technically grounded for tabular CDSS models with SHAP monitoring. Its extension to imaging AI with Grad-CAM introduces the contested faithfulness of gradient-based saliency methods. Its extension to LLM chatbots with attention map monitoring rests on the contested assumption that attention weights are faithful explanations. The framework should not be treated as equally mature across all claimed application contexts; the technical readiness level decreases substantially from CDSS to imaging to LLM to IoMT edge deployments.

# 11. FUTURE RESEARCH DIRECTIONS

The XaaD framework opens five high-priority research avenues that together constitute an emerging research agenda for explanation-based healthcare AI security.

## 11.1 Empirical Proof-of-Concept Validation

The most urgent future research contribution is an empirical proof-of-concept evaluation of XaaD's detection claims. A minimum viable study would use a public healthcare dataset such as MIMIC-III or the NIH Chest X-ray14 dataset, train a representative clinical AI model, simulate two or three attack types from Table 1 (data poisoning, adversarial input, and backdoor), generate SHAP or Grad-CAM explanations under clean and attacked conditions, and quantify drift using the metrics specified in Algorithm 1. The evaluation should report detection rate, false positive rate under benign distribution shift, latency overhead, and a comparison against performance-metric monitoring as a baseline.

## 11.2 Integration with OOD Detection and Uncertainty Quantification

Future work should develop composite AI assurance architectures that combine XaaD's reasoning-layer monitoring with OOD detection at the input layer and uncertainty quantification at the output layer. Such a composite approach would provide multi-layer defense coverage and allow empirical comparison of each component's contribution to detection performance. Conformal prediction methods offer particularly promising complementarity with XaaD, as they provide statistical guarantees on output reliability under distribution shift that explanation-based monitoring alone cannot provide.

## 11.3 Self-Adaptive Explanation Baselines

Current XaaD baselines require governed human-supervised updates. Future research should develop self-adaptive baseline mechanisms that autonomously distinguish clinically motivated explanation shifts from adversarial ones, using causal inference and clinical ontology alignment to update baseline without human intervention while maintaining security sensitivity.

## 11.4 Fairness and Subgroup Sensitivity in Baseline Construction

Explanation baselines may vary substantially across patient subgroups defined by age, sex, disease prevalence, site, imaging modality, and socioeconomic status. Future research must develop baseline construction methodologies that explicitly account for subgroup heterogeneity, ensure that XaaD's monitoring does not normalize inequitable reasoning patterns, and assess whether drift detection performance differs across demographic subgroups.

## 11.5 Standardization and Open Implementation

The most impactful near-term contribution would be an open XaaD standard specifying explanation baseline formats, drift detection thresholds, audit log schemas, and Clinical Change Log protocols that healthcare AI vendors, regulators, and organizations could adopt as a common interoperability framework. Open-source reference implementations would additionally address the deployment equity gap identified in Section 5.7, enabling resource-constrained institutions to access XaaD-compatible monitoring tooling without custom development.

## CONCLUSION

This chapter introduced Explainability-as-a-Defense, a conceptual framework and theory-building contribution that proposes repositioning explainable AI outputs as potential real-time cybersecurity signals for healthcare AI systems. Its five original conceptual contributions are the formal establishment of explanation outputs as security observables, the definition of explanation drift as a mathematically specified candidate cybersecurity signal, the XaaD five-layer architecture as a proposed deployable clinical security overlay, the XaaD Security Score as a proposed real-time model integrity metric, and a structured mapping between adversarial attack types and explanation anomaly signatures. These contributions are offered as a conceptual research agenda, not as demonstrated engineering results; none of the detection claims presented have been empirically validated, and empirical proof-of-concept evaluation is the highest-priority future work identified in Section 10. The chapter argues that the transparency infrastructure already present in responsible healthcare AI deployments may contain a latent security capability that, if validated, could be operationalized at manageable additional cost, offering a potentially achievable convergence of explainability and defense. Realizing this potential requires interdisciplinary collaboration across cybersecurity researchers, XAI specialists, clinical informaticists, and regulators, as well as empirical validation studies, open implementation work, and regulatory guidance on baseline governance and forensic evidence standards.

## NOTE

This chapter presents XaaD, Explainability-as-a-Defense, a novel framework that repositions explainable AI outputs, including SHAP, LIME, Grad-CAM, and attention maps, as real-time cybersecurity signals for healthcare AI systems. By defining explanation drift as a measurable deviation from a validated baseline, XaaD is designed to enable detection of adversarial attacks at the AI reasoning layer where conventional security tools have no visibility. The chapter introduces a five-layer deployable architecture, the XaaD Security Score as a real-time integrity metric, and a drift taxonomy linking attack classes to explanation anomaly signatures, demonstrated across clinical decision support, medical chatbots, IoMT, federated learning, and cross-hospital threat intelligence scenarios. Security, privacy, ethical, and regulatory implications are examined alongside key implementation challenges and future research priorities. Ultimately, XaaD establishes that the transparency infrastructure already present in responsible healthcare AI deployments contains a latent security capability, offering a practically achievable convergence of explainability and defense.

## ACKNOWLEDGMENT

This research received no specific grant from any funding agency in the public, commercial, or not-for-profit sectors.

## REFERENCES

Abbas, S. R., Abbas, Z., Zahir, A., & Lee, S. W. (2024). Federated learning in smart healthcare: A comprehensive review on privacy, security, and predictive analytics with IoT integration. *Sensors (Basel)*, *24*(3), 868. DOI: 10.3390/s24030868 PMID: 38339586

Abdul Razak, M. S., Nirmala, C. R., Sreenivasa, B. R., Lahza, H., & Lahza, H. F. M. (2023). A survey on detecting healthcare concept drift in AI/ML models. *Frontiers in Artificial Intelligence*, *5*, 955314. DOI: 10.3389/frai.2022.955314 PMID: 37139355

Alvarez-Melis, D., & Jaakkola, T. S. (2018). On the robustness of interpretability methods. ICML Workshop on Human Interpretability in Machine Learning. https://arxiv.org/abs/1806.08049

American Hospital Association. (2025). Report: Health care had most reported cyberthreats in 2024. AHA News. https://www.aha.org/news/headline/2025-05-12-report-health-care-had-most-reported-cyberthreats-2024

American Hospital Association (AHA). (2024). A look at 2024's health care cybersecurity challenges. https://www.aha.org/news/aha-cyber-intel/2024-10-07-look-2024s-health-care-cybersecurity-challenges

Baniecki, H., & Biecek, P. (2024). Adversarial attacks and defenses in explainable artificial intelligence: A survey. *Information Fusion*, *107*, 102303. DOI: 10.1016/j.inffus.2024.102303

Bienefeld, N., Keller, E., & Grote, G. (2024). Human-AI teaming in critical care: A comparative analysis of data scientists' and clinicians' perspectives on AI augmentation and automation. *Journal of Medical Internet Research*, *26*, e50130. DOI: 10.2196/50130 PMID: 39038285

Chen, Y., & Esmaeilzadeh, P. (2024). Generative AI in medical practice: In-depth exploration of privacy and security challenges. *Journal of Medical Internet Research*, *26*, e53008. DOI: 10.2196/53008 PMID: 38457208

Dzindolet, M. T., Pierce, L. G., Beck, H. P., & Dawe, L. A. (2024). From trust in automation to trust in AI in healthcare: A 30-year longitudinal review and an interdisciplinary framework. PMC. https://pmc.ncbi.nlm.nih.gov/articles/PMC12562135/

Elhaddad, M., & Hamam, S. (2024). AI-driven clinical decision support systems: An ongoing pursuit of potential. *Cureus*, *16*(4), e57728. DOI: 10.7759/cureus.57728 PMID: 38711724

European Parliament & Council of the European Union. (2024). Regulation (EU) 2024/1689 — Artificial Intelligence Act. Official Journal of the European Union. https://eur-lex.europa.eu/legal-content/EN/TXT/?uri=CELEX:32024R1689

Feki, I., Ammar, S., Kessentini, Y., & Philip, K. (2023). Federated learning for IoMT applications: A standardization and benchmarking framework. *IEEE Communications Magazine*, *61*(6), 36–42. DOI: 10.1109/MCOM.001.2200055

Gambetti, A., Han, Q., Shen, H., & Soares, C. (2025). A survey on human-centered evaluation of explainable AI methods in clinical decision support systems. arXiv preprint arXiv:2502.09849.

Gerke, S., Minssen, T., Cohen, G., & Tobia, K. P. (2025). Ethical and legal considerations in healthcare AI: Innovation and policy for safe and fair use. *Royal Society Open Science*, *12*(5), 241873. Advance online publication. DOI: 10.1098/rsos.241873 PMID: 40370601

Gomez, C., Unberath, M., & Huang, C.-M. (2024). Human-AI collaboration is not very collaborative yet: A taxonomy of interaction patterns in AI-assisted decision making. *Frontiers of Computer Science*. Advance online publication. DOI: 10.3389/fcomp.2024.1521066

He, Y., Zhang, J., Shan, H., & Wang, G. (2024). Survey on adversarial attack and defense for medical image analysis: Methods and challenges. *ACM Computing Surveys*. Advance online publication. DOI: 10.1145/3702638

Hinder, F., Vaquet, V., & Hammer, B. (2024). One or two things we know about concept drift — A survey on monitoring in evolving environments. *Frontiers in Artificial Intelligence*, *7*, 1330257. DOI: 10.3389/frai.2024.1330257 PMID: 38962502

Journal, H. I. P. A. A. (2025). The biggest healthcare data breaches of 2024. https://www.hipaajournal.com/biggest-healthcare-data-breaches-2024/

Kaviani, S., Khokhar, A. A., & Sharifzadeh, M. (2022). Adversarial attacks and defenses on AI in medical imaging informatics: A survey. *Neurocomputing*, *492*, 278–307. DOI: 10.1016/j.neucom.2022.04.051

Konnoth, C. (2024). AI and data protection law in health. In Solaiman, B., & Cohen, I. G. (Eds.), *Research Handbook on Health, AI and the Law*. Edward Elgar Publishing., DOI: 10.4337/9781802205657.ch07

Lundberg, S. M., & Lee, S. I. (2017). A unified approach to interpreting model predictions. *Advances in Neural Information Processing Systems, 30*, 4765–4774.

MarketsandMarkets. (2025). Artificial intelligence in healthcare market — global forecast to 2030. https://www.marketsandmarkets.com/Market-Reports/artificial-intelligence-healthcare-market-54679303.html

Naiseh, M., Al-Thani, D., Jiang, N., & Ali, R. (2023). How the different explanation classes impact trust calibration: The case of clinical decision support systems. *International Journal of Human-Computer Studies, 169*, 102941. DOI: 10.1016/j.ijhcs.2022.102941

National Institute of Standards and Technology. (2023). Artificial intelligence risk management framework (AI RMF 1.0) (NIST AI 100-1). DOI: 10.6028/NIST.AI.100-1

Noor, F., Bano, S., Shafiq, M., & Iqbal, M. W. (2025). Unveiling explainable AI in healthcare: Current trends, challenges, and future directions. *Wiley Interdisciplinary Reviews. Data Mining and Knowledge Discovery, 15*(2), e70018. Advance online publication. DOI: 10.1002/widm.70018

Oke, F., Bolaji, O., & Umakor, M. (2025). Building AI-ready infrastructure for U.S. healthcare: A product management perspective. *World Journal of Advanced Research and Reviews, 27*(2), 588–603. DOI: 10.30574/wjarr.2025.27.2.2892

Ouanes, K., & Farhah, N. (2024). Effectiveness of AI in clinical decision support systems and care delivery. *Journal of Medical Systems, 48*(1), 74. DOI: 10.1007/s10916-024-02098-4 PMID: 39133332

Pfitzner, B., Steckhan, N., & Arnrich, B. (2021). Federated learning in a medical context: A systematic literature review. *ACM Transactions on Internet Technology, 21*(2), 1–38. DOI: 10.1145/3412357

Qureshi, A. S.. (2024). Advancing healthcare systems: A tri-tier architecture using data communication, AI data generative and regulation and compliance standards. *Expert Systems: International Journal of Knowledge Engineering and Neural Networks*. Advance online publication. DOI: 10.1111/exsy.13742

Ribeiro, M. T., Singh, S., & Guestrin, C. (2016). "Why should I trust you?": Explaining the predictions of any classifier. Proceedings of the 22nd ACM SIGKDD International Conference on Knowledge Discovery and Data Mining, 1135–1144. DOI: 10.1145/2939672.2939778

Riggi, J. (2024). A look at 2024's health care cybersecurity challenges. American Hospital Association. https://www.aha.org/news/aha-cyber-intel/2024-10-07-look-2024s-health-care-cybersecurity-challenges

Sahiner, B., Chen, W., Lu, L., Ko, Y., & Hung, L. Y. (2023). Strategies for detecting and mitigating dataset shift in machine learning for health predictions. *Journal of Biomedical Informatics*. Advance online publication. DOI: 10.1016/j.jbi.2025.104818

Salih, A., Galazzo, I. B., Raisi-Estabragh, Z., Petersen, S., Menegaz, G., & Radeva, P. (2024). A perspective on explainable artificial intelligence methods: SHAP and LIME. *Advanced Intelligent Systems*. Advance online publication. DOI: 10.1002/aisy.202400304

Security, I. B. M. (2023). Cost of a data breach report 2023. IBM Corporation. https://www.ibm.com/reports/data-breach

Sezgin, E. (2024). Redefining virtual assistants in health care: The future with large language models. *Journal of Medical Internet Research*, *26*, e53225. DOI: 10.2196/53225 PMID: 38241074

Slack, D., Hilgard, S., Jia, E., Singh, S., & Lakkaraju, H. (2020). Fooling LIME and SHAP: Adversarial attacks on post hoc explanation methods. Proceedings of the AAAI/ACM Conference on AI, Ethics, and Society, 180–186. DOI: 10.1145/3375627.3375830

Sommer, R., & Paxson, V. (2010). Outside the closed world: On using machine learning for network intrusion detection. *Proceedings of the IEEE Symposium on Security and Privacy*, 305–316. DOI: 10.1109/SP.2010.25

Stallings, W., & Brown, L. (2018). *Computer security: Principles and practice* (4th ed.). Pearson Education.

Thiyagarajan, A., . . .. (2025). The role of artificial intelligence in safeguarding patient privacy in healthcare systems. PMC. https://pmc.ncbi.nlm.nih.gov/articles/PMC12244842/

Topol, E. J. (2019). High-performance medicine: The convergence of human and artificial intelligence. *Nature Medicine*, *25*(1), 44–56. DOI: 10.1038/s41591-018-0300-7 PMID: 30617339

U.S. Food and Drug Administration. (2021). Artificial intelligence/machine learning (AI/ML)-based software as a medical device (SaMD) action plan. https://www.fda .gov/media/145022/download

Vadillo, J., Santana, R., & Lozano, J. A. (2025). Adversarial attacks in explainable machine learning: A survey of threats against models and humans. *Wiley Interdisciplinary Reviews. Data Mining and Knowledge Discovery*, *15*(1), e1567. Advance online publication. DOI: 10.1002/widm.1567

## KEY TERMS AND DEFINITIONS

**Adversarial Machine Learning (AML):** A class of cybersecurity attacks that exploit vulnerabilities in machine learning models by manipulating training data, model inputs, or model parameters to cause erroneous, harmful, or adversary-controlled outputs.

**AI Circuit Breaker:** A safety mechanism within the XaaD architecture that automatically suspends AI model inference and activates human-only clinical fallback protocols when the XaaD Security Score exceeds a critical threshold.

**Explanation Baseline:** A validated reference distribution of explanation vectors generated from a clinical AI model's pre-deployment inference set under known-good conditions.

**Explanation Drift:** A formally defined cybersecurity signal in which the divergence between a clinical AI model's runtime explanation vector and its validated baseline distribution exceeds a statistically defined threshold in a manner not attributable to documented clinical population changes.

**Explainability-as-a-Defense (XaaD):** A novel cybersecurity paradigm introduced in this chapter that repositions explainable AI outputs, including SHAP values, LIME approximations, Grad-CAM heatmaps, and attention maps, from transparency artifacts into active, real-time security signals.

**Grad-CAM (Gradient-weighted Class Activation Mapping):** A model-specific explainability technique for convolutional neural networks that generates spatial heatmaps indicating which regions of an input image most strongly influenced the model's prediction.

**LIME (Local Interpretable Model-Agnostic Explanations):** A model-agnostic post-hoc explainability method that approximates a complex machine learning model's behavior in the local neighborhood of a specific input using a simpler, interpretable surrogate model.

**SHAP (SHapley Additive exPlanations):** A post-hoc explainability method grounded in cooperative game theory that assigns each input feature a Shapley value representing its marginal contribution to a specific model prediction.

**XaaD Security Score (XSS):** A composite real-time metric computed by XaaD's Layer 3 that quantifies the degree to which a clinical AI model's current explanation output deviates from its validated baseline.

# Chapter 4
# Trends and Convergence in Healthcare Cybersecurity Literature

**Amanpreet Kaur**
http://orcid.org/0009-0004-1966-0006
*Apex Institute of Management, Chandigarh University, India*

**Sharneet Jagirdar**
http://orcid.org/0000-0001-5716-6368
*Apex Institute of Management, Chandigarh University, India*

## ABSTRACT

*This study analyses five decades of research at the intersection of computing, informatics, and organisational studies to trace trends in qualitative (e.g., discourse analysis, ethnography) and quantitative (e.g., experimental design, statistical modelling) methods. Emphasizing methodological pluralism, it bridges positivist and constructivist paradigms using a pragmatism-triangulation-bibliometrics framework (co-citation, co-word analysis) to map the evolution of computational research. It identifies emerging domains, such as AI ethics, reinforcement learning, and experimental designs for new technologies. Findings highlight how interdisciplinary methods are shaped by innovations from machine learning to quantum computing. Recommendations emphasise sustainable technology, ethical AI, and hybrid methods that balance both academic rigour and real-world relevance.*

DOI: 10.4018/979-8-3373-9119-9.ch004

## INTRODUCTION

Few industries have been subjected to the forces of digital transformation as profoundly as the healthcare sector. The widespread adoption of electronic health records, telemedicine software, cloud-based data infrastructure, and AI-assisted diagnostics has redefined care delivery in fundamental ways, enabling real-time data communication, remote monitoring, and quicker clinical judgment. However, this very interconnection that enables these gains has also exposed hospitals and health systems to a wide range of cyber threats that were not anticipated by previous generations of healthcare administrators.

Health organizations occupy a particularly vulnerable position in the cyber threat environment. Unlike most commercial organizations, hospitals hold sensitive and high-value personal data, including clinical histories, insurance records, and prescription data, and their operational continuity is directly linked to patient safety. This makes them a target not only for financially motivated attackers but also for state actors seeking to disrupt critical infrastructure. Healthcare systems now face a wide range of attack types, including ransomware that can paralyze hospital networks by encrypting databases, phishing attacks targeting clinical personnel, vulnerabilities in networked medical devices, and insider threats arising from inadequate access controls.

The WannaCry ransomware attack of May 2017 remains one of the most high-profile examples of a cybersecurity breach within the healthcare domain. On 12 May 2017, the malware spread rapidly through NHS networks, disrupting routine clinical services across England. Around 80 NHS trusts were affected, nearly 19,000 appointments had to be cancelled, and five hospitals diverted ambulances because they could no longer admit emergency patients safely (Ghafur et al., 2019). In many hospitals, staff returned to paper records and manual processes as IT systems became unavailable. Telephone services were also affected, making communication more difficult during an already challenging situation. The incident highlighted the extent to which routine healthcare services had become dependent on digital systems across the NHS.

The attack also brought attention to several long-standing weaknesses in NHS cybersecurity practices. WannaCry made use of the EternalBlue vulnerability, even though Microsoft had released a patch approximately two months earlier. Many organizations had not installed the update, while some NHS trusts were still using Windows XP, despite the operating system no longer receiving standard support. The incident highlighted differences in patch management practices, incident response arrangements, and communication procedures across NHS organizations (Ehrenfeld, 2017; Ghafur et al., 2019). Although these failures did not precipitate the attack, they did influence the scale of its impact within the healthcare system.

Following the attack, cybersecurity became a greater priority within the NHS. Additional funding was allocated to improve cybersecurity infrastructure, NHS Digital expanded its CareCERT programme, and trusts became subject to more regular cybersecurity assessments. Security requirements were also strengthened across the system. However, the single biggest lesson learned from the WannaCry attack was that healthcare cybersecurity could not be regarded merely as a technical issue. Technology played a role, but so did governance, leadership, preparedness, and decision-making. The attack demonstrated that weaknesses in digital systems can have direct consequences for patient safety. While bibliometric findings help identify major themes within the literature, the WannaCry case provides a practical example of the challenges frequently discussed in healthcare cybersecurity research (Ghafur et al., 2019; Ehrenfeld, 2017).

Scholarly production in this area has grown considerably in response. Research on cybersecurity in health settings has expanded over the past two decades across computer science, health informatics, public policy, information systems, and management studies. What has not kept pace with this growth is systematic synthesis. The existing literature tends to concentrate on discrete issues: a specific type of threat, a particular regulatory framework, or a given technology. Relatively little work has been done to illuminate the broader intellectual architecture of the field, its central themes, how those themes have evolved, and who is conducting research in what collaborative groupings (Coventry and Branley, 2018; Wasserman and Wasserman, 2022; Jalali and Kaiser, 2018).

Bibliometric analysis addresses this gap. Rather than summarizing individual studies, it examines quantitative patterns across large bodies of scholarly literature, including keyword co-occurrence, co-authorship, and publication trends, to reveal structural properties that cannot be observed at the level of single studies. This approach can identify the intellectual core of a field, trace the rise and fall of research topics over time, and map the collaborative networks through which knowledge flows. Used alongside visualization tools such as VOSviewer, it provides a spatial representation of these connections accessible to both researchers and policymakers. The present study applies these methods to healthcare cybersecurity research using a Scopus dataset spanning nearly thirty years. Its aim is not to explain what has been written but to expose the architecture of the field: its dominant themes, its historical development, its collaborative geography, and the gaps that current research has yet to address (Jalali et al., 2019; Ahouanmenou et al., 2022).

## RESEARCH OBJECTIVES

The main idea of this chapter is a systematic bibliometric analysis of the published literature on the topic of healthcare cybersecurity, which includes the years 1997 to June 2026. Healthcare cybersecurity overlaps with a range of challenging academic traditions, and its literature has become large and complicated enough to be subject to systematic structural analysis. The paper focuses specifically on such thematic areas as cyber-threat management, response to ransomware and data breaches, AI-based security management, regulatory compliance, and health information system protection, which are the primary intellectual domain of the industry.

One of the secondary intentions is to trace the change of these themes throughout the time. The paper is divided into the chronological order by which cybersecurity research priorities are reacting to significant changes in technology: the infiltration of networked medical devices, the use of cloud computing infrastructure, and adoption of machine learning tools in clinical practice, and how individual incidents (such as massive cyberattacks) have shifted the academic focus. Through tracing this historical development, the chapter demonstrates a discipline that has shifted toward a reactive and incident-oriented research level to a proactive and systems-oriented scholarship (Nair and Saha, 2023; Ewoh and Vartiainen, 2024).

Social organization of the literature production in this field is also considered in the chapter: who are the authors and institutions in central positions, what national research community is most productive, how to organize international collaboration. Since cybersecurity threats are also transnational and because the digital health infrastructure remains globally interconnected, geographic architecture of the research community can be a significant object of scrutiny. Last but not least, the chapter will seek to indicate the fruitful future through the identification of yet unexplored themes in the literature to date, such as the ethics of AI in clinical cybersecurity, the capacity of security in low-resource health systems, or the combination of governance frameworks and technical security architectures (Jalali et al., 2019; Bhuyan et al., 2020).

## LITERATURE REVIEW

Cybersecurity in healthcare has become a major subject of scholarly interest over the past two decades, with the literature reflecting the growing scale of threats to digitalized health systems. Early investigations focused primarily on network security principles and encryption protocols needed to protect confidential patient information in hospital information systems. As the attack surface expanded through the adoption of electronic health records, cloud computing, and networked diagnostic devices, scholarly inquiry extended to cover ransomware response, IoT device protection, AI-powered intrusion detection, and regulatory frameworks for maintaining compliance across institutional and national boundaries. The WannaCry attack of 2017 marked a significant turning point, accelerating a shift in how researchers framed cybersecurity: rather than a purely technical support function, it came to be understood as an organizational and governance challenge, with growing attention to how healthcare organizations could maintain service delivery during and after a cyberattack (Coventry and Branley, 2018; Jalali and Kaiser, 2018).

Bibliometric analysis has become a fully developed tool of conducting a systematic study of the structure and development of research areas. Influence is best captured by citation analysis, which is due to the fact that in the world of contemporary bibliometric data collection methods, such as co-citation analysis, bibliographic coupling, co-word analysis, and thematic mapping, the relational architecture of a whole field of study is exposed. Particularly co-word analysis has been effective in identifying new research frontiers in the field of cybersecurity: the use of blockchain in health data integrity, the implementation of machine learning in anomaly-detection systems, and the coming of age of governance frameworks to deal with institutional cyber risk. These structural relationships are then visualised with software like VOSviewer, which spatialises these connections so that anyone can see these networks of intellectual connection as well as researchers and policy-makers (van Eck and Waltman, 2010; Moral-Munoz et al., 2020).

The high interdisciplinarity of the field of healthcare cybersecurity is what makes it a unique research topic and bibliometric mapping in this context bring a specific value. The topic is based on computer science, health informatics, public policy, information systems management, and clinical practice, implying that parallel streams of literature have been formed without much cross-referencing. The systematic approaches to bibliometrics provide one of the methods to combine these parallel streams to the coherent representation of the field, discovering the intellectual centers of gravity of the field as well as the conceptual bridges and collaboration networks between otherwise separate scholarly communities (Jalali et al., 2019; Nobanee et al., 2023; Dotsenko and Kuzmenko, 2023).

Methodologically, this study is grounded in a pragmatic paradigm that draws upon elements of both positivist and constructivist perspectives without being fully aligned with either tradition. The bibliometric component reflects a positivist orientation by systematically examining publication trends, citation networks, keyword co-occurrences, and centrality measures to identify patterns in the development and organization of knowledge within the field. These quantitative indicators provide a structured means of mapping the intellectual landscape and understanding the evolution of scholarly contributions over time. At the same time, the study adopts an interpretivist perspective in the analysis and explanation of thematic clusters, shifts in research priorities, and the formation of scholarly communities. The interpretation of these patterns extends beyond numerical outputs and requires contextual understanding of the literature and its development. This dual perspective is particularly relevant in the context of healthcare cybersecurity and ransomware research, where technical dimensions intersect with organizational, managerial, and patient-safety concerns. A ransomware attack, for instance, may be examined as a technological event through quantitative evidence, yet its broader implications can only be fully understood through qualitative interpretation. As highlighted by Paul et al. (2021) in the SPAR-4-SLR framework, a pragmatic stance prioritizes the research problem when determining methodological choices rather than adhering rigidly to a single philosophical position. Consistent with this approach, the present study integrates bibliometric evidence with interpretive analysis to develop a richer and more comprehensive understanding of the literature. By combining quantitative mapping with qualitative insights, the study is able to contextualize emerging patterns, explain their significance, and generate findings that contribute meaningfully to both theory and practice.

## RESEARCH METHODOLOGY

The bibliometric analysis is made with the SPAR-4-SLR framework developed by Paul et al. which presents the process of systematic literature review in terms of three stages of gathering, structuring, and evaluating. This framework is employed due to its emphasis on methodological transparency and replicability is especially significant when undertaking a bibliometric review of an interdisciplinary research that has intertwined subjects of an engineering study and clinical science study, in addition to policy study.

The bibliometric analysis is compiled with the help of Scopus database due to its ability to cover the whole range of peer-reviewed literature and their metadata framework which fits the bibliometric software. Moreover, this database is a good choice in particular when performing a bibliometric analysis of an interdisciplinary domain like healthcare cybersecurity since it encompasses a diverse variety of fields of expertise, which have been involved in this domain of research. The search in the database includes the years 1997 to June 2026, and it was done to embrace the timeframe of when this sector of cybersecurity started to be taken seriously in regards to digital health security.

The search query was created as a result of refining the search query, through the published recommendations on how to design a Boolean query in bibliometric studies and prior literature that has discussed the topic of healthcare data security, threat management with AI and regulatory governance in health environments:

*(TITLE-ABS-KEY("healthcare cybersecurity" OR "medical cybersecurity" OR "health information security" OR "hospital cyber security" OR "healthcare data breach" OR "ransomware in healthcare") AND ("artificial intelligence" OR "AI" OR "machine learning" OR "intrusion detection" OR "anomaly detection" OR "cyber resilience") AND (("regulatory compliance" OR "data protection" OR "HIPAA" OR "GDPR" OR "governance" OR "cyber risk management")))*

The three-part Boolean structure was designed to capture studies that explicitly address cybersecurity within a health context, incorporate technological approaches to threat detection or mitigation, and engage with governance or regulatory dimensions of digital health security. This combination was chosen to identify literature that addresses healthcare cybersecurity comprehensively rather than from a single disciplinary perspective; studies addressing only one or two of these dimensions were considered outside the scope of this review.

The exclusion criteria covered editorials, errata, notes, and retracted publications for the purposes of analytical work. These document types were identified in the dataset and retained for descriptive reporting in Table 1 to provide a complete picture of the source material; the analytical stages of the study focused on peer-reviewed journal articles, review articles, and conference papers as the primary scholarly corpus.

The evaluation step involved two software packages namely Biblioshiny with bibliometrix package and VOSviewer. The analyses included yearly patterns of scientific output, count of global and local citation, and networks of authors and institutional collaboration, key word co-occurrence visualization, bibliographic coupling, co-citation analysis, thematic mapping with Callon measures of centrality and density, and theme evolution in five time slices that represent almost thirty years. The SPAR-4-SLR has methodological rigour and achieves this through the use of clear delimitations between review stages. Limitations such as database bias, keyword bias and the omission of non indexed literature have been recognized as inherent limitations that cut across any bibliometric frameworks of this type.

## RESULTS

*Table 1. Descriptive Analysis*

| Description | Results |
|---|---|
| MAIN INFORMATION ABOUT DATA | |
| Timespan | 1997:June 2026 |
| Sources (Journals, Books, etc) | 878 |
| Documents | 1366 |
| Annual Growth Rate % | 12.04 |
| Document Average Age | 4.42 |
| Average citations per doc | 12.76 |
| References | 9645 |
| DOCUMENT CONTENTS | |
| Keywords Plus (ID) | 5319 |
| Author's Keywords (DE) | 2917 |
| AUTHORS | |
| Authors | 4100 |
| Authors of single-authored docs | 170 |
| AUTHORS COLLABORATION | |
| Single-authored docs | 173 |
| Co-Authors per Doc | 3.45 |
| International co-authorships % | 20.5 |
| DOCUMENT TYPES | |
| Article | 547 |
| Book | 18 |
| book chapter | 153 |
| conference paper | 515 |
| conference review | 29 |
| Editorial | 8 |
| Erratum | 1 |
| Letter | 11 |
| Note | 21 |
| Retracted | 3 |
| Review | 56 |
| short survey | 4 |

Spanning from 1997 to June 2026, the dataset comprises 1,366 documents from 878 unique publication sources, with an annual growth rate of 12.04% reflecting the field's rapid expansion in response to escalating cybersecurity challenges in health infrastructures worldwide. The average document age of 4.42 years points to a fast-moving field where new contributions continually emerge rather than one settling into established consensus. Average citations per document stand at 12.76, supported by a reference pool of 9,645 unique sources. The 4,100 contributing authors average 3.45 co-authors per document, consistent with the collaborative and interdisciplinary character of the field. International co-authorship at 20.5% underscores the broadly shared nature of healthcare cybersecurity as a global challenge. Document types span journal articles (547), conference papers (515), book chapters (153), and reviews (56), a distribution typical of fields where innovations first circulate through conference venues before receiving extended treatment in peer-reviewed journals.

## Co-occurrence Network Analysis:

*Figure 1. Co-occurrence Network (Abstract)*

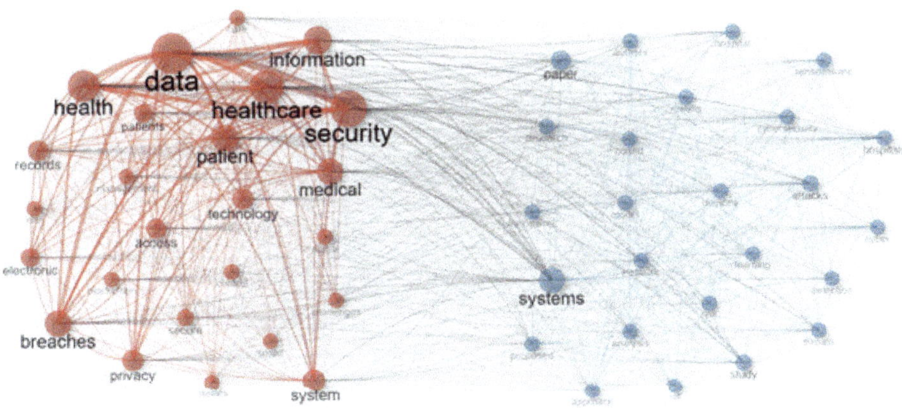


The analysis of abstract keywords using the co-occurrence analysis (Figure 1) indicates that two structural clusters are present in the intellectual architecture of healthcare cybersecurity research. The former, and, by far, the most prevalent cluster, revolves around the keywords such as data, healthcare, security, patient, privacy and breaches. The level of interconnection in this cluster is an indicator of conceptual maturity: the security of patient data has been an internally stable issue throughout the history of the profession.

The second set revolves around such keywords as systems, cybersecurity, attack, detection, learning, model, and IoT. The dominance of the word systems in this cluster is one significant change in the direction of guarding the separate data storage facilities to handling and guaranteeing complete hospital ecosystems against advanced attacks. The keywords of machine learning as well as the inclusion of the term IoT indicate the introduction of AI to the field of cybersecurity and an increasing worry about networked medical devices as a source of attack. The keywords, which are used in both of the clusters, include security, systems, and healthcare, which means that the domain is not subdivided into rival sub-agendas but it is actively striving to achieve an integrated research agenda.

Bibliographic Coupling: The bibliographic coupling makes use of citations, reference lists, and references to measure the similarity between documents.

## Bibliographic Coupling & Citation Analysis:

*Figure 2. Clustering by Coupling Map*

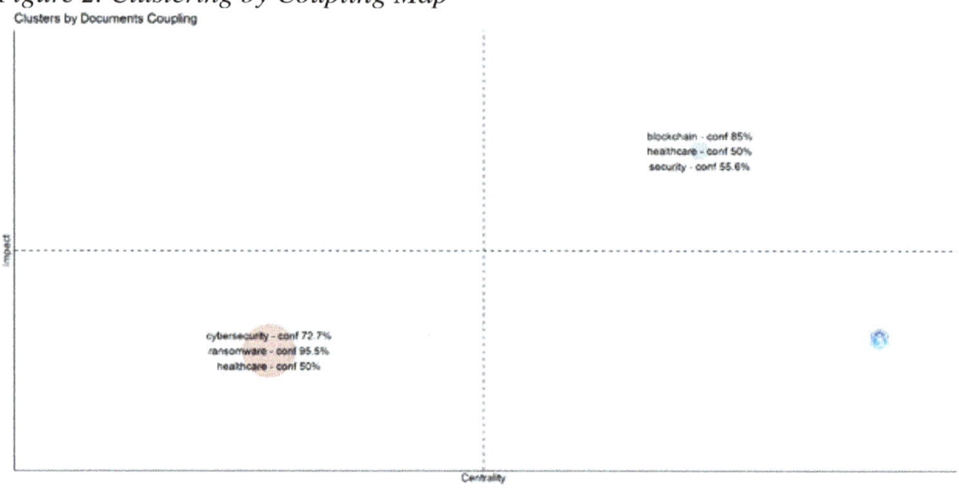


The bibliographic coupling map (Figure 2) groups documents according to the degree to which they share common references, plotting each cluster along two dimensions: centrality, which reflects how closely a cluster connects to the wider body of literature, and impact, which captures the average citation influence of the documents within each cluster.

Two primary clusters are identifiable. The first, positioned in the upper-right quadrant and therefore high in both centrality and impact, is anchored by the keywords blockchain (confidence 85%), healthcare (confidence 50%), and security (confidence 55.6%). The placement of this cluster indicates that documents linking blockchain technology with healthcare security represent a prominent and well-cited strand of the literature. The high confidence value for blockchain suggests it is the most defining characteristic of this cluster, consistent with sustained research interest in decentralised data security solutions during the period covered by the dataset.

The second cluster, located below the impact midpoint at moderate centrality, is defined by cybersecurity (confidence 72.7%), ransomware (confidence 95.5%), and healthcare (confidence 50%). The very high confidence value for ransomware indicates that documents in this cluster are strongly and distinctively associated with ransomware-related research. The cluster's below-average impact score may reflect the tendency for incident-focused technical studies to appear in conference proceedings rather than peer-reviewed journals, which typically attract fewer citations. Despite its lower impact, the cluster's moderate centrality confirms that ransomware research is well integrated into the broader healthcare cybersecurity literature.

A third, smaller cluster appears at high centrality but low impact, suggesting a body of work that is structurally connected to the main research network but has not yet accumulated substantial citation influence, possibly representing emerging or methodologically specialised work not yet widely adopted by citing authors.

The overall pattern suggests two relatively distinct intellectual traditions within healthcare cybersecurity: one oriented toward technological innovation and data governance, and another driven by incident response and threat analysis. The limited overlap between clusters reflects the tendency for these two research communities to draw on different foundational literatures, consistent with the thematic fragmentation noted elsewhere in this study.

Note: Confidence values reported alongside cluster keywords reflect the degree of association between a keyword and its assigned cluster as calculated by the Biblioshiny bibliometrix package. They indicate the probability that a given keyword belongs to its assigned cluster rather than to an alternative cluster within the same analysis.

*Figure 3. Thematic Map*

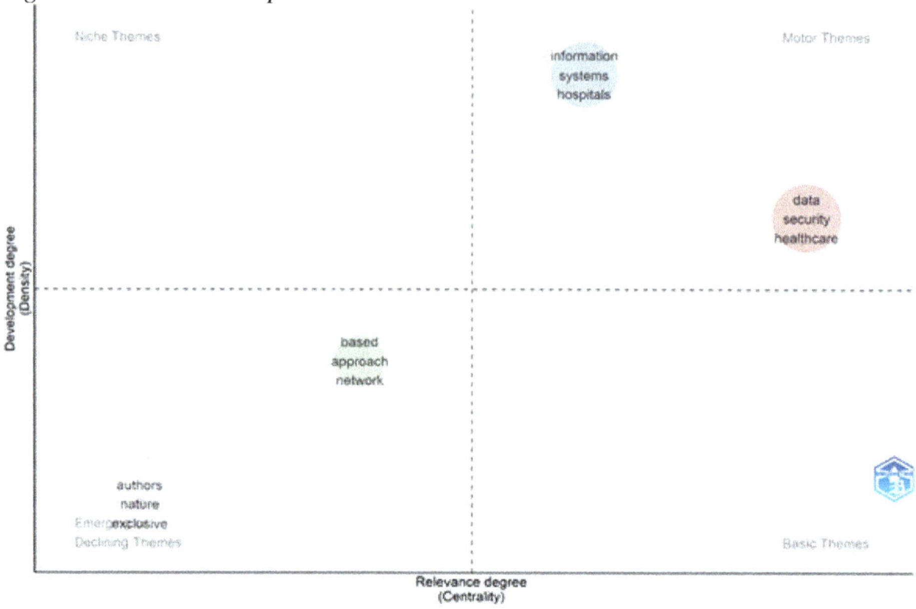


*Figure 4. Thematic Map – Network*

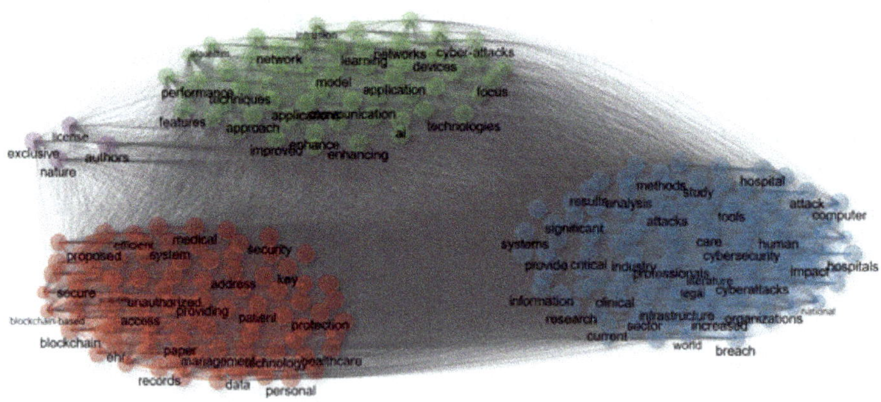

As demonstrated in (Figures 3,4), the terms used in the context of healthcare cybersecurity are very diverse, as the sphere is multi-dimensional. The terms healthcare, security, data, systems, hospitals, attacks, and cybersecurity are frequently used which indicates a high level of attention given to the digital health infrastructure protection and patient information systems.

The presence of other widely occurring words such as blockchain, protection, access, privacy, unauthorized, and medical records denotes the significance of safe data exchange, confidentiality and identity management within a healthcare setting. Meanwhile, such terms as attacks, breach, ransomware, detection, learning, model, and IoT underline the technical nature of research in the field of cybersecurity. The keywords imply that it is now more focused on artificial intelligence, intrusion detection systems, and protection of connected medical devices.

The occurrence of the terms concerned with learning and algorithms, along with models, signify the growing popularity of the predictive analytics and AI-driven approaches in the fields of healthcare cybersecurity as well. Such solutions are also becoming a significant component of the contemporary hospital security systems.

Based on the thematic mapping, data security healthcare seems to be a motor theme with a high level of relevance, and high development. It means that the preservation of healthcare data is a topical and well-developed field of study. Equally, the information systems hospitals theme is equally ranked as high and it can be considered as an indicator of the increasing interest in cybersecurity at the system level in healthcare institutions.

Conversely, such topics as based approach networks are placed under the emerging category that proposes that network-based security models are under development. The other themes that are less central and dense are defining niche or underdeveloped research areas.

The most predominant data security healthcare cluster at the cluster level has a high idea development and significance. The integrated healthcare infrastructure security is evidenced by the shift in the information systems hospitals cluster. The blockchain protection access cluster is relevant and less mature, which means that it is in development. The network approach based cluster reflects new technical approaches like intrusion detection systems.

The studies of healthcare cybersecurity have gone through various phases. It started with its emphasis on ensuring the safety of patient data and proceeded to adopt a hospital information system and has since advanced to more complex technologies like blockchain and artificial intelligence. This development can be viewed as an indication of a discipline that has grown into a more integrated and technology-focused paradigm of cybersecurity.

*Figure 5. Thematic Evolution Map – Abstract*

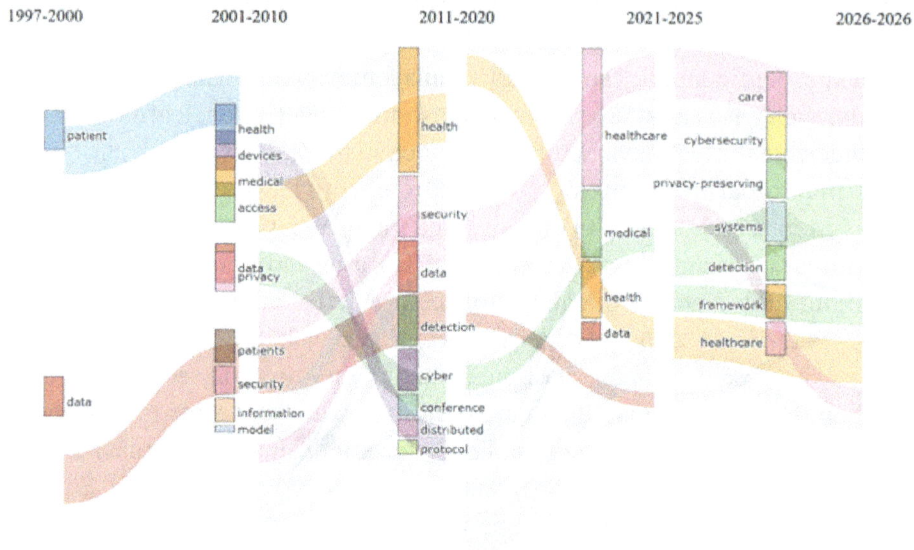


The information offered in (Figure 5) reveals a very broad spectrum of the terms that could be applied to healthcare cybersecurity as it is a multi-dimensional condition. The keywords often used (healthcare, security, data, systems, hospitals, attacks, and cybersecurity) mark the high interest in the digital health infrastructure and patient information systems protection. It is also indicative of how much weight is placed on the security of hospital systems and confidential medical information.

Such other names as blockchain, protection, access, unauthorized, privacy, and medical records imply that there is increasing concern regarding the safety of data exchange, confidentiality, and access control in healthcare. Meanwhile, the words attacks, breach, ransomware, detection, learning, model, and IoT demonstrate the technical character of the profession and the necessity of cybersecurity mechanisms. It is likely that the use of predictive analytics and AI-based security systems will continue to grow in hospitals because the use of AI-related words, such as learning, model, algorithm, and techniques, is increasing.

The theme data security healthcare has been represented as a motor theme having high centrality, as well as development. This is to mean that healthcare data protection is fairly established and at the center of the study zone. Likewise, the information systems hospital theme is also quite developed and can be attributed to an increased interest in the system-level security in healthcare institutions.

Conversely, the theme of based approach networks is in the emerging category, which implies that network based security models are new and are yet to achieve full maturity. Nature's exclusive theme of the authors is found to be a niche domain with little centrality and growth, meaning that not much research is paid to it.

The most dominant cluster of data security healthcare clusters is centralized and dense at the cluster level. It pays attention to such aspects as protection of patient data, breach prevention, and compliance with regulations. The shift to the integrated hospital cybersecurity infrastructure is denoted by the information systems hospitals cluster. The blockchain protection access cluster is very relevant and less mature meaning that it is in its developmental stages. The cluster that is based on the network approach is new research in the technical field, including intrusion detection and AI-based cybersecurity models.

In general, the thematic framework demonstrates a distinct development of healthcare cybersecurity research. It has shifted to a concern with basic data protection to system-level security and currently advanced technologies like blockchain and artificial intelligence. This shows that the essential focus has changed towards higher proactive and technology-driven security models as opposed to reactive measures.

The current state of healthcare cybersecurity research extends to the field of data protection, infrastructure security, and technological innovation, which can be viewed as indicative of the maturity of the field and its increased role in the digitalized medical system.

*Figure 6. Thematic Evolution Map – Time Slice 1*

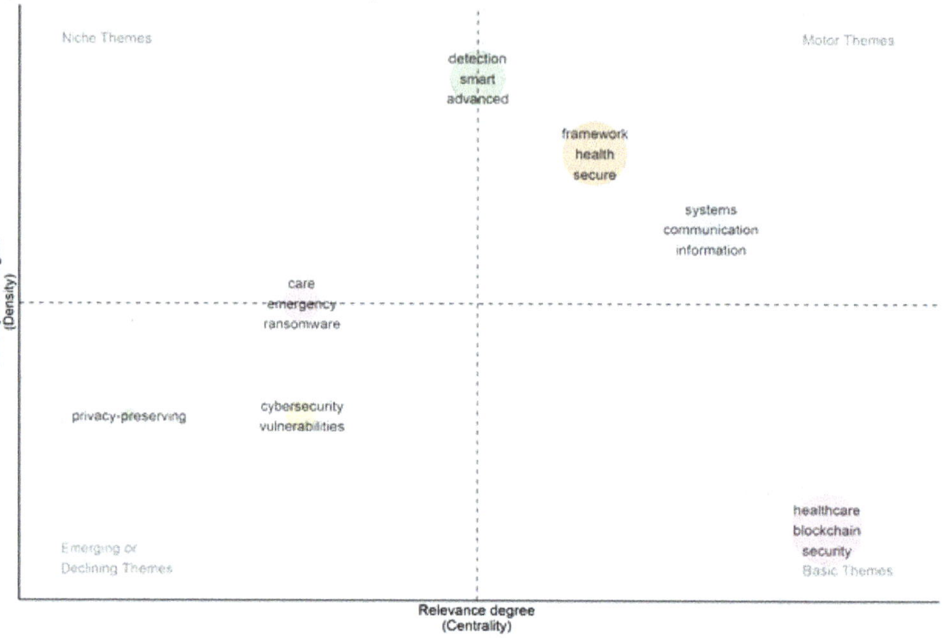


The first time slice maps the early intellectual architecture of healthcare cybersecurity research, a period when the field was establishing its foundational concerns before major disruptive incidents reshaped its priorities. The dominant cluster, combining systems, communication, and information, sits firmly in the Motor Themes quadrant, indicating that securing hospital communication networks and health information systems was the defining preoccupation of researchers at this stage. The widespread adoption of electronic health records and networked hospital infrastructure had created an urgent demand for research into communication security, data transfer protocols, and system-level protection, and the literature responded accordingly.

The framework-health-secure cluster also shows high density alongside moderate-to-high centrality, suggesting that governance frameworks and security designs specific to healthcare were already beginning to take shape as a coherent body of knowledge, though still developing somewhat separately from the technical infrastructure research.

The detection-smart-advanced cluster occupies the niche quadrant, high in internal density but low in centrality. Advanced detection systems and AI-assisted security tools were already being explored by specialist researchers, but had not yet connected with the broader governance or infrastructure conversations taking place in the field. The emergence of care-emergency-ransomware as a loosely organized cluster is worth noting: ransomware appears here as a growing concern, but one that had not attracted the sustained theoretical attention it would receive after 2017. Privacy-preserving mechanisms appear in the declining or emerging quadrant, suggesting that standalone privacy discourse was beginning to be absorbed into larger frameworks. Blockchain security registers as a Basic Theme, widely referenced but not yet conceptually mature.

Overall, the findings suggest a field that was still establishing its technical foundations, with governance and detection research present but not yet integrated into a common research agenda.

*Figure 7. Thematic Evolution Map – Time Slice 2*

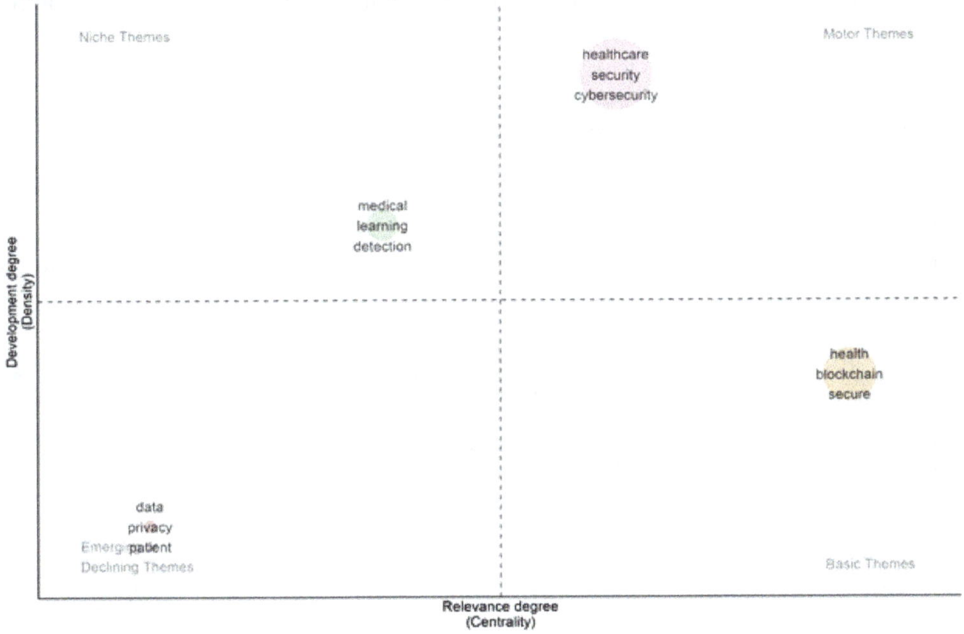


By the second time slice, the intellectual landscape had begun to shift. Where the first period was defined by foundational infrastructure concerns, this period shows security and healthcare moving toward closer integration, with governance considerations starting to carry greater weight alongside technical themes.

The healthcare-security cluster emerges as the dominant force, centralized and dense, reflecting the increasing convergence of clinical priorities with cybersecurity concerns. This cluster encompasses not only data protection and network configuration but also institutional responses to cyber risk, hospital-level policy, and patient data governance as an integrated concern.

Blockchain registers more prominently here than in the first slice, appearing as a moderately developed cluster. Its growth during this period reflects broader interest in decentralized data systems, though the gap between academic attention and actual deployment remained significant. The detection-learning cluster, combining AI and machine learning themes with active security monitoring, shows moderate centrality and moderate density, suggesting that AI-driven cybersecurity was gaining traction as a research area without having yet achieved the prominence it would later develop.

Rather than introducing entirely new themes, this period was characterized by the further development of themes that had already emerged in the earlier stage. Research communities were beginning to organize around distinct approaches, including institutional security governance, AI-based detection, and blockchain-based data protection. Although the field was becoming more diverse, these research communities remained largely disconnected from one another.

*Figure 8. Thematic Evolution Map – Time Slice 3*

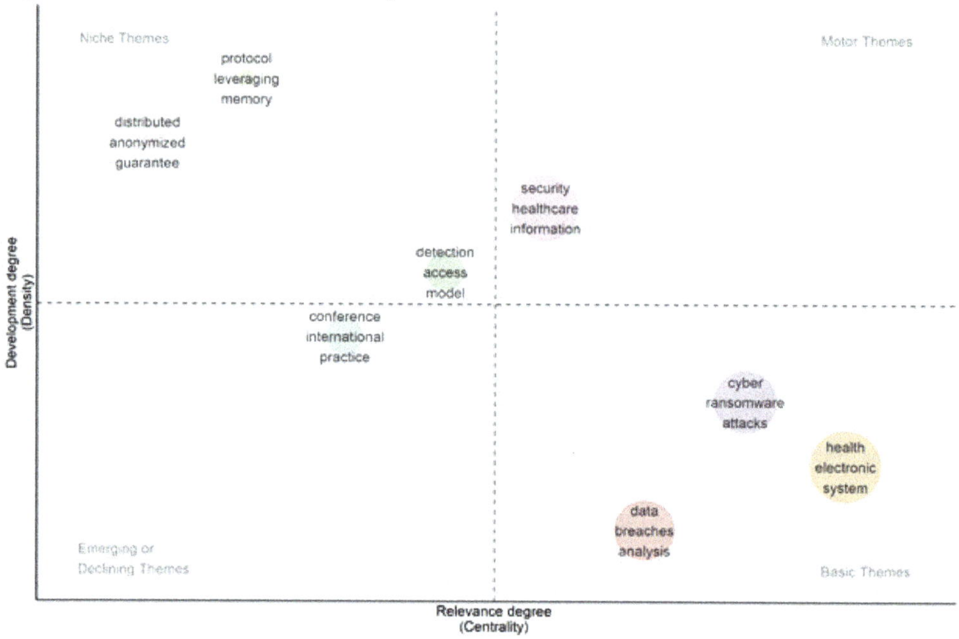


The third time slice carries the clearest imprint of real-world events. This period coincides with the aftermath of major cyberattacks on health systems, and the thematic structure of the research reflects this directly. For the first time, cyber, ransomware, and attacks appear as Basic Themes, meaning they are highly central to the research network even if their theoretical development remains incomplete. Ransomware had crossed from a niche technical concern into a mainstream research priority.

The Motor Themes quadrant is dominated by the security-healthcare-information cluster, which by this point represents a well-developed and influential body of research. The presence of health-electronic-system and data-breaches-analysis as Basic Themes confirms that hospital digital infrastructure and breach analysis were major active concerns, driven by the volume of reported incidents during this period.

The niche quadrant contains notably technical clusters: protocol, leveraging, and memory alongside distributed, anonymized, and guarantee. These suggest that technical specialists were working on advanced security architecture and anonymization systems, but that this work remained disconnected from the governance-oriented mainstream. The detection-access-model cluster in the emerging quadrant hints at security modelling work that was still taking shape.

A notable feature of this period is the reactive nature of its research agenda. Themes are organized around incident types and breach categories rather than governance outcomes. The thematic structure suggests that research during this period was strongly influenced by ongoing cyber incidents, resulting in a substantial body of applied work oriented toward immediate challenges rather than broader governance frameworks.

*Figure 9. Thematic Evolution Map – Time Slice 4*

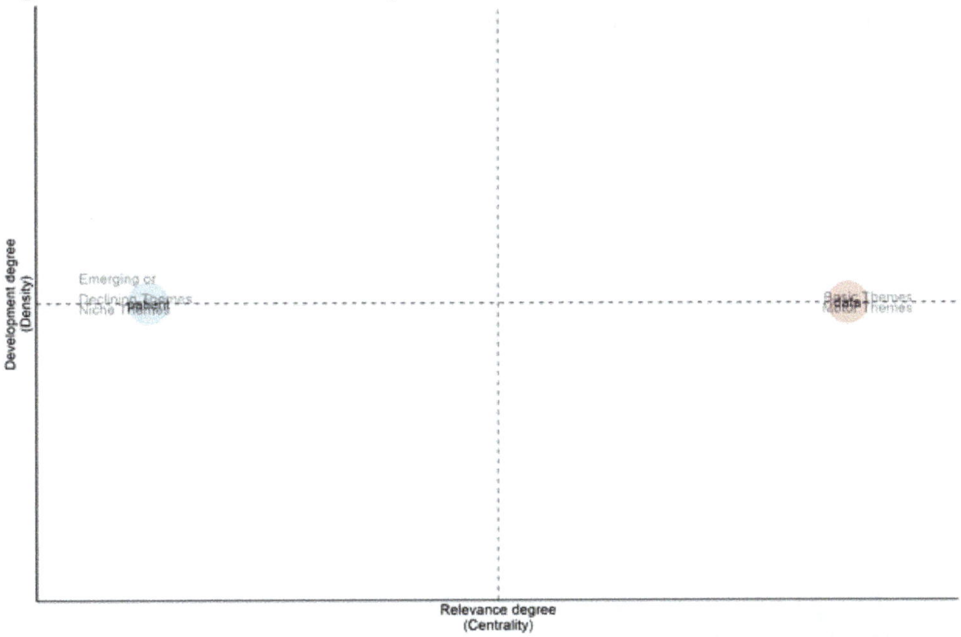


By the fourth time slice, the reactive posture visible in the previous period had begun to give way to a more systematic approach. The Motor Themes quadrant now includes security-hospital-risk as a consolidated cluster, alongside model-assignment-authoring and information-assurance-management. These are not simply technical themes; they describe the institutionalization of cybersecurity risk governance within healthcare organizations, with structured frameworks, accountability models, and formal assurance practices becoming central research concerns.

These findings indicate a shift in how the research community conceptualized healthcare cybersecurity challenges. Earlier periods focused primarily on identifying threats and understanding their mechanisms. In contrast, this period increasingly emphasized how organizations should be structured to manage those threats over time.

The Basic Themes quadrant includes devices-internet-issues and health-electronic-legal, pointing to two developing concerns: the security challenges posed by IoMT devices and the legal and regulatory frameworks governing digital health data. Both themes had high centrality but relatively low density, indicating that they were widely referenced but not yet theoretically consolidated. The declining or emerging quadrant is particularly informative, as data breaches, privacy, and network themes show reduced density. This pattern suggests that standalone breach-response discourse was increasingly being incorporated into broader governance-oriented discussions rather than remaining independent areas of inquiry.

*Figure 10. Thematic Evolution Map – Time Slice 5*

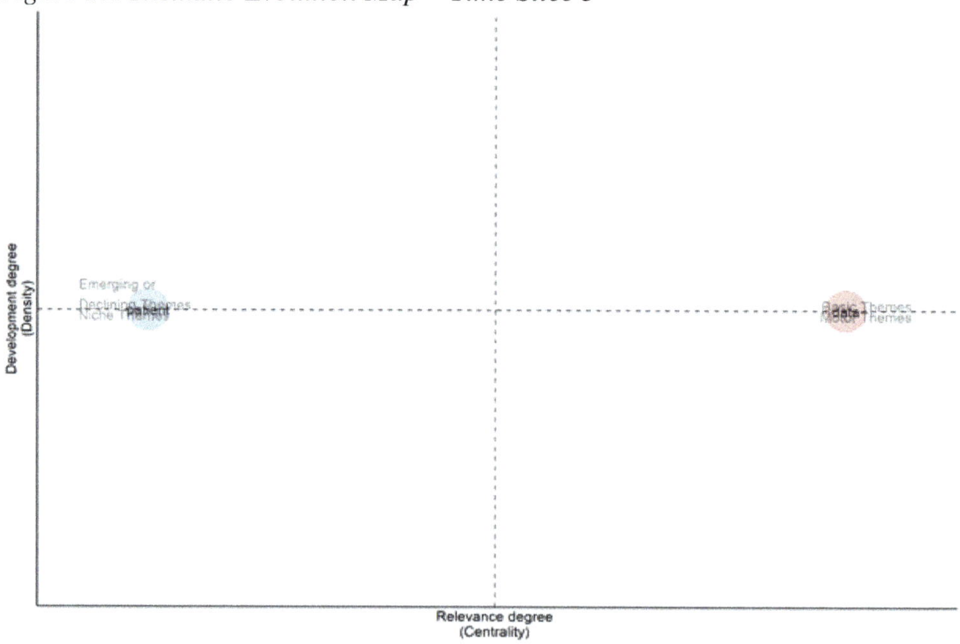

The fifth time slice presents a markedly different picture from its predecessors. Where earlier maps showed multiple clusters organized around distinct themes, this final period is characterized by consolidation. Only two principal clusters are visible, and the dominant one sits at the boundary between Basic and Motor Themes, indicating a research field that has largely resolved its thematic fragmentation and converged around a coherent macro-level concern.

This convergence reflects the cumulative development of the field over nearly three decades. Themes that appeared separately in earlier periods, including technical security infrastructure, governance frameworks, institutional risk management, AI-based detection, and regulatory compliance, increasingly converged into a broader conception of healthcare cybersecurity as a strategic, system-wide priority rather than a technical specialty.

The smaller cluster in this slice sits at the Niche and Emerging boundary, indicating that certain methodological or technical sub-domains have not yet been fully absorbed into the central conversation. These may gain prominence in the next phase of research, or they may reflect transitional themes that are losing relevance as the field settles.

The final slice suggests that healthcare cybersecurity has evolved from a collection of specialized research streams into a more coherent field with a shared intellectual focus. The consolidation visible here indicates that future research may be built upon a more stable foundation than was available to earlier scholars working across relatively disconnected sub-domains.

A search of keywords that involve healthcare cybersecurity (Figure 11-15) indicates that a strong tendency is present in the development of the digital health protection and integration of technology. As an example, the keyword that we identified as the most prevalent was eHealth record having 422 instances, indicating that the safety of EHR systems is the very heart of healthcare cybersecurity studies.

Other keywords that appeared the most of the time were observed to be the following: health care (304 occurrences) and network security (303 occurrences), which implies that the topic of healthcare cybersecurity research is very specific to the systemic and infrastructure-based component of cybersecurity in the healthcare environment. The fact that such dominant keywords as cyber security have 270 occurrences, and human has 270 occurrences indicates that the studies of healthcare cybersecurity are not only focused on technical aspects of cybersecurity, but also on the human aspect of cybersecurity in hospitals.

The keywords of the technological nature including blockchain (257 occurrences), cyber security (219 occurrences), and computer security (210 occurrences) indicate that research on healthcare cybersecurity identifies much focus on the concept of decentralized technology and secure computing paradigm in healthcare environments.

*Figure 11. Most Relevant Sources*

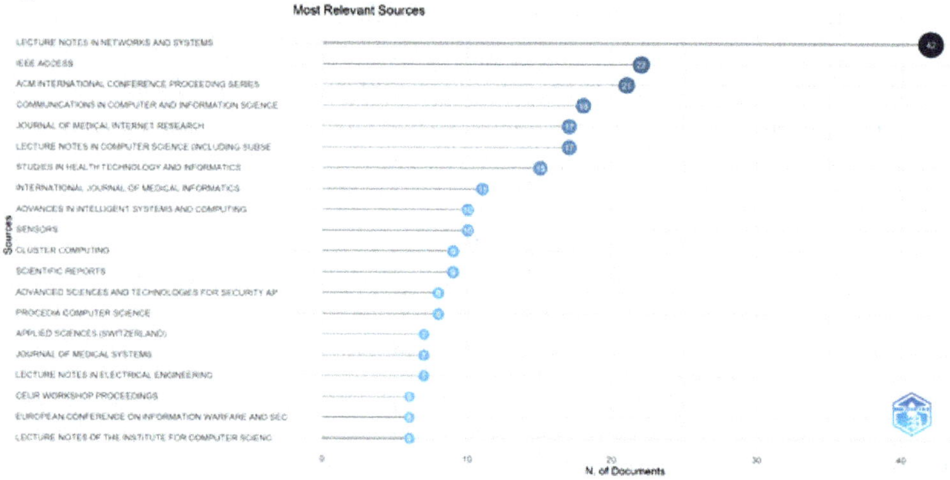


*Figure 12. Most Relevant Authors*

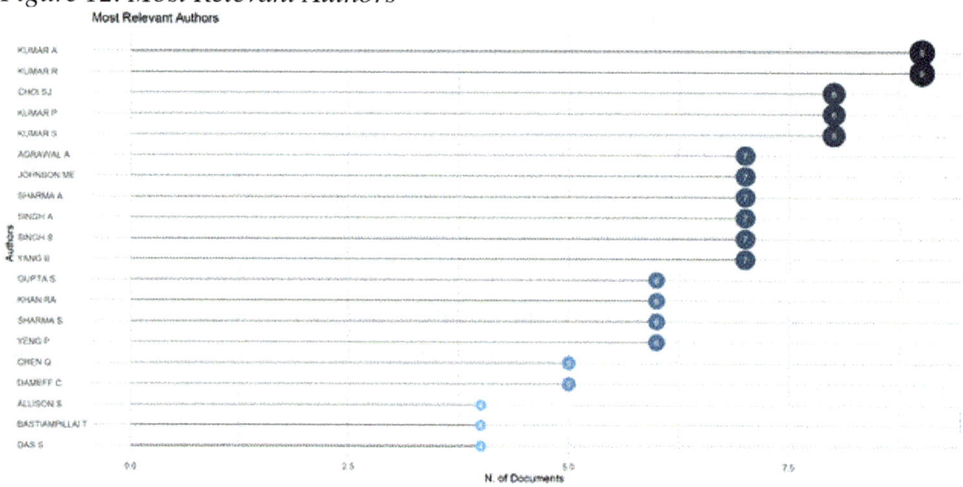

*Figure 13. Most Relevant Affiliations*

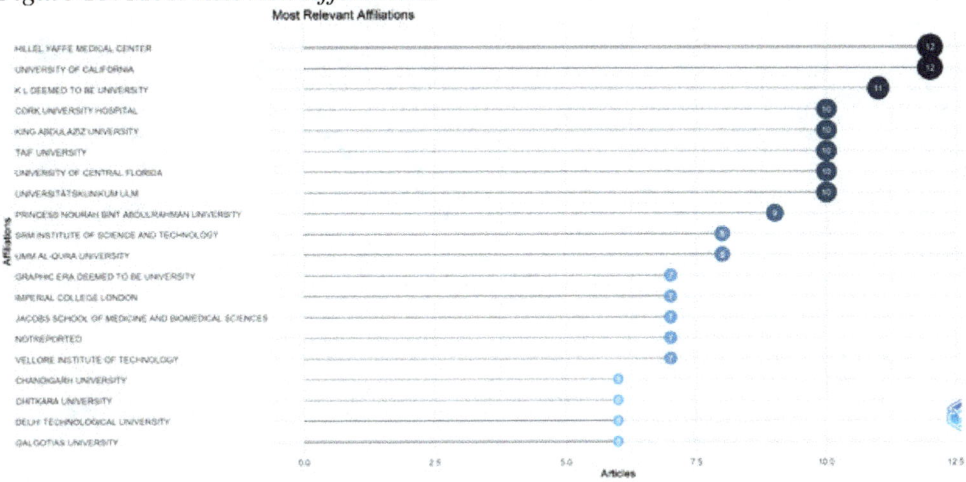


*Figure 14. Most Global Cited Document*

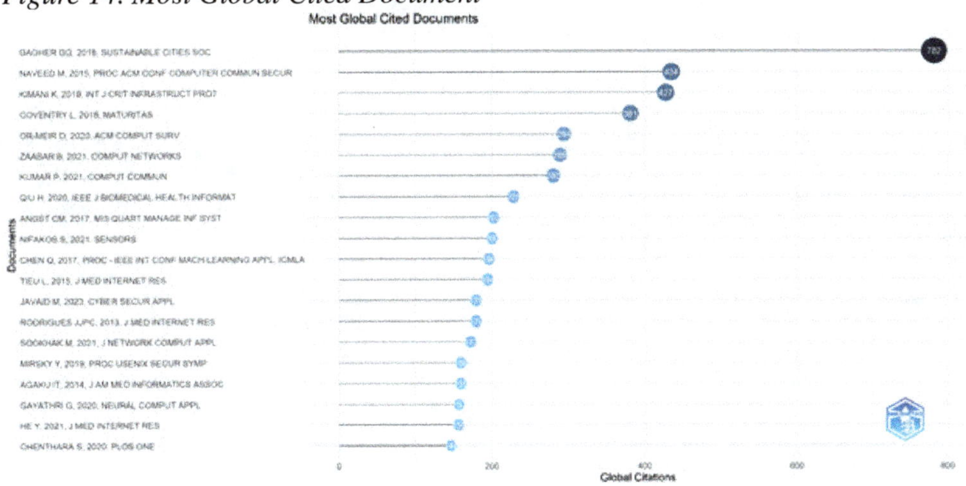

*Figure 15. Most Frequent Words*

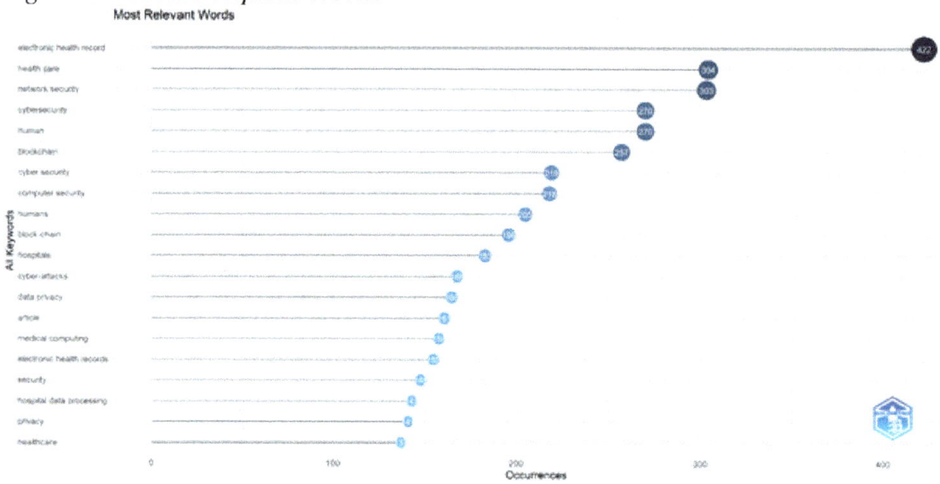


*Figure 16. Trend Topics*

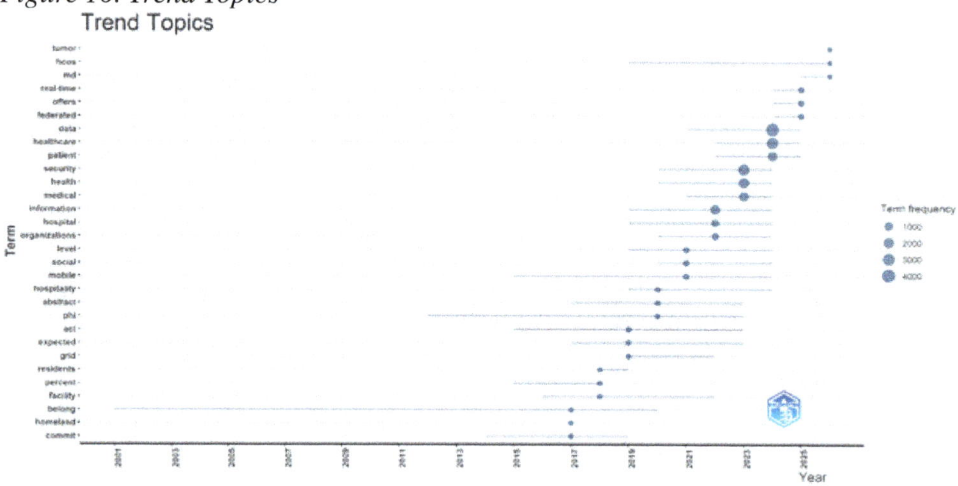


The frequency data (Figure 16) indicates that the pattern of healthcare cybersecurity research has undoubtedly shifted, particularly since the year 2018, with the growth rate increasing further in 2020 and further. The use of several words is also becoming common, and it is the indicator of the dynamism of the process of digital healthcare protection and integration.

The simple words related to healthcare, including the terms healthcare, patient, health, medical, hospital, and information, have shown an increasing trend since

2019 to 2024. This higher rate of these basic healthcare related words is an indication of the heightened interest on the safety of digital healthcare systems and the safety of patient-focused information systems.

The words dealing with security, e.g., security, data, and federated, have increased in growth at a higher rate since 2020. The term federated is particularly remarkable in this regard, given that its frequency of usage is amplified by the amplified interest in federated learning models and architectures in the framework of healthcare cybersecurity.

The emergence of the words "real-time" and "mobile" are also another indicator of the greater relevance of dynamic monitoring systems, telehealth solutions, and mobile health applications. Interestingly, such terminology as phi (Protected Health Information) became popular in the period between 2012 and 2020, which centered the issues of compliance-related aspects of the topic.

Nevertheless, the recent years have shown the tendency toward more generic system-related topics such as healthcare, patient, federated, etc., which possibly signals the transition of the confined compliance-related aspects to a more coherent digital governance strategy.

Homeland, facility, residents, percent are also terms that were used more in the period between 2001 and 2016, which might also imply that the first steps towards the topic of healthcare cybersecurity were policy-related over AI or technology-related.

The emergence of such words as offers, md, hcos (Health Care Organizations), tumor, etc. indicates that there is a trend to use the topic of cybersecurity in the specialized context.

In general, the analysis of the trends above represents three significant temporal shifts:

Early Phase (1997-2015): Policy, infrastructure and facilities discussions.

Middle Phase (2016-2019): The talks about going big, patient data security, and security in the organization.

Recent Phase (2020-2025): debates on the expedited growth of federated learning systems, real-time surveillance systems, mobile health security, AI based healthcare and cybersecurity structures.

Based on the above analysis, it is evident that a move has been done towards dynamic protection systems, as opposed to the existence of the static protection systems. The recent growth in federated systems has been due to the significance of AI systems in healthcare cybersecurity.

The research on healthcare cybersecurity has evolved through the initial interest in the field of protection of data to more elaborate, technology-based strategies, which reflect the overall evolution of health systems in the digital arena worldwide.

*Figure 17. Factorial Analysis*

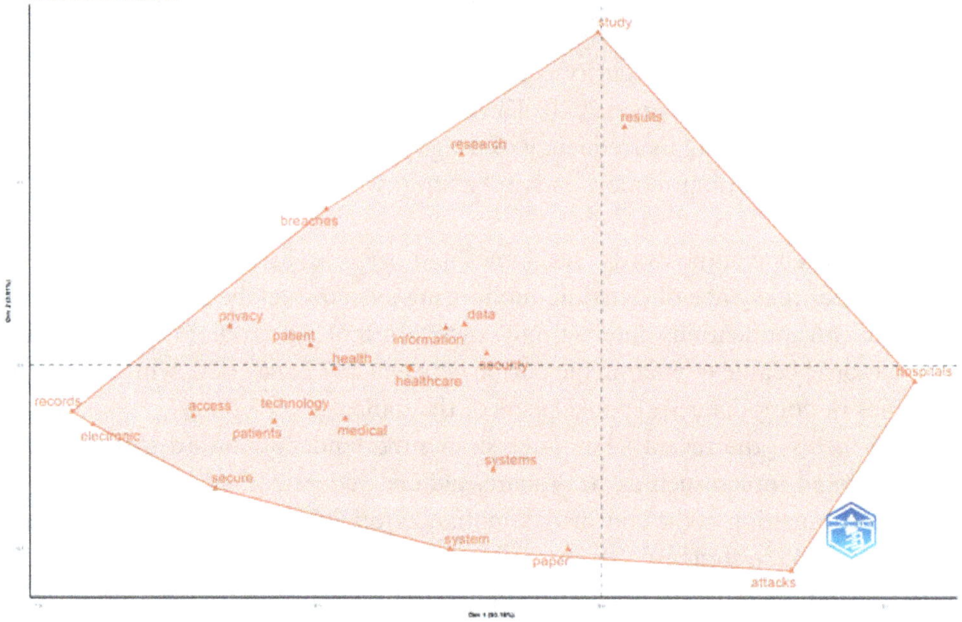


Figure 17, which is the Conceptual Structure Map created with the help of Multiple Correspondence Analysis, gives a two-dimensional perspective of the intellectual framework of the research on healthcare cybersecurity. The two axes indicate the change in the themes and the way the varied concepts are connected or distanced. The horizontal axis differentiates patient data oriented topics with general system level issues regarding cybersecurity, whereas the vertical axis separates governance related themes with operational and technical research.

Healthcare, health, security, data, information, and medical are the key terms closely clustered at the centre of the map. This is because this central positioning implies that the majority of research is constructed based on the protection of medical data and health information systems.Data and security are closely related to healthcare, which reflects their firm interconnection in the sphere.

On the left, one can see such terms as records, electronic, privacy, patient, access, secure, and breaches that create a cluster of terms dedicated to patient data protection. This is an indication of initial studies that focused on electronic health records and privacy issues. The fact that breaches are still present implies that there will still be focus on other negative factors, like ransomwares and data leakages in this sector.

The words on the right (including hospitals, attacks, and systems) suggest that one shifts towards institutional and infrastructure-level security. This topic focuses on practical cyber threats to healthcare organizations and underscores the increased attention to operational cybersecurity issues.

The terminologies in the lower section imply systems and technical focus that focuses on system design, security architecture, and infrastructure modelling. This is an indication of a shift in the safeguarding of individual records to the safeguarding of the complete healthcare systems.

The upper part entails such terms as research, study and results, which denote the analytical and methodological aspect of the sphere. It means that healthcare cybersecurity is an academic field that is becoming more mature.

In general, the map presents three key areas, including patient data protection, institutional system protection, and governance and analytical research. It also demonstrates a distinct change of looking at the issue of privacy and records alone to a more comprehensive and all-encompassing system in healthcare in relation to cybersecurity. This indicates that the discipline is increasingly going into convergence and integrates the technological, organizational and analytical points of view.

*Figure 18. Co-Citation Network*

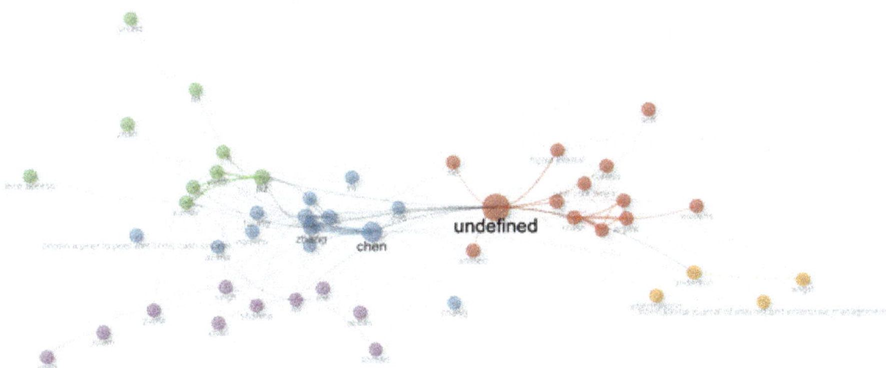


The co-citation network (Figure 18) maps the degree to which authors and sources within the healthcare cybersecurity literature are cited together across the dataset. When two items are frequently referenced in the same publications they appear in close proximity within the network, and clusters reflect communities of work that share a common intellectual foundation.

Four primary clusters are visible. The blue cluster, anchored by authors including Chen, Zhang, Kumar, Huang, and Nguyen, represents the most densely connected community and reflects a technical research tradition associated with AI-based security systems, intrusion detection, and network defence within healthcare environments. The high internal connectivity of this cluster indicates that these authors are regularly cited together, suggesting a coherent body of work with shared methodological and thematic foundations.

The green cluster, including Liu, Yang, Zhao, Lin, and Javaid, forms a distinct co-citation community associated with emerging technology applications in healthcare security, including blockchain and decentralised systems. The purple cluster, comprising Singh, Sharma, Ali, Khan, Abbas, and Ahmad, represents a research community whose members are frequently co-cited in studies addressing data protection and access management in clinical settings.

The red cluster is notable for the prominence of an 'undefined' node, which represents references that could not be fully parsed by the bibliometric software, likely due to inconsistent citation formatting in the Scopus source records. This cluster also includes grey literature and policy sources such as the HIPAA Journal and Cureus, indicating that a portion of healthcare cybersecurity research draws on non-traditional citation sources alongside peer-reviewed literature. A smaller orange cluster reflects a distinct governance-oriented strand of the literature with limited overlap with the other communities.

Overall, the co-citation network reveals that healthcare cybersecurity research draws on several intellectually distinct traditions that remain partially compartmentalised. While some cross-cluster citation activity is visible, the clusters are predominantly self-referential, indicating that the field has not yet converged around a single unified foundational literature.

*Figure 19. Historiograph*

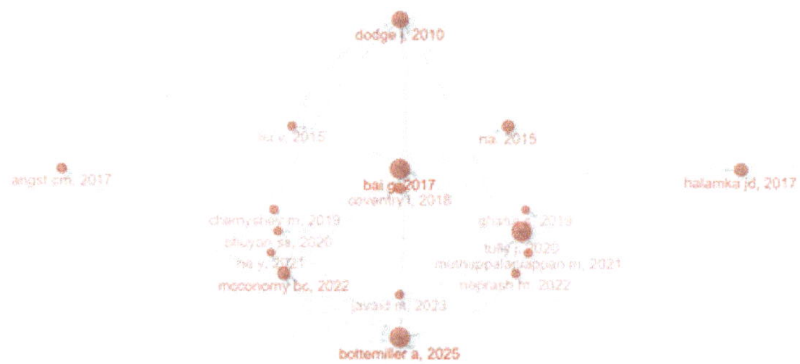


Figure 19 (historiography) illustrates the chronological progression of the study on the topic of healthcare cybersecurity by drawing citation links among the most notable works. Unlike the co-citation analysis, it focuses on the manner in which the knowledge has evolved over the years and the manner in which the past studies contributed to the formation of the future ones.

The pioneer research works had an effect on the discipline during the first stage (1997-2015). Further literature was rooted in these premises and overall ideas of cybersecurity used in the healthcare setting. It was an initial stage of establishment of technical knowledge.

The second step (2017-2019) is a sign of the shift towards institutional and governance aspects. The major studies of that period involved risk management, IT governance of healthcare, and questions related to policies, and in this regard, Coventry and Branley (2018) turn critical of the role of connecting technical research with organizational issues.

The field went through a phase of operation and practice growth between 2020 and 2023 and a broad and manifold research emerged. The time is related to the increased activity of research because of real-life cyberattacks, especially ransomware. The primary topics are the resilience of hospitals, breach analytical, policy response, and the use of artificial intelligence in cybersecurity. Bhuyan et al. (2020) presented a foundation with regard to amending the existing culture of healthcare cybersecurity to prevention strategies rather than response actions.

Recent work is more indicative of the emerging trends in the field, since it suggests the further focus on future strategies, countries policy, and the improvement of digital health protection systems, but it is also an extension of prior research.

Balance of the historiographic trend suggests that the studies of healthcare cybersecurity have been cumulative in nature with one step of the research being based on a prior step of the research. The field has expanded to go further than the technical basis to institutional and operational questions more generally, and has grown exponentially since 2019. This fact reveals that cybersecurity has gained increasing importance in the evolving healthcare system in the digital space.

*Figure 20. Authors Collaboration Network*

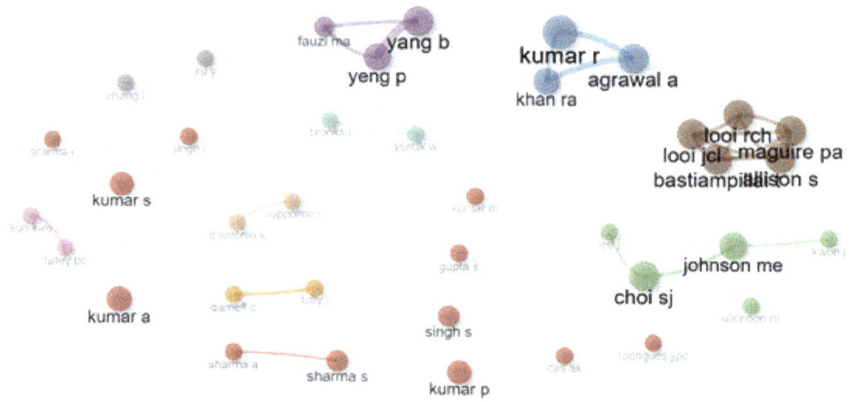


The author collaboration network (Figure 20) reflects the connection between the scholars that operate in the sphere of cybersecurity in healthcare based on the co-authoring. The nodes are the authors and the cooperation is represented by the links. It is observable that the network has several autonomous research groups that are semi-autonomous and this indicates a decentralized system of research that is partially interconnected.

One of the big clusters includes Kumar A, Kumar S, Kumar P, Sharma A, Sharma S and Singh S. This kind of an organization is very cooperative within the group, i.e. there is much co-authorship and even similar institutional or regional backgrounds. Another group of Kumar R, Agrawal A and Khan RA where close collaboration may be observed may be discussed which supports special and aimed research work.

A different group consisting of Choi SJ, Johnson ME, Kwon J and Alkinnon M portrays systematic collaboration, maybe across institutions or disciplines. Johnson ME appears to be a mediating figure between this cluster. Smaller teams, e.g., Loo JCL, Maguirre PA, and Allison S, and Yang B, Yeng P, and Fauzi MA possess a high number of internal connections but a lower number of external connections and one can even propose that they are conducting niche research.

Some of them are loosely intertwined or independent authors, e.g. Zhang L, Xu Y, Kumar M, and Gupta S. This may refer to new scientists or scholars whose contribution falls under the new fields in the field. Smaller collaborations among small groups of authors are also signs that there was early or discovery research.

The network is usually highly modular i.e. it is broken into various clusters. The sphere of collaboration between groups is high, but the relationships between groups are weak. It implies that the active work on research groups exists but the greater collaboration between different groups is in its infancy.

The other research areas that are portrayed by the structure are also artificial intelligence, governance, blockchain and system security. However, the number of links between clusters is not very large, which proves that the field is somewhat fragmented. The further exposure of these groups to each other would make the integration of different approaches to research more effective.

To be more precise, the collaboration network suggests that the research of the field of healthcare cybersecurity is growing increasingly higher, but it is not turning into the fully-integrated one. The local research communities are strongly established and global cooperation is on the rise, which indicates that the discipline is gradually becoming more interconnected and mature.

*Figure 21. Countries Collaboration World Map*

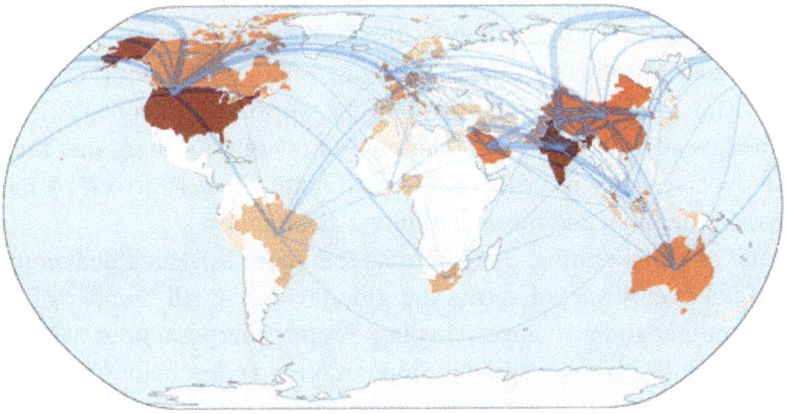

The Countries Collaboration World Map (Figure 21) shows the world trend of the research collaboration on healthcare cybersecurity. The high number of the colors indicates the publishing of the works, and this is the collaboration of the countries, the lines.

The US is the leading global hub, and the study is the most fruitful, and the quantity of international relationships is the highest. It is well related and this means that it is central to the world research shaping. India and China are the other countries on the list, which have proven to be significant in terms of their production and the further development of the global community, especially in areas like AI-driven security and digital health. The United Kingdom, the European countries of Germany and Italy have been highly cooperative with each other forming a tight knit network in the area.

The collaboration between North America and Europe is noted to have a distinct mode of collaboration in that there are in-depth and normal partnerships. The leading fields of such partnerships include healthcare IT governance, AI-based cybersecurity and hospital resilience. India, China, and Australia are among the countries that have been quickly intensifying their cooperation in the Asia-Pacific direction, which is linked to the intensive development of digital healthcare and the increasing role in research activities.

It is a moderate cooperation in the Middle East that is often linked with India, Europe, and the United States which could be most likely attributed to the growing investments in digital healthcare and cybersecurity. South America and certain parts of Africa on the contrary have low levels of collaboration indicating emergent research participation.

Overall, the international network has the characteristics of a core-periphery organization, with the United States as the core. North America and Europe are highly integrated in terms of integration with Asia-Pacific being reinforced and much slower integration with other parts of the world. This can be justified by the fact that the level of international collaboration is high, meaning that the issue of healthcare cybersecurity is a global research inquiry that is driven by the shared challenges, digitization, and the shared interests in policy.

The trend of collaborating also indicates that there exists a global connectivity of research not evenly spread across the globe with a small number of countries sourcing the output and influence. This implies that there is a need to have greater engagement, enhanced cross-regional cooperation and coordination of international cybersecurity policy.

## DISCUSSION

### Key Findings

The bibliometric study has resulted in making important discoveries in the context of the development of the sphere of health care cybersecurity. The research has established that the area of health care cybersecurity has ceased being a side-technical concern to attaining the level of strategic centrality in the digital transformation of health.

The analysis indicates that the structurally most central and most impacting theme areas are the healthcare security systems as indicated by the high values of centrality of the different thematic maps. The use of the key terms, e.g., electronic health records, network security, cybersecurity, and data protection has been identified to occupy central positions in the co-occurrence network maps. This implies the predominance of the existing study area on the security of patient information, hospital security, and the cyber resilience of healthcare facilities.

In addition, the centrality of the word analysis showed that cybersecurity in the hospital level and risk management on the institutional level are important. According to the thematic evolution analysis, it can be stated that the initial terms associated with privacy are replaced by the terms associated with system resilience, ransomware, and governance. The abundance of such terms as hospital, attack, systems, and resilience indicates that more and more researchers are drawn to the issue of cybersecurity threats in hospitals (Wasserman and Wasserman, 2022; Nair and Saha, 2023; Jalali et al., 2019).

Besides, the outcome of the historiographic analysis coupled with citation network analysis also demonstrates the existence of cumulative intellectual progression. The prior background literature was closer to technical security structures and algorithms but later studies involved institutional regulation, AI detection algorithms, and policy reactions towards cyber threats. These findings verify that healthcare cybersecurity as an academic discipline has matured into an interdisciplinary discipline, which encompasses computer science, health informatics, and risk management.

Other themes that emerged, including the idea of federated learning, blockchain, and privacy, also show that recent studies in the sphere of healthcare cybersecurity are focused on more advanced, decentralized, and AI-driven cybersecurity methods. These motifs are becoming increasingly common, and it may prove that more people are interested in collaborative data security, particularly because of the growing demands of healthcare networks in terms of digitization and interoperability.

The prominence of artificial intelligence and blockchain within the bibliometric dataset raises an important question. It remains unclear whether this reflects technologies that are being actively adopted across healthcare systems or topics that attracted heightened attention from researchers and funding bodies during a particular period.

Evidence supports both interpretations. AI-based applications such as anomaly detection systems and intrusion detection tools have moved beyond conceptual discussion in several settings, while federated learning addresses an important challenge related to privacy-preserving data sharing across healthcare networks. In these areas, the strong presence of AI within the literature is likely associated with developments occurring in practice.

The case of blockchain is more nuanced. Publications related to blockchain increased substantially between 2017 and 2020, a period during which the technology attracted considerable interest from researchers, funders, and publishers across multiple sectors. Many proposed healthcare blockchain applications have faced significant implementation challenges, with a number of high-profile initiatives failing to progress beyond pilot stages. This observation does not diminish the value of the research itself; however, it suggests that publication activity and real-world deployment do not necessarily advance at the same pace. Academic attention may be influenced by novelty and funding opportunities as much as by demonstrated clinical demand.

This distinction is important when interpreting the findings of the present study. Measures such as keyword frequency and co-occurrence analysis capture the level of attention a topic receives within the scientific literature rather than its rate of implementation, clinical uptake, or demonstrated effectiveness. A research theme may become highly visible because it remains contested or unresolved, not necessarily because it has been widely adopted in practice. Future studies that combine bibliometric evidence with implementation data from healthcare organizations may provide a clearer understanding of whether prominent research themes represent enduring changes in the field or concentrated periods of academic interest.

The findings of the collaboration analysis also verify that the level of global integration in healthcare cybersecurity research is moderate, USA, India, China, and European countries are big research clusters. Nevertheless, the co-authorship network also demonstrates that the clusters of collaboration are more closed off to one another, with little connecting them (Pratama et al., 2025; Nobanee et al., 2023; Dotsenko and Kuzmenko, 2023).

Notably, the study also highlights several areas that have received comparatively less attention in the existing literature. While a significant proportion of research has focused on technical detection systems, cyber threats, and institutional resilience, there remains a need for greater attention to human factors in healthcare cybersecurity, cybersecurity capacity-building in low- and middle-income countries, the long-term effectiveness of cybersecurity policies, and the integration of AI ethics into clinical cybersecurity practices.

Overall, the findings suggest that healthcare cybersecurity research has grown rapidly over the past decade and has become increasingly interdisciplinary in nature. The field has gradually moved beyond a narrow focus on technical protection towards broader concerns related to system resilience, governance, and AI-enabled security approaches. However, the limited interaction between some thematic research areas and geographical research communities indicates that opportunities still exist for stronger knowledge sharing and collaboration across the field. Addressing these gaps may contribute to a more comprehensive understanding of healthcare cybersecurity and support the development of more effective and sustainable security strategies (Khurana et al., 2024; Nobanee et al., 2023; Jalali et al., 2019; Nifakos et al., 2021).

## Implications for Practice and Policy

The findings of this study have implications for both healthcare practice and policy development. The bibliometric evidence indicates that healthcare cybersecurity research has increasingly emphasized governance, organizational resilience, and risk management rather than treating cybersecurity solely as a technical function. This pattern suggests that healthcare organizations may benefit from combining technical safeguards with broader governance mechanisms, including leadership oversight and cross-departmental coordination. In practice, this may involve strengthening governance structures, conducting regular risk assessments that incorporate human factors, and establishing incident response procedures before security incidents occur.

Human factors continue to represent an important cybersecurity consideration in clinical environments. Across the literature, staff behaviour remains associated with cybersecurity vulnerabilities, including password management practices, susceptibility to phishing attacks, and awareness of risks related to connected medical devices. As a result, context-specific and regularly updated training programmes may provide a practical and cost-effective approach to reducing organizational risk.

The collaboration network analysis also points to a research community that remains relatively fragmented across regions. Because cybersecurity threats routinely cross national boundaries, greater international cooperation remains important for addressing shared risks. Areas for collaboration may include threat intelligence sharing, the development of common minimum security standards, and coordinated approaches to incident response during large-scale cyber incidents.

Another issue evident within the bibliometric findings is the concentration of research output in a limited number of high-income countries. While low- and middle-income healthcare systems face many of the same cybersecurity challenges, they often operate with fewer resources and more limited response capacity. These settings remain comparatively underrepresented within the literature. This suggests an opportunity for policymakers, funding agencies, and international health organizations to support cybersecurity capacity-building initiatives through investments in infrastructure, workforce development, and locally relevant research.

## Theoretical Framework:

The theoretical framework provides the basis of healthcare cybersecurity research with the combination of various viewpoints. Because this area relates to technology, governance, and healthcare management, there are several theories applied to comprehend the way in which research themes are evolving.

The interaction of technology with human or organizational aspects is emphasized in the socio-technical systems theory. Systems such as electronic health records, telemedicine, and connected medical devices are operating in complicated settings that include institutions, policies, and professionals in the healthcare sector. There are technical vulnerabilities that can cause cybersecurity risks, and other human vulnerabilities like poor governance or ignorance. Thus, successful security is achieved by matching technology with organizational practice.

Institutional theory is an explanation of the way organizations achieve practices because of the pressures by regulation and social expectations. Healthcare organizations operate within very strict environments with data security being a critical issue. Laws like HIPAA, GDPR and national policies compel organizations to adopt standard cybersecurity practices. This can be seen in studies that emphasize on governance, compliance as well as risk management.

The cyber resilience viewpoint deals with how systems are able to manage and recuperate cyber threats. This perspective focuses more on adaptability and continuity as compared to the traditional approaches, which lay emphasis on prevention. Resilience is particularly critical in the healthcare sector since a cyberattack may interfere with important services and impact patient safety. Consequently, studies are gradually shifting their interest towards system-level protection, AI-based detection, and resistant digital infrastructures.

These views combined give a complete ideology on healthcare cybersecurity. The socio-technical theory describes the interactions of the systems, the institutional theory pays attention to the regulatory impact, and the cyber resilience focuses on adaptive security. Their combination provides the explanation of research topics convergence regarding technology, governance, and organizational resilience in healthcare cybersecurity (Ewoh et al., 2025; Ewoh and Vartiainen, 2024; Komaragiri et al., 2025).

## Conceptual Framework:

The conceptual framework of the present study establishes the key variables that define the evolution and the extent of studies on healthcare cybersecurity.

According to the bibliometric analysis, the following four key elements make up the framework:

To begin with, the advancement in healthcare technology has led to the enhancement of healthcare services by introducing electronic health records, telemedicine, cloud technology and IoMT devices among others. Nevertheless, there is also the introduction of new risks within the healthcare sector due to the introduction of the new technologies. This has led to the emergence of new cybersecurity solutions, such as the introduction of artificial intelligence-based cybersecurity tools, blockchain technology based on cybersecurity, encryption technology among others.

Second, the evolution of the cyber threat has also played a crucial role in the evolution of the studies on healthcare cybersecurity. The nature of information applied in the healthcare sector makes healthcare institutions the target of cyber attacks, including ransomware attacks, data breaches, and phishing attacks.

Third, the research in the field is also influenced by institutional governance and regulations. Policies have been set by governments to facilitate the security of information in regards to cybersecurity. Therefore, the studies within the domain pay more attention to the models of governance.

Finally, interdisciplinary research also helps the development of the sphere. Cybersecurity in health care touches upon various disciplines such as computer science, healthcare management, and public policy. This helps in the formulation of more elaborate security systems.

As it has been mentioned above, the future of healthcare cybersecurity research lies in the interconnection between technology, threats, governance, and interdisciplinary collaboration (Ewoh et al., 2025; Komaragiri et al., 2025; Garcia-Perez et al., 2022).

## CONCLUSION

This bibliometric review shows how the topic of healthcare cybersecurity has developed through the years, becoming less technical and more interdisciplinary, with the orientation at governance, resilience, and innovative technologies. The study employs bibliometric methods (co-occurrence analysis, co-citation analysis and thematic mapping) to analyze the intellectual landscape and patterns of development in the field using 1,366 publications published in almost 30 years. The results define three significant stages. Its early stage (1997-2015) focused on technical protection of electronic health records and hospital systems, and North America and Europe played a powerful role. This is in line with previous studies that have focused on system-level security and data safeguarding (Coventry & Branley, 2018; Jalali and Kaiser, 2018).

The second stage (2017-2019) is an indication of transition to governance, risk management, and regulatory compliance. This change was conditioned by significant cyber attacks, e.g., ransomware (e.g., WannaCry), which revealed the ineffectiveness of strictly technical solutions.

Since 2020, the industry has grown up, incorporating new technologies such as artificial intelligence and blockchain and making cybersecurity one of the central areas of healthcare regulation and strategic planning. This step focuses on the development of resilient and adaptive health care systems that can deal with the emerging cyber threats.

This research project will be useful in providing a systematic review of the area, establishing critical research groups, triadic patterns, and research gaps. Such systematic reviews are critical towards theory development and future research direction.

It is also interesting to note that such understudied topics are AI ethics in clinical cybersecurity, cybersecurity capacity in resource-constrained environments, and cross-border governance structures.

On the whole, the future of healthcare resilience to cybercrime must be viewed as the combination of technological advancement, regulatory policies, and organizational readiness (Jalali et al., 2019; Argaw et al., 2019; Nair and Saha, 2023).

## REFERENCES


Ahouanmenou, S., Van Looy, A., & Poels, G. (2022). Information security and privacy in hospitals: A literature mapping and review of research gaps. *Informatics for Health & Social Care*, *48*(1), 30–46. DOI: 10.1080/17538157.2022.2049274 PMID: 35300555

Argaw, S., Bempong, N., Eshaya-Chauvin, B., & Flahault, A. (2019). The state of research on cyberattacks against hospitals and available best practice recommendations: A scoping review. *BMC Medical Informatics and Decision Making*, *19*(1), 10. DOI: 10.1186/s12911-018-0724-5 PMID: 30634962

Bhuyan, S., Kabir, U., Escareno, J., Ector, K., Palakodeti, S., Wyant, D., Kumar, S., Levy, M., Kedia, S., Dasgupta, D., & Dobalian, A. (2020). Transforming healthcare cybersecurity from reactive to proactive: Current status and future recommendations. *Journal of Medical Systems*, *44*(5), 98. DOI: 10.1007/s10916-019-1507-y PMID: 32239357

Coventry, L., & Branley, D. (2018). Cybersecurity in healthcare: A narrative review of trends, threats and ways forward. *Maturitas*, *113*, 48–52. DOI: 10.1016/j.maturitas.2018.04.008 PMID: 29903648

Dotsenko, T., & Kuzmenko, M. (2023). Cyber fraud as a threat to the sustainable development of the health care system: A systematic bibliometric analysis. *Stalyi rozvytok ekonomiky*. https://doi.org/DOI: 10.32782/2308-1988/2023-47-7

Ehrenfeld, J. M. (2017). WannaCry, cybersecurity and health information technology: A time to act. *Journal of Medical Systems*, *41*(10), 104. DOI: 10.1007/s10916-017-0752-1 PMID: 28540616

Ewoh, P., & Vartiainen, T. (2024). Vulnerability to cyberattacks and sociotechnical solutions for health care systems: Systematic review. *Journal of Medical Internet Research*, *26*, e46904. DOI: 10.2196/46904 PMID: 38820579

Ewoh, P., Vartiainen, T., & Mantere, T. (2025). Sociotechnical cybersecurity framework for securing health care from vulnerabilities and cyberattacks: Scoping review. *Journal of Medical Internet Research*, *27*, e75584. DOI: 10.2196/75584 PMID: 40838797

García-Pérez, A., Cegarra-Navarro, J., Sallos, M., Martínez-Caro, E., & Chinnaswamy, A. (2022). Resilience in healthcare systems: Cyber security and digital transformation. *Technovation*, *121*, 102583. DOI: 10.1016/j.technovation.2022.102583

Ghafur, S., Kristensen, S., Honeyford, K., Martin, G., Darzi, A., & Aylin, P. (2019). A retrospective impact analysis of the WannaCry cyberattack on the NHS. *NPJ Digital Medicine*, *2*(1), 98. DOI: 10.1038/s41746-019-0161-6 PMID: 31602404

Jalali, M., & Kaiser, J. (2018). Cybersecurity in hospitals: A systematic, organizational perspective. *Journal of Medical Internet Research*, *20*(5), e10059. DOI: 10.2196/10059 PMID: 29807882

Jalali, M., Razak, S., Gordon, W., Perakslis, E., & Madnick, S. (2019). Health care and cybersecurity: Bibliometric analysis of the literature. *Journal of Medical Internet Research*, *21*(2), e12644. DOI: 10.2196/12644 PMID: 30767908

Khurana, P., Narula, S., Tiwari, N., Kapoor, R., & Arora, M. (2024). Mapping the cybersecurity research: A comprehensive bibliometric analysis. *International Journal of Experimental Research and Review*, 46, 016. https://doi.org/DOI: 10.52756/ijerr.2024.v46.016

Komaragiri, S., Alla, S., Duvall, T., Karahan, S., Bheesetty, N., & Chattu, V. (2025). A governance-centric framework for strengthening healthcare cybersecurity: A systems perspective. *International Conference on Cyber Warfare and Security*. https://doi.org/DOI: 10.34190/iccws.20.1.3374

Moral-Munoz, J. A., Herrera-Viedma, E., Santisteban-Espejo, A., & Cobo, M. J. (2020). Software tools for conducting bibliometric analysis in science: An up-to-date review. *El Profesional de la Información*, *29*(1). Advance online publication. DOI: 10.3145/epi.2020.ene.03

Nair, S., & Saha, S. (2023). Advancements in cyber security and information systems in healthcare from 2004 to 2022: A bibliometric analysis. *2023 International Conference on Intelligent Systems, Advanced Computing and Communication (ISACC)*, 1–6. https://doi.org/DOI: 10.1109/ISACC56298.2023.10084049

Nifakos, S., Chandramouli, K., Nikolaou, C. K., Papachristou, P., Koch, S., Panaousis, E., & Bonacina, S. (2021). Influence of human factors on cyber security within healthcare organisations: A systematic review. *Sensors (Basel)*, *21*(10), 3523. DOI: 10.3390/s21155119 PMID: 34372354

Nobanee, H., Alodat, A., Bajodah, R., Al-Ali, M., & Darmaki, A. (2023). Bibliometric analysis of cybercrime and cybersecurity risks literature. *Journal of Financial Crime*, *30*(6), 1736–1754. Advance online publication. DOI: 10.1108/JFC-11-2022-0287

Paul, J., Lim, W. M., O'Cass, A., Hao, A. W., & Bresciani, S. (2021). Scientific procedures and rationales for systematic literature reviews (SPAR-4-SLR). *International Journal of Consumer Studies*, *45*(4), O1–O16. DOI: 10.1111/ijcs.12695

Pratama, I., Widyantara, I., Linawati, L., & Gunantara, N. (2025). Bibliometric analysis of AI-based prototype proposal for user security awareness in healthcare. *JOIV: International Journal on Informatics Visualization*, *9*(3), 982. Advance online publication. DOI: 10.62527/joiv.9.3.3319

van Eck, N. J., & Waltman, L. (2010). Software survey: VOSviewer, a computer program for bibliometric mapping. *Scientometrics*, *84*(2), 523–538. DOI: 10.1007/s11192-009-0146-3 PMID: 20585380

Wasserman, L., & Wasserman, Y. (2022). Hospital cybersecurity risks and gaps: Review (for the non-cyber professional). *Frontiers in Digital Health*, *4*, 86222. DOI: 10.3389/fdgth.2022.862221 PMID: 36033634

# Chapter 5
# Designing Cyber-Resilient AI Pipelines for Healthcare Software From Data Ingestion to Clinical Deployment

**Afsheen Mansoor**
http://orcid.org/0000-0002-1666-2987
*Shaheed Zulfiqar Ali Bhutto Medical University, Islamabad, Pakistan*

**Emaan Mansoor**
*Islamic International Dental College, Riphah International University, Islamabad, Pakistan*

**Ezza Mansoor**
*Islamic International Dental College, Riphah International University, Islamabad, Pakistan*

**Efrah Mansoor**
*Islamic International Dental College, Riphah International University, Islamabad, Pakistan*

**Mobeen Ghulam Ahmed**
*Department of Pharmacology, Faculty of Pharmaceutical Sciences, Government College University, Faisalabad, Pakistan*

**Adnan Afzal**
http://orcid.org/0009-0001-4359-5695
*Government College University, Faisalabad, Pakistan*

**Imrana Amir**
http://orcid.org/0000-0001-7304-2816
*Department of Zoology, University of Mianwali, Mianwali, Pakistan*

**Hafiz Aamir Ali Kharl**
http://orcid.org/0000-0002-7365-2937
*Narcotics Forensic Laboratory, Anti-Narcotics Force, Ministry of Interior and Narcotics Control, Islamabad, Pakistan*

DOI: 10.4018/979-8-3373-9119-9.ch005

**Muhammad Nouman Arif**
*Department of Pharmacy, Iqra University H-9 Campus, Islamabad, Pakistan*

**Amina Arif**
*Department of Basic and Applied Chemistry, Faculty of Sciences and Technology (FOST), University of Central Punjab, Pakistan*

**Hira Bukhat**
*University of Mianwali, Mianwali, Pakistan*

## ABSTRACT

*Healthcare software is one of the places where artificial intelligence is being employed as an effort to assist the decision, diagnoses, and healthcare efficiency in healthcare operations among others. Nevertheless, AI pipelines are also new cyber threats because they use sensitive data and inter-connect clinical systems and their models. This chapter examines design of cyber-resilient artificial intelligence (AI) pipelines of healthcare software with a full AI software lifecycle of growing datasets and data pre-processing to model development, validation and deployment to clinical use. It highlights some of the most significant threats such as data poisoning, adversarial attacks and system compromise, and technical, governance and ethical methods to additionally ensure the system resilience. The focus is put on patient safety, regulatory compliance and trust, seen through the AI-enabled clinical environments lens.*

## INTRODUCTION TO CYBER RESILIENCE IN HEALTHCARE AI SYSTEMS

The artificial intelligence being brought over to healthcare software changed not only the process of clinical data processing but also the process of informed decision-making and care delivery (Alowais et al., 2023). Intelligent systems powered by AI now have significance in the field of diagnostics, clinical decision support, medical imaging, patient monitoring, and operations optimization (Reddy et al., 2019). These systems possess complicated pipelines where sensitive information is absorbed in comparison with health, inputting data on multifaceted algorithms of data processing and the results of the processing are directly sent to the clinical (Namli et al., 2024). Although this change is also marked by certain substantial advantages in regards to efficiency, precision and personalization of care, it also puts the healthcare artificial intelligence systems at risk of diverse cyber threats. As a result, cyber resilience is set as a basic requirement in the design and implementation of AI pipeline for healthcare software (Ahmed et al., 2023). Cyber resilience is not only cyber security but countering cyber security i.e. to overcome cyber security defensives. In relation to its concept of healthcare AI systems, cyber resilience designates the capability to anticipate, withhold, restore and adapt to a cyber incident, keeping the clinical functionality intact (Sharma, 2024). This is an important distinction to be made, because the healthcare environment is mission critical; a system downtime, or corrupting data or manipulating the data and outcomes of AI algorithms, can directly affect patient safety and clinical outcomes (Furrow, 2020). Setting up a cyber resilient AI pipelines therefore requires a holistic approach in all phases of the AI lifecycle that addresses not only data security, but also system robustness, systems operating continuity and trustworthiness of all AI (Davahli et al., 2021). Healthcare AI pipelines are particularly vulnerable due to the fact how much of the access data is large volumes of heterogeneous and sensitive data (Esther, 2025). Electronic health records, medical images, laboratory results, genomic data and real-time signals from medical devices are all constantly taking in data from within the AI systems. These data sources are often obtained from other institutions and external providers which means more exposure to data poisoning, unauthorised access and integrity attacks (Chen et al., 2025). Moreover, healthcare data are extremely valuable for targets for cybercriminals, and thus AI pipelines make for attractive attack surfaces for ransomware attacks, data model manipulation attacks, and data exfiltration (Esther, 2025). Another defining challenge is the complexity of the systems itself - AI systems. Unlike traditional software, AI models find patterns within data and could have unpredictable behaviours with funny inputs or changes in its distribution. Adversarial attacks - when intentionally crafted input causes the model to output something that it otherwise would not - are a serious threat in a clinical case. For example, small changes in medical images, or in patient records could be used to make incorrect diagnoses or treatment recommendations. Cyber resilience in healthcare AI must therefore not only take into account both traditional IT threats, but also weaknesses that are specific to AI and may shake the claim to reliability and trust of the models for clinical use (Finlayson et al., 2019).

*Figure 1. Cyber Resilience in Healthcare Ai Systems*

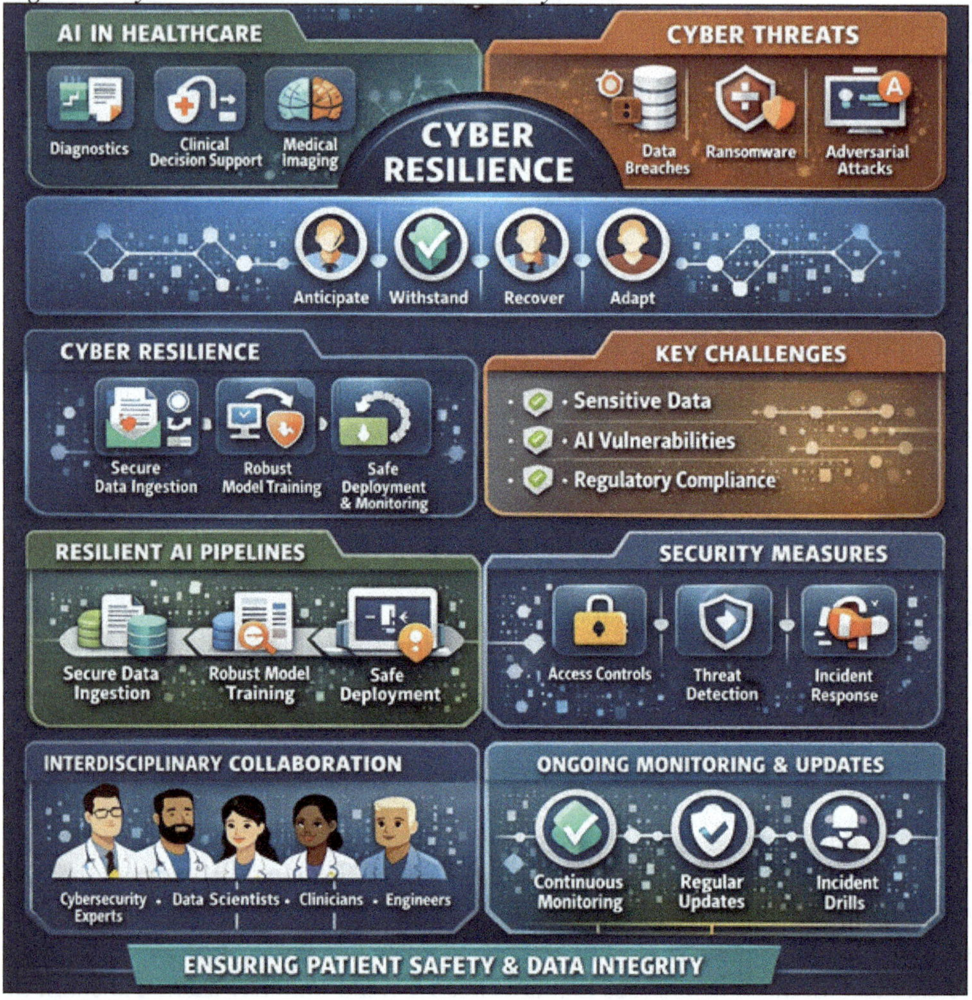


It is even more significant due to regulatory and ethical considerations, therefore, making cyber resilience even more significant. The healthcare software is highly regulated concerning patient and clinical safety, privacy as well as data privacy. In this case, a breach using AI systems may result in legal consequences, loss of credibility of an institution, and loss of trust of a patient in one (Dupont, 2019). Compliance can be further enhanced using the cyber resilient design that will guarantee the level of security, auditability as well as accountability via the AI pipeline, such as the process of data ingestion and its clinical deployment. This strategy complies with the broader concept of security by design, which adheres to a proactive risk management strategy, rather than a reactive mitigation one (Wasif, 2024). Clinical environment of implementation: There are additional restrictions on healthcare AI due to the manner of environment of its implementation (He et al., 2019). AI systems should be connected to electronic health record systems, clinical processes, and medical equipment and can often be required to be connected in real time. Any outcome of an interruption as a factor of cyber incidents may guarantee that there will be a delay in care or clinicians will be overworked or unsafe prescriptions will be presented (Barbieri et al., 2023). Cyber resilience below is in ensuring that AI systems will gracefully break down and maintain core functionality and permit human control even with unfavourable circumstances. This is vital mostly in high stakes situations like when individuals are in intensive care units, emergency departments and diagnostic labs (Whig et al., 2024). The need of interdisciplinary collaboration is developed during the designing of cyber-resilient AI Transects. Cybersecurity experts, data scientists, clinicians, software engineers and regulatory specialists will be required to work around the painting of the picture of risks and acceptable trade-offs between performance, usability and security. Cyber resilience is neither a technical force nor an ability, but an ongoing process involving both governance and technology, and organizational culture (Sahinoglu, 2016). The constant monitoring, updating of the models, planning and training users of the incident response are all the aspects of resilient healthcare Artificial Intelligence systems. Besides this, the use of cloud computing is increasing, third-party AI services and interoperability healthcare platforms that present limitations in the form of dependencies that must be effectively handled (Agapito & Cannataro, 2023). Otherwise, strong AI pipelines can be compromised by vulnerabilities in their supply chain supply chain, insecure APIs and poor configuration of cloud resources. Cyber-resilient design is concerned with being visible and having control over these dependencies such that failure or attacks on one component of the system do not result in a knock on effect on the rest of the system (Kaul & Khurana, 2021). To conclude, cyber resilience is a set of standards in the development of trustful and safe AI pipeline in healthcare software. With the AI systems playing a progressively larger role in clinical decisions making and patient outcomes, however, their resilience and recoverability in the event of a cyber threat also become as important as the possibility of the AI system to produce a prediction (Namli et al., 2024). Developing resiliency throughout the AI lifecycle - between the data ingestion and training the AI model, its deployment, and ongoing monitoring, health care organizations can gain the greatest value of the utilization of the AI, ensuring patient safety, data integrity, and clinical trust (Sharma, 2024).

## Critical Review of Existing Cyber Resilience Frameworks

Several cybersecurity and AI governance frameworks have been proposed to improve security and trustworthiness in digital healthcare systems. The NIST Cybersecurity Framework provides comprehensive risk management guidance; however, it was not specifically designed to address AI-specific threats such as adversarial attacks, model poisoning, and data drift. Similarly, Zero Trust Architecture enhances identity verification and access control but provides limited guidance for AI lifecycle management in clinical environments.

More recently, the NIST AI Risk Management Framework (AI RMF) has introduced principles for trustworthy AI development. Nevertheless, many existing frameworks focus on isolated aspects of security, governance, or compliance rather than integrating cyber resilience across the complete healthcare AI pipeline. Furthermore, limited attention has been given to aligning cybersecurity controls with clinical workflows and patient safety requirements.

Therefore, there remains a need for a lifecycle-oriented cyber-resilience framework that combines data security, model robustness, operational continuity, governance, and regulatory compliance within healthcare AI ecosystems.

## HEALTHCARE DATA INGESTION AND THREAT LANDSCAPE

Data ingestion is the point of attack of AI pipelines in healthcare software and is one of the most important stages from the point of view of cyber-resilience. Healthcare AI systems take in data from other sources which may be diverse and distributed such as electronic health records, medical imaging systems, laboratory information systems, wearable devices and connected medical equipment (Namli et al., 2024). These data streams are required for training, validating, and executing AI models but they are also a prime attack surface for cyber threats to wreak havoc with the integrity of the systems before the downstream security counter-measures are implemented (FAVINO et al., 2025). Designing resilient AI pipelines therefore requires the preparing team to have a good understanding of the healthcare data ingestion ecosystem and its related threat landscape. Healthcare data ingestion environments are noisy, and, in fact, complex (Esther, 2025). Data comes from many different vendors, institutions and geographical locations, and can massage data to many different standards, formats and interfaces. Interoperability protocols and application programming interfaces do offer open data exchange but open possibilities for an attack if not properly secured (Rao et al., 2019). Little or no authentication (authenticating users) - insecure application programming interfaces (APIs) - misconfigured data transfer channels - unauthorized access to information - interception of sensitive health information Given the high value of healthcare data, ingestion layers are common targets of cyberattacks, which are intended to steal and/or ransom, or disrupt systems (Kaul & Khurana, 2021). One of the largest dangers at the data ingestion stage is data poisoning. In this kind of attack, adversaries intentionally add malicious or corrupted data to training data sets or operational data sets in a bid to manipulate the behaviour of AI models. In the healthcare industry, the consequences of data poisoning can be serious - making biased predictions regarding risk, making wrong diagnoses or unsafe clinical recommendations (Schwarzschild et al., 2021). Since AI models connect between trends within consumed data, thousands of even minor manipulations of information may be missed as the models continue to get corrupted over time. Ingestion pipelines that are resilient to cyber-attacks should also have a way of verifying the authenticity, integrity and consistency of data prior to AI systems utilizing the data (Alevizos & Dekker, 2024).

## Healthcare Data Ingestion and Cyber Threat Landscape in AI-Driven Systems

Below is a **clear, structured table** that summarizes the key threats discussed in your text, their sources, impacts, and resilience-focused mitigation strategies.

*Table 1. Threat Landscape in Healthcare Data Ingestion for AI Systems*

| Threat Category | Description | Primary Sources / Attack Vectors | Potential Impact on AI & Clinical Systems | Cyber-Resilient Mitigation Strategies |
|---|---|---|---|---|
| **Insecure Data Sources** | Healthcare AI systems ingest data from diverse, distributed, and heterogeneous sources | EHRs, imaging systems, labs, wearables, connected medical devices | Data integrity loss, system compromise before downstream security | Source validation, standardized interfaces, secure interoperability protocols |
| **Insecure APIs & Interfaces** | Poorly secured APIs enable unauthorized access and data interception | Open APIs, misconfigured interfaces, lack of authentication | Data leakage, system manipulation, exposure of sensitive health data | Strong authentication, API gateways, role-based access control |
| **Data Poisoning Attacks** | Injection of malicious or corrupted data into training or operational datasets | Compromised data feeds, insider threats, third-party sources | Biased predictions, misdiagnosis, unsafe clinical recommendations | Data validation, anomaly detection, provenance tracking |
| **Unauthorized Access & Privacy Violations** | Weak access controls expose sensitive patient information | Cloud environments, data transfer channels, identity mismanagement | Legal penalties, ethical violations, loss of trust in AI systems | Encryption in transit and at rest, identity and access management (IAM) |

continued on following page

*Table 1. Continued*

| Threat Category | Description | Primary Sources / Attack Vectors | Potential Impact on AI & Clinical Systems | Cyber-Resilient Mitigation Strategies |
|---|---|---|---|---|
| **Wearable & IoT Device Compromise** | Resource-constrained devices lack strong security protections | Wearables, remote monitoring sensors, edge devices | Manipulated real-time data affecting monitoring and predictive models | Endpoint security, device authentication, continuous integrity checks |
| **Supply Chain Threats** | Compromised vendors or third-party components introduce malicious data | External data suppliers, software libraries, platform updates | Silent corruption of ingestion pipelines, reduced system resilience | Vendor risk assessment, dependency transparency, secure updates |
| **Availability vs. Security Trade-off** | Excessive security controls may disrupt real-time data flows | Latency-heavy authentication, rigid access policies | Delayed clinical decisions, degraded system performance | Adaptive security, rate limiting, graceful degradation mechanisms |

Unauthorized accesses to data and violation of privacy are quite an enormous threat, as well. Ingesting of healthcare data is frequently involving the movement of personal identifiable and sensitive clinical information among networks and cloud environments. Without access controls or identity management systems, or in case they are not good, attackers may have access to raw data of patients. Such violations are not only offensive to the legal and ethical duties such as; furthermore, it causes the deficiency of trust towards AI-enabled health software (Sloan & Warner, 2017). More precisely, under the resilience view, a secure ingestion view demands good encryption along the transmission path, good authentication and active monitoring of abnormal access pattern. One should also be the fact that the utilization of real-time data sources, such as wearable devices and /or remote monitoring systems, are also a risk factor that is increasingly becoming topical. Such devices are possible to be less powerful in their computation and have less strict security measures and thus are more vulnerable to be compromised. The manipulated sensor data would help in the diffusion of A.I. pipelines and will be involved in clinical decision-making process, especially through monitoring and predictive applications. The endpoint-oriented cyber-resilient ingestion strategies should thus put security in mind too, and the reliability of devices, not the centralized data repositories themselves (Tao et al., 2019). Another threat that is increasing during the stage of data ingestion is that of supply chain threats. Healthcare artificial intelligence systems are based on the reception of third-party data suppliers, software libraries, and external platforms. Compromised vendors or malicious updates - without being attacked by a threat actor the healthcare organization itself, there is a potential of having compromised or corrupted data being introduced into ingestion pipelines. Transparency into data provenance, vendor security practice, and software dependency are also the factors that help to minimize risks and raise resiliency. The other regalia is to find a certain balance between availability and security. The data flows in the healthcare systems should be stalemate and encourages real-time decision making yet the violent security controls may cause latency or friction on the operation (Jabarulla & Lee, 2021). Cyber-resilient constructions are preoccupied with adaptive protection systems so as to guarantee the availability of the data as well as dynamically respond to a security menace. This involves automatic trace of threat, rate control and fallbacks which might result to the safe degradation of functionality as opposed to a complete breakdown in the event of an incident (Verma et al., 2025). Regulatory and Compliance Requirements Assist in defining the Threat Landscape There are also additional regulatory and compliance requirements which drives the threat landscape. The processes of data ingestion must be in line with healthcare data protection regulations and standards; whereby confidentiality, integrity and availability of data must be secured. The inability to obtain the ingress pipelines may lead to the penalties in terms of regulations, and failure to perform (Shandilya et al., 2024). Asking the correct questions and keeping the rules, Cyber resilience can assist in compliance with available auditability, monitoring and incident response facilities that are hard-coded into ingestion architectures that are susceptible to cyber-attack with a ripple effect on the model performance and clinical safety. It is necessary to have knowledge of the threat environment of data poisoning, unauthorized access, device compromise and supply chain to build systems resiliently. With strong validation to ensure the placement of ingestion layers, encryption, monitoring and adaptive defence, healthcare organizations can strengthen the basis of AI-based pipelines-and defend the upstream clinical applications(Ilori et al., 2022) .

## Real-World Case Study: NHS WannaCry Ransomware Attack

A notable example highlighting the importance of cyber resilience in healthcare occurred during the WannaCry ransomware attack in 2017, which affected the United Kingdom's National Health Service (NHS). The attack disrupted hospital operations, cancelled thousands of appointments, and restricted access to critical patient information systems. Although the incident did not specifically target AI systems, it demonstrated how cyber disruptions can directly impact clinical workflows and patient care. This case emphasizes the necessity of resilient healthcare infrastructures capable of maintaining operational continuity during cyber incidents.

## SECURE DATA PREPROCESSING AND FEATURE ENGINEERING FOR AI MODELS

The security of data preprocessing and feature engineering is a major bridge between the acceptance of raw data from healthcare in the production of a A.I. model (HOSSAIN et al., 2023). At this stage, heterogeneous clinical data is cleaned, normalized, transformed and transformed into features which have a direct effect on the behaviour of the model. While the issue of preprocessing is more of technical / analytical nature, this is also a huge cybersecurity and resilience issue (Wang et al., 2024). Any compromise while performing preprocessing may silently drift all the way through the AI pipeline and impact the training and validation process of the model as well as the ultimate clinical deployment(Namli et al., 2024). Designing cyber-resilient healthcare AI systems therefore dictates to incorporate security, integrity and robustness controls into proceedings in the fields of preprocessing and feature engineering. Healthcare data preprocessing pipelines that work with sensitive data from a number of data sources, including structured data, unstructured clinical data, medical images, and times series sensor data (Athinaiou, 2022). These datasets often contain missing values, noise and inconsistencies which have to be processed before modelling. However, the processing routines are vulnerable and might be exploited by your adversaries by giving them a batch of malformed or malicious data that might generate errors in the preprocessing or bypass validation routines or distort the feature distributions. Without such protections, such manipulations might avoid detection at the cost of compromising that of models or injecting hidden bias in making clinical decisions (Verma et al., 2025). One great risk that is posed during the process of preprocessing data is the silent corruption of data. Errors that are introduced during data cleaning, data transformation or data merging can introduce changes in clinical meaning without causing obvious system failures (Felix & Lee, 2019). In a cyber context it is even possible for an attacker to purposely exploit such vulnerabilities by creating inputs in such a way as to skew preprocessing logic and end up with skewed features or mislabelled results. Cyber-resilient pipelines need therefore to have powerful validation checks, schema enforcement and consistency checks at each preprocessing step to ensure that transformed data accurately reflect the context of their original clinical origin(s). Feature engineering on its own introduces other security problems (Aslan et al., 2023). Features are the abstraction of raw data, and is what determines directly what the AI models learn. Malicious manipulation of the feature extraction logic can introduce bias, suppress important signals and amplify noise, in particular in a manner that is difficult to trace using standard performance metrics. In healthcare applications such manipulation can have serious consequences such as patient risk being under-estimated or a wrong classification for the severity of a disease. The feature engineering tasks should be done using version control, access restrictions and detailed documentation as not to get unauthorized changes and enabled traceability (Daga & Groth, 2024).

*Figure 2. Secure Data Preprocessing and Feature Engineering for Ai Models*

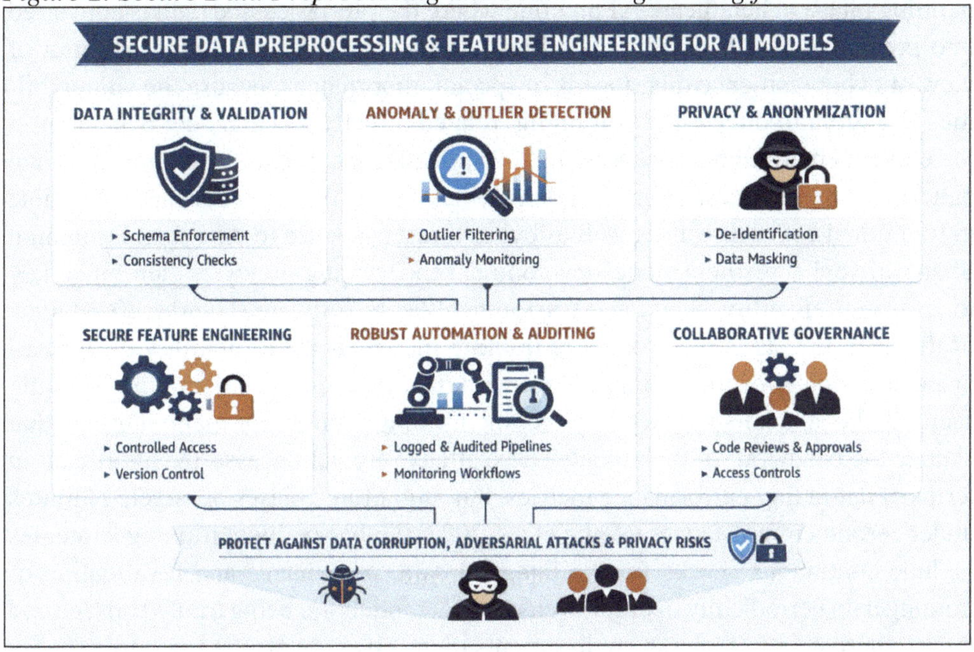


The use of automated tools for preprocessing and feature engineering business offers an even higher level of efficiency and risk. While the use of automation in the development process of AI reduces the time required to develop AI, it can also lead to a lack of transparency as it hides the decision points. If preprocessing pipes are incorrectly performed, the mistakes of machine systems can also be easily propagated throughout large datasets (Sharma et al., 2024). Cyber resilience in this aspect is focused on controlled automation in which the preprocessing workflows are monitored, logged and audited constantly. This is visible enough to the organization and gives them the capability to detect and track back where the anomaly from and take the action before these errors are no longer propagated to the downstream models (Felix & Lee, 2019). Data anonymization and privacy preserving preprocessing is also a crucial part of secure feature engineering for healthcare sector. It may not be possible to remove or convert personally identifiable information to not only adhere to regulations but also use the data ethically. However, badly designed anonymization techniques may still allow to re-identify the data or to create security loopholes which can be exploited by attackers (Srijayanthi & Sethukarasi, 2023).

## CYBER-RESILIENT MODEL DEVELOPMENT AND TRAINING STRATEGIES

Model development and training are considered as the heart part of intelligence-building phase in healthcare AI pipeline where the pre-processed data is converted into predictive and decision capabilities (Addisu et al., 2025). From the point of view of cyber resilience this stage is of special importance, because the vulnerabilities that are introduced in this training, related directly to the model behaviour in the clinical environment (Sobb et al., 2025). Unlike traditional software, statistical patterns AI models learn from their data, which means that their data are vulnerable to traditional cyber threats as well as cyber threats specific to AI cyber. Designing Shapeshift cyber resilient model development and training strategies therefore is key to ensuring reliability, safety and trust in healthcare software (Gundu, 2024). One of the main threats in the process of training models is the availability of infected or incorrect data for the training. Even with data ingestion and data preprocessing secured, the attackers may try to affect the training with minor manipulations that change the behaviour of the model. These attacks are not necessarily significant in terms of degrading performance metrics, but might force biases or targeted failures under certain circumstances (Wang et al., 2022). Cyber-resilient training strategies include continuous checks for the integrity data, provenance and revalidation of training data periodically in order to ensure that models are being trained on true and representative data. Training environments themselves are also not safe from cyber threats. Often health care AI models are trained using high-performance computing resources, cloud platforms or by shared research infrastructure (Doukas, 2025).

*Table 2. Cyber-Resilience Strategies Across AI Model Development, Training, and Validation in Healthcare*

| AI Pipeline Stage | Key Cyber Threats | Description of Risk | Potential Clinical / System Impact | Cyber-Resilient Strategies |
|---|---|---|---|---|
| **Model Development & Training** | Poisoned or corrupted training data | Minor data manipulations introduce bias or targeted failures without degrading overall performance metrics | Unsafe predictions, biased clinical decisions, silent model corruption | Data provenance tracking, integrity verification, periodic revalidation of datasets |
| **Training Infrastructure Security** | Unauthorized access to training environments | Misconfigured cloud/ HPC platforms, weak credentials, vulnerable dependencies | Manipulation of code, hyperparameters, or model weights | Strong identity and access management, execution isolation, restricted privileges |
| **Model Parameter Integrity** | Tampering with model weights and parameters | Altered parameters lead to compromised inference behavior | Unsafe or unreliable clinical outputs | Secure storage, encryption, controlled access to model artifacts |
| **Adversarial Input Attacks** | Crafted malicious inputs | Fake medical images or altered patient records designed to deceive models | Misdiagnosis, incorrect risk stratification, unsafe recommendations | Adversarial training, data augmentation, robustness stress testing |
| **Model Robustness** | Sensitivity to small perturbations | Minor input changes cause large output deviations | Clinically significant errors from subtle manipulations | Robustness evaluation, adversarial testing, perturbation analysis |
| **Model Complexity & Opacity** | Lack of interpretability | Highly complex models are difficult to audit or investigate after failure | Undetected compromise, reduced clinician trust | Explainable AI (XAI), interpretable model architectures, audit-friendly design |
| **Traditional Model Validation** | Limited performance-only validation | Accuracy metrics fail to detect cyber or adversarial vulnerabilities | False sense of safety before deployment | Expanded validation including security and resilience testing |
| **Adversarial Validation** | Stealthy adversarial manipulation | Inputs designed to mislead models without obvious data tampering | Hidden failure modes in live clinical systems | Purposeful adversarial testing, failure-mode analysis |

continued on following page

*Table 2. Continued*

| AI Pipeline Stage | Key Cyber Threats | Description of Risk | Potential Clinical / System Impact | Cyber-Resilient Strategies |
|---|---|---|---|---|
| **Data Drift & Distribution Shifts** | Changes in real-world data over time | Evolving clinical practices or demographics exploited by attackers | Gradual performance degradation, unsafe predictions | Continuous validation, drift detection, adaptive retraining |
| **Lifecycle Monitoring** | One-time validation mindset | Models degrade after deployment without detection | Long-term safety and reliability risks | Continuous monitoring, automated alerts, adaptive corrective actions |

Misconfigured access controls, insecure credentials or HQT or vulnerable dependencies can allow an attacker to mess with the training code, hyperparameters or model weights. To counteract these dangers, credible Meet designs have to be well lined up secure training atmosphere with solid identity management, execution separation and restricted access control to model things (Almaiah et al., 2024). The protection of the confidentiality and integrity of model parameters are particularly important with the fact that flawed models can lead to unsafe clinical outputs. Another important facet of cyber resilient model development is robust to adversarial behaviour (Javed et al., 2024). Healthcare AI systems might be vulnerable to adversarial inputs when applications are deployed, which are artificially generated inputs (e.g., fake medical images, fake patient records) that are intentionally designed to fool models. Training strategies that can include measures to assess robustness such as data augmentation, adversarial training, stress testing, can help to withstand such attacks. While no model has perfect inviolability, resilience based training minimises the likelihood that minute perturbations will cause clinically significant error (Zbrzezny & Grzybowski, 2023). Model complexity and explainability are also subjects of cyber resilience. Highly complex models might be so good at prediction but hard to interpret, audit or validate. This opacity may make it difficult to see why things have gone wrong, and it would be difficult to detect if a model has been compromised (Islam et al., 2025). Cyber-resilient strategies encourage a trade-off of performance for interpretability, particularly in the case of high stakes clinical application. Transparent model architectures along with explainable artificial intelligence techniques provide for a reinforcement of security reviews, regulatory adherence and clinician trust (Cadet et al., 2021).

## AI MODEL VALIDATION, ROBUSTNESS, AND ADVERSARIAL DEFENSE

Model validation is one of the most important defences against dangerous behaviour in healthcare artificial intelligence pipelines and the chances of such behaviour are even lower if it is tested by an effective validation model before being put into practice in various clinical scenarios (Alevizos & Dekker, 2024). From the point of view of cyber-resilience, validation is more than the standard measures of performance and is understood to include robustness testing, security testing and the resilience against adversarial manipulation (Javed et al., 2024). Because the ability of healthcare AI systems to have direct impacts on clinical decisions is real, validity failures can pose significant risk to patients and organizations. And the design of resilient frameworks for validation is key to ensuring trust and safety throughout the AI lifecycle (Verma et al., 2025). Traditional validation of a model in healthcare is focused on accuracy, sensitivity, specificity and generalisability across patient populations. While all of these metrics are necessary, they do not go far enough to identify vulnerabilities related to cyber. Models might be good on datasets that are common in non-adversarial environments and subject to adversarial influences, changes in data distribution or subtle manipulations or attacks exploiting weaknesses that the model has learned (Prateek & Rathore, 2025). Cyber-resilient validation strategies include stress testing and assessment of model robustness to reflect the behaviour of models under abnormal or hostile conditions which might arise in the real-world situation in clinical settings (Cascella et al., 2023).

*Figure 3. Ai Model Validation, Robustness, And Adversarial Défense*

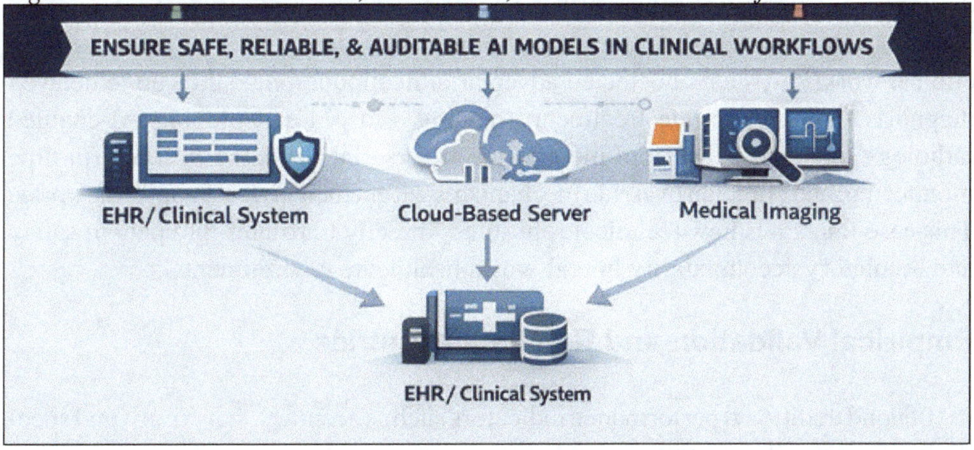

Adversarial attacks act as a threat that is now major in healthcare AI systems. These attacks involve carefully crafted inputs which are designed to mislead models in ways which can't reveal themselves as tangibly tampering with the model (Finlayson et al., 2019). In medical imaging, for example, small changes at the pixels level can alter diagnostic prediction and in the case of structured data, small changes in clinical variables can alter clinical risk scores (Bi et al., 2019). Cyber-resilient validation involves adversarial testing in which the models are fed with purposefully manipulated inputs, to see if the models show susceptibility and the failure mode. Awareness of these vulnerabilities can help the software developer secure the coffins before the vulnerability outside their control culminates in a live system (Javed et al., 2024). Robustness to data drift and changes in data distribution is another aspect of validation which is important. Healthcare data changes over time due to the changing clinical practice, patient demographics, as well as data collection technology (Wasif, 2024). Attackers can exploit this variability to include malicious patterns to reduce the performance of the model. Continuous validation and monitoring can help in detecting the unexpected changes in input data or behaviour of the output and taking corrective actions right from the earliest stages. Cyber resilient pipelines have a different approach to validation in that they do not consider it a one-time checkpoint, but rather a process that continues in order to maintain validity (Biggio et al., 2013).

## Real-World Clinical Illustration

A practical example of these risks can be observed in medical imaging systems where deep learning models are deployed for tumour detection. Studies have demonstrated that minimal pixel-level perturbations in radiological images can significantly alter model predictions without being detectable to clinicians. In a clinical workflow, such undetected adversarial manipulation could lead to delayed diagnosis or inappropriate treatment planning. Hospitals deploying AI-enabled radiology tools must therefore incorporate adversarial validation testing, runtime monitoring, and clinician override mechanisms within their governance frameworks. This case illustrates how technical robustness directly translates into patient safety and regulatory accountability in real-world healthcare environments.

## Empirical Validation and Resilience Metrics

Beyond traditional performance indicators such as accuracy, sensitivity, and specificity, cyber-resilient healthcare AI systems require additional validation metrics. These include adversarial robustness scores, data integrity verification rates, drift detection thresholds, mean time to detection (MTTD) of anomalies, and mean time to recovery (MTTR) following system disruptions. In operational clinical settings, resilience should also be measured through system uptime, fail-safe activation success rates, and clinician override frequency. Integrating these quantitative indicators into validation protocols enables healthcare institutions to objectively assess not only predictive performance but also operational reliability and patient safety compliance.

## SECURE DEPLOYMENT AND INTEGRATION OF AI MODELS IN CLINICAL SYSTEMS

Secure deployment is the movement from the more structured development phases of artificial intelligence AI models into a real clinical environment where AI models are in contact with clinicians and patients and with the necessary clinical and healthcare infrastructure (Fahim et al., 2025). This stage can be characterized as one of the most sensitive points in the AI pipeline because here is where vulnerabilities that were penetrated at the deployment or integration phase can impinge directly upon the safety of the patient and continuity of operations (Esther, 2025). From a cyber-resilience point of view, it critical that deployment can make AI models secure, reliable and auditable and seamlessly-integrated into complex clinical workflows. Healthcare AI Models are often deployed in Electronic Health Record system, clinical decision support or medical imaging software or even as the cloud-based service. These environments are very interconnected and often to do with legacy systems with different security maturities (Corbin et al., 2023). Poorest of these would be poor integration points that make AI model erode, mishandling data flow and integration may expose the data and AI model to unauthorized access, manipulation or misuse (Hudson, 2024). Cyber-resilient deployment is focused on strengthening security around interfaces, authentication, encryption processes into the clinical systems and data, and data and model outputs as they are moved from the clinical systems (Athinaiou, 2022). Model integrity during deployment time is a major issue. In order to change the behaviour without being detected, attackers may try to tamper the model binaries and configuration files or runtime parameters (Kruegel et al., 2005). Secure deployment strategies spanning integrity checks and digital signatures, and controlled distribution mechanisms to ensure that only verified and approved versions of the model are executed in clinical environments are other strategies (Micheal, 2025). These are done in order to limit the potential for replacement or corruption of the model which may lead to unsafe clinical recommendations (Al Qudah et al., 2025). Operational resilience is also important critically in the clinical environment where downtime or a deterioration in the performance of a system may have serious consequences for the delivery of care. AI systems have to fail in a safe manner so they can keep themselves degrading gracefully in the event of cyber, network outage, or unexpected errors (Parise et al., 2020). Cyber Resilient Deployment incorporates elements of redundancy, fail flares and explicit communication pathways such as point of care escalation, deployed protocols to enable clinicians to continue provision of care, with alternate workflows or similar clinic based human judgement, in the absence of or compromise of an AI system (Quinn, 2025). Depiction of deployed AI systems to centralize AMS data for central monitoring of the various components and leaf's to log any finalities of urban work that needs to be classified and mapped for monitoring purposes (Chauhan et al., 2025). Runtime monitoring is a technique that can detect any anomalous behaviour like strange pattern of the input, unexpected distribution of the output or an abnormal access attempt etc. Comprehensive Logging Aids in Forensic Analysis and Accountability Comprehensive logging can be beneficial for organizations in the context of forensic analysis and accountability. These capabilities are important to help establish trust in AI-assisted clinical decision making (Pichan et al., 2018).

## GOVERNANCE, COMPLIANCE, AND ETHICAL CONSIDERATIONS IN HEALTHCARE AI SECURITY

The institutional reason why governance, compliance, and ethics negatively affect cyber-resilient AI pipeline in healthcare software is that of an institutional nature (Abubakari, 2024). Technical safeguards are highly essential, but in themselves do not suffice to guarantee safe and reliable use of AI in clinical settings. Healthcare artificial intelligence systems belong to heavily regulated and ethically sensitive settings, breaches of which may put patient confidence at stake, evoke a clash between the law and negatively influence clinical safety (Ellahham et al., 2020). Cyber resilience thus requires governance framework in order to balance between technical design, regulatory demands and ethics in the AI lifecycle. Good governance starts with good understanding on accountability (Abubakari, 2024). When dealing with the healthcare human AI pipeline, the task division usually takes place between data providers, software developers, clouding vendors and clinical organisations (Gajula, 2025). Without clearly defined roles it becomes difficult to determine the responsibilities of security failures, biased outputs or misuse of the system (Loscocco et al., 1998). Cyber resilient governance frameworks ensure ownership for both the data stewardship and performance including security monitoring and performance incident response models (Abubakari, 2024). This clarity plays a key role in helping to implement timely decision-making in the face of cyber events and the regulation and institutional trust. Regulatory Compliance Regulatory Compliance, a fundamental factor in healthcare AI security. Healthcare software must be in line with data protection, patient safety and medical device regulations with stringent requirements on confidentiality, integrity and availability (Folorunso et al., 2024). AI pipelines can also have other meanings, including that models may be changing over time and have potentially non-transparent ramifications to model-based clinical decisions (Alevizos & Dekker, 2024). Cyber resilient governance guarantees that compliance checks are included in all stages of the pipeline to ensure that the manner in which data is handled, updating that model and putting it into action are in line with the expectations put forward by the individual regulations (Abubakari, 2024). On-going documentation, audit trails and evidence of validation in support of accountability and regulatory review. This plays further role on how to handle governance in healthcare AI security. AI systems are often prejudiced, obscure the decision process, or even create a reliance so strong on the recommendation of the automation systems (Ranjitsingh & Rao, 2025). From a cybersecurity perspective, manipulated or misinterpreted AI outputs are difficult to deal with from an ethical standpoint due to the issues created by harm to patients and loss of autonomy (Ausaf & Khan). Governance frameworks must therefore help to enable transparency, explainability and human oversight, and ensure that clinicians bear responsibility for the final decisions. Ethical principles of AI underline cyber resiliency as it guarantees the need for promoting freedom from blind trusting of any automated systems and urging caution while considering the results of AI (Akbar et al., 2024).

*Table 1.*

| Security Requirement | HIPAA | GDPR | Cyber Resilience Control |
|---|---|---|---|
| Data Confidentiality | ✓ | ✓ | Encryption |
| Access Management | ✓ | ✓ | IAM |
| Audit Logging | ✓ | ✓ | Monitoring & Logging |
| Incident Response | ✓ | ✓ | Security Operations |
| Data Integrity | ✓ | ✓ | Validation Controls |

Healthcare AI systems must comply with regulatory frameworks such as HIPAA in the United States and GDPR within the European Union. These regulations require organizations to ensure confidentiality, integrity, availability, accountability, and transparency of healthcare data. Cyber-resilient AI architectures support compliance by embedding encryption, auditability, access controls, monitoring mechanisms, and incident response procedures throughout the AI lifecycle.

## Human Factors and Clinical Workflow Integration

While technical safeguards are essential, cyber resilience in healthcare AI also depends on human and organizational factors. Clinicians remain ultimately responsible for patient care decisions and therefore must understand the capabilities and limitations of AI-assisted systems. Excessive reliance on automated recommendations may introduce automation bias, while poor usability may reduce clinician adoption.

Healthcare organizations should implement training programs, clinician-centered interface design, human-in-the-loop validation mechanisms, and continuous feedback systems. Integrating cyber resilience with clinical workflows ensures that AI systems support rather than disrupt healthcare delivery, particularly during cyber incidents or system failures.

# FUTURE DIRECTIONS FOR CYBER-RESILIENT AI IN CLINICAL SOFTWARE ECOSYSTEMS

The future of healthcare AI will not only be that of more powerful and higher-performing algorithms, but it will also encompass the capability of AI systems to secure and be reliably available to operate within large growing complex clinical software environments (Alotaibi, 2025). Cyber resiliency will be one of the characteristics of the reliable healthcare AI as the cyber threats are always a step forward with the increased sophistication and magnitude. Future opportunities in this area include concentrating on the proactive and adaptive solutions/systems that include the security, resilience and clinical safety through design up to deployment interfaces (Alhidaifi et al., 2024). The shift towards the adaptive and self-healing pipelines would be one of the significant trends of the AI pipelines in the future. The next generation of healthcare AI systems will probably have security controls regarding continuous monitoring, automated detection of anomalies and dynamic response mechanisms, as opposed to being purely founded on static security controls (Chakraborty, 2025). Such facilities will enable AI pipes to identify data poisoning, adversarial actions or breach of the AI system in real time and adjust functions accordingly to guarantee safety. Such adaptive resilience is important in clinical situations in which uninterrupted service, as well as patient safety, are of paramount importance (Anderson et al., 2020). A combination of cyber resilience and explainable and trustworthy AI will also decide the fate of clinical software ecosystems. As use of the AI systems become more autonomous, the tendency of clinicians and regulators would require more transparency into how models make decisions and how it reacts to abnormal conditions (Islam et al., 2025). Explainable AI techniques combined with security monitoring will help to unlock the suspicious model behaviour, encourage human supervision and increase the trust in AI-assisted clinical decisions (Juang et al., 2022). Another direction that is important is to strengthen the supply chain of healthcare AI's resilience. With the familiarity of a pipeline and its dependencies (dependencies of open-source code), future pipelines will depend more on shared datasets, inspectional models and the subordinate cloud services and third-party software components. Cyber-resilient ecosystems will require standardised security certifications, perpetual vendor risk assessment and provenance tracking of data and models, amongst others. These measures will reduce the hidden dependency and make sure that vulnerabilities introduced upstream of the planned clinical system do not compromise downstream systems (Williams et al., 2012).

While prior literature has largely focused on individual components of AI security—such as data encryption, adversarial defense, or regulatory compliance—fewer studies integrate these elements into a unified resilience framework that explicitly aligns with clinical workflows. The current body of research often treats cybersecurity as a technical add-on rather than a clinical safety imperative. This chapter advances the discussion by synthesizing technical safeguards, governance structures, and operational continuity into a lifecycle-based resilience model tailored specifically for healthcare AI systems.

## Cyber Resilience Challenges in Generative AI and Large Language Models

The increasing adoption of Generative AI and Large Language Models (LLMs) in healthcare introduces new cybersecurity challenges. Clinical chatbots and AI assistants may be vulnerable to prompt injection attacks, model inversion attacks, training data leakage, hallucinated medical recommendations, and unauthorized disclosure of sensitive patient information.

Future cyber-resilient healthcare architectures must incorporate secure prompt validation, retrieval security controls, model monitoring, explainability mechanisms, and governance frameworks specifically designed for LLM-enabled clinical systems. Addressing these emerging threats will be critical for ensuring safe and trustworthy deployment of generative AI technologies in healthcare environments.

## Economic and Operational Considerations

Implementing cyber-resilient AI pipelines requires substantial investment in cybersecurity infrastructure, governance mechanisms, workforce training, and continuous monitoring capabilities. However, these investments must be balanced against the financial consequences of cyber incidents, including operational downtime, regulatory penalties, reputational damage, and patient safety risks. Future healthcare organizations should adopt cost-benefit assessment models to evaluate resilience investments and prioritize controls based on clinical impact and organizational risk exposure.

## CONCLUSION

One of the secrets of secure and reliable integration of artificial intelligence into healthcare software is designing Cyber Resilient AI Pipelines. Since AI systems will increasingly touch upon clinical choices and patient outcomes, they could be disastrous in case there are weaknesses anywhere in the pipeline, even at the upper end of the pipeline in the data ingestion to the deployment of the systems in the clinical environment. It has been demonstrated in this chapter that cyber resilience must be viewed as having to be more holistic as it goes beyond cybersecurity efforts and incorporates elements of data integrity, model robustness, operational continuity and governance across the AI lifecycle. Healthcare AI pipelines that are cyber-resistant comprise safeguarded data consumption/swallowing, safeguarded and directed data preprocessing workflows, safeguarded and managed model learning plans and complete validation to adversarial and functional assaults. A quote of safe deployment practices and continued monitoring could be provided as follows: Another significant challenge is such security of artificial intelligence practices when implemented in a clinical and real-world system. Governance and ethical systems that characterize accountability, assist in regulatory compliance and ensure clinician accountability are equally crucial. These non-technical elements are auxiliary to the technical defences to form a meet between security of AI use and patient safety, transparency and trust. Another aspect that the chapter brings out is that the concept of cyber resilience cannot be a fixed objective but rather a process. Clinical environment, healthcare practices, and the nature of cyber threats are in the process of constant change and defence needs to be dynamic, the results of frequent audit and event control must be addressed. There are new techniques like privacy preserving learning, explainable box AI and resilient supply format management that are expected to further provide defines to healthcare AI ecosystems. The final outcome - through cyber-resilient artificial intelligence pipelines, the healthcare organizations will be able to both enjoy the benefits of artificial intelligence and overcome the threat. With resiliency added to the design, development and implementation of healthcare software, it is possible to provide healthcare with reliable, ethical and secure clinical care with the use of AI technologies. This combined method is necessitated to facilitate the possibility of AI to be utilized in the rest of the healthcare system in the long term with confidence.

## REFERENCES


Abubakari, P. (2024). *Human factors matter: the intersection of cybersecurity governance, and culture in risk management of critical infrastructure*. Pepperdine University.

Addisu, E. G., Yirga, T. G., Yirga, H. G., & Yehuala, A. D. (2025). Transfer learning-based hybrid VGG16-machine learning approach for heart disease detection with explainable artificial intelligence. *Frontiers in Artificial Intelligence*, *8*, 1504281. DOI: 10.3389/frai.2025.1504281 PMID: 40070809

Agapito, G., & Cannataro, M. (2023). An overview on the challenges and limitations using cloud computing in healthcare corporations. *Big Data and Cognitive Computing*, *7*(2), 68. DOI: 10.3390/bdcc7020068

Ahmed, A., Xi, R., Hou, M., Shah, S. A., & Hameed, S. (2023). Harnessing big data analytics for healthcare: A comprehensive review of frameworks, implications, applications, and impacts. *IEEE Access : Practical Innovations, Open Solutions*, *11*, 112891–112928. DOI: 10.1109/ACCESS.2023.3323574

Akbar, W., Ullah, M., Hussain, T., Haq, M. I. U., Ullah, I., Adhikari, D., & Khan, R. (2024). Cybersecurity Challenges and Strategies for Safe Artificial General Intelligence. In *Future Tech Startups and Innovation in the Age of AI* (pp. 209–236). CRC Press.

Al Qudah, A. M., Al-haddad, L., & Aljabali, A. (2025). Combatting medical corruption: A global review of root causes, consequences, and evidence-based interventions. *International Journal of Innovative Research and Scientific Studies*, *8*(2), 968–985. DOI: 10.53894/ijirss.v8i2.5397

Alevizos, L., & Dekker, M. (2024). Towards an AI-enhanced cyber threat intelligence processing pipeline. *Electronics (Basel)*, *13*(11), 2021. DOI: 10.3390/electronics13112021

Alhidaifi, S. M., Asghar, M. R., & Ansari, I. S. (2024). A survey on cyber resilience: Key strategies, research challenges, and future directions. *ACM Computing Surveys*, *56*(8), 1–48. DOI: 10.1145/3649218

Almaiah, M. A., Saqr, L. M., Al-Rawwash, L. A., Altellawi, L. A., Al-Ali, R., & Almomani, O. (2024). Classification of Cybersecurity Threats, Vulnerabilities and Countermeasures in Database Systems. *Computers, Materials & Continua*, *81*(2), 3189–3220. DOI: 10.32604/cmc.2024.057673

Alotaibi, B. (2025). *A Review of Resilient IoT Systems: Trends*. Challenges, and Future Directions.

Alowais, S. A., Alghamdi, S. S., Alsuhebany, N., Alqahtani, T., Alshaya, A. I., Almohareb, S. N., Aldairem, A., Alrashed, M., Bin Saleh, K., Badreldin, H. A., Al Yami, M. S., Al Harbi, S., & Albekairy, A. M. (2023). Revolutionizing healthcare: The role of artificial intelligence in clinical practice. *BMC Medical Education*, *23*(1), 689. DOI: 10.1186/s12909-023-04698-z PMID: 37740191

Anderson, J., Ross, A., Back, J., Duncan, M., Snell, P., Hopper, A., & Jaye, P. (2020). Beyond 'find and fix': Improving quality and safety through resilient healthcare systems. *International Journal for Quality in Health Care : Journal of the International Society for Quality in Health Care*, *32*(3), 204–211. DOI: 10.1093/intqhc/mzaa007 PMID: 32108882

Aslan, Ö., Aktuğ, S. S., Ozkan-Okay, M., Yilmaz, A. A., & Akin, E. (2023). A comprehensive review of cyber security vulnerabilities, threats, attacks, and solutions. *Electronics (Basel)*, *12*(6), 1333. DOI: 10.3390/electronics12061333

Athinaiou, M. (2022). *Model-based Management of Cyber Resiliency for Healthcare Systems* University of Brighton]. Ausaf, H., & Khan, M. Threats by Artificial Intelligence to Human Health and Human Existence.

Barbieri, C., Neri, L., Stuard, S., Mari, F., & Martín-Guerrero, J. D. (2023). From electronic health records to clinical management systems: How the digital transformation can support healthcare services. *Clinical Kidney Journal*, *16*(11), 1878–1884. DOI: 10.1093/ckj/sfad168 PMID: 37915897

Bi, W. L., Hosny, A., Schabath, M. B., Giger, M. L., Birkbak, N. J., Mehrtash, A., Allison, T., Arnaout, O., Abbosh, C., Dunn, I. F., Mak, R. H., Tamimi, R. M., Tempany, C. M., Swanton, C., Hoffmann, U., Schwartz, L. H., Gillies, R. J., Huang, R. Y., & Aerts, H. J. W. L. (2019). Artificial intelligence in cancer imaging: Clinical challenges and applications. *CA: a Cancer Journal for Clinicians*, *69*(2), 127–157. DOI: 10.3322/caac.21552 PMID: 30720861

Biggio, B., Fumera, G., & Roli, F. (2013). Security evaluation of pattern classifiers under attack. *IEEE Transactions on Knowledge and Data Engineering*, *26*(4), 984–996. DOI: 10.1109/TKDE.2013.57

Cadet, E., Etim, E. D., Essien, I. A., Ajayi, J. O., & Erigha, E. D. (2021). The role of reinforcement learning in adaptive cyber defense mechanisms. *International Journal of Multidisciplinary Research and Growth Evaluation*, *2*(2), 544–559. DOI: 10.54660/.IJMRGE.2021.2.2.544-559

Cascella, M., Cascella, A., Monaco, F., & Shariff, M. N. (2023). Envisioning gamification in anesthesia, pain management, and critical care: Basic principles, integration of artificial intelligence, and simulation strategies. *Journal of Anesthesia, Analgesia and Critical Care*, *3*(1), 33. DOI: 10.1186/s44158-023-00118-2 PMID: 37697415

Chakraborty, S. (2025). Beyond ETL: How AI Agents Are Building Self-Healing Data Pipelines. *Journal of Computer Science and Technology Studies*, *7*(3), 741–756. DOI: 10.32996/jcsts.2025.7.3.81

Chauhan, B. V., Vedrtnam, A., Wyche, K. P., & Verma, S. (2025). Review on Artificial Intelligence in the Environmental Monitoring. *Prospects of Artificial Intelligence in the Environment*, 29-60.

Chen, Y.-M., Hsiao, T.-H., Lin, C.-H., & Fann, Y. C. (2025). Unlocking precision medicine: Clinical applications of integrating health records, genetics, and immunology through artificial intelligence. *Journal of Biomedical Science*, *32*(1), 16. DOI: 10.1186/s12929-024-01110-w PMID: 39915780

Corbin, C. K., Maclay, R., Acharya, A., Mony, S., Punnathanam, S., Thapa, R., Kotecha, N., Shah, N. H., & Chen, J. H. (2023). DEPLOYR: A technical framework for deploying custom real-time machine learning models into the electronic medical record. *Journal of the American Medical Informatics Association : JAMIA*, *30*(9), 1532–1542. DOI: 10.1093/jamia/ocad114 PMID: 37369008

Daga, E., & Groth, P. (2024). Data journeys: Explaining AI workflows through abstraction. *Semantic Web*, *15*(4), 1057–1083. DOI: 10.3233/SW-233407

Davahli, M. R., Karwowski, W., Fiok, K., Wan, T., & Parsaei, H. R. (2021). Controlling safety of artificial intelligence-based systems in healthcare. *Symmetry*, *13*(1), 102. DOI: 10.3390/sym13010102

Doukas, N. (2025). Reliability-based design optimization for cyber survivability. In *Reliability Assessment and Optimization of Complex Systems* (pp. 363–411). Elsevier. DOI: 10.1016/B978-0-443-29112-8.00029-3

Dupont, B. (2019). The cyber-resilience of financial institutions: Significance and applicability. *Journal of Cybersecurity*, *5*(1), tyz013. DOI: 10.1093/cybsec/tyz013

Ellahham, S., Ellahham, N., & Simsekler, M. C. E. (2020). Application of artificial intelligence in the health care safety context: Opportunities and challenges. *American Journal of Medical Quality : The Official Journal of the American College of Medical Quality*, *35*(4), 341–348. DOI: 10.1177/1062860619878515 PMID: 31581790

Esther, D. (2025). Securing Sensitive Health Data in AI Pipelines.

Fahim, Y. A., Hasani, I. W., Kabba, S., & Ragab, W. M. (2025). Artificial intelligence in healthcare and medicine: Clinical applications, therapeutic advances, and future perspectives. *European Journal of Medical Research*, *30*(1), 848. DOI: 10.1186/s40001-025-03196-w PMID: 40988064

FAVINO. R., CONTE, N., DE, M. A., GARCIA, M. E., MONTANARI, E., PAGANINI, A., SANGIORGI, M., & SFALAGKIARIS, C. E. (2025). Emerging risks and opportunities for EU internal security stemming from new technologies.

Felix, E. A., & Lee, S. P. (2019). Systematic literature review of preprocessing techniques for imbalanced data. *IET Software*, *13*(6), 479–496. DOI: 10.1049/iet-sen.2018.5193

Finlayson, S. G., Bowers, J. D., Ito, J., Zittrain, J. L., Beam, A. L., & Kohane, I. S. (2019). Adversarial attacks on medical machine learning. *Science*, *363*(6433), 1287–1289. DOI: 10.1126/science.aaw4399 PMID: 30898923

Folorunso, A., Wada, I., Samuel, B., & Mohammed, V. (2024). Security compliance and its implication for cybersecurity. *World Journal of Advanced Research and Reviews*, *24*(01), 2105–2121. DOI: 10.30574/wjarr.2024.24.1.3170

Furrow, B. R. (2020). The limits of current AI in health care: Patient safety policing in hospitals. *Ne. UL Rev.*, *12*, 1.

Gajula, M. (2025). Empowering Healthcare Professionals: The Role of Cloud-Native Data Engineering in Human-AI Collaboration. *Journal of Computer Science and Technology Studies*, *7*(4), 417–426. DOI: 10.32996/jcsts.2025.7.4.50

Gundu, T. (2024). Learn, unlearn and relearn: Adaptive cybersecurity culture model. International Conference on Cyber Warfare and Security

He, J., Baxter, S. L., Xu, J., Xu, J., Zhou, X., & Zhang, K. (2019). The practical implementation of artificial intelligence technologies in medicine. Nature Medicine, 25(1), 30–36. PubMed

HOSSAINESRAT ZAHAN SNIGDHASHOHONI MAHABUB. (2023). AI-Driven Data Optimization: Automating Cleaning, Feature Engineering, and Augmentation for Superior Machine Learning Performance in Digital Health Care System. *Journal of Computer Science and Technology Studies*, *5*(4), 218–228. DOI: 10.32996/jcsts.2023.5.4.23

Hudson, J. (2024). Artificial Intelligence and Cybersecurity Integration: Modern Database Techniques for Securing AI Models.

Ilori, O., Lawal, C. I., Friday, S. C., Isibor, N. J., & Chukwuma-Eke, E. C. (2022). Cybersecurity auditing in the digital age: A review of methodologies and regulatory implications. *Journal of Frontiers in Multidisciplinary Research*, *3*(1), 174–187. DOI: 10.54660/.IJFMR.2022.3.1.174-187

Islam, S., Basheer, N., Papastergiou, S., Ciampi, M., & Silvestri, S. (2025). Intelligent dynamic cybersecurity risk management framework with explainability and interpretability of AI models for enhancing security and resilience of digital infrastructure. *Journal of Reliable Intelligent Environments*, *11*(3), 12. DOI: 10.1007/s40860-025-00253-3 PMID: 40656511

Jabarulla, M. Y., & Lee, H.-N. (2021). A blockchain and artificial intelligence-based, patient-centric healthcare system for combating the COVID-19 pandemic: Opportunities and applications. Healthcare

Javed, H., El-Sappagh, S., & Abuhmed, T. (2024). Robustness in deep learning models for medical diagnostics: security and adversarial challenges towards robust AI applications. Artificial Intelligence Review, 58(1), 12.

Juang, W.-C., Hsu, M.-H., Cai, Z.-X., & Chen, C.-M. (2022). Developing an AI-assisted clinical decision support system to enhance in-patient holistic health care. *PLoS One*, *17*(10), e0276501. DOI: 10.1371/journal.pone.0276501 PMID: 36315554

Kaul, D., & Khurana, R. (2021). AI to detect and mitigate security vulnerabilities in APIs: Encryption, authentication, and anomaly detection in enterprise-level distributed systems. *Eigenpub Review of Science and Technology*, *5*(1), 34–62.

Kruegel, C., Kirda, E., Mutz, D., Robertson, W., & Vigna, G. (2005). Automating mimicry attacks using static binary analysis. USENIX Security Symposium

Loscocco, P. A., Smalley, S. D., Muckelbauer, P. A., Taylor, R. C., Turner, S. J., & Farrell, J. F. (1998). The inevitability of failure: The flawed assumption of security in modern computing environments. In Proceedings of the 21st national information systems security conference

Micheal, D. (2025). Comprehensive Survey of Security Techniques in the Post-Digital Era: From Intrusion Detection to Blockchain-Based Assurance Models.

Namli, T., Anıl Sınacı, A., Gönül, S., Herguido, C. R., Garcia-Canadilla, P., Muñoz, A. M., Esteve, A. V., & Ertürkmen, G. B. L. (2024). A scalable and transparent data pipeline for AI-enabled health data ecosystems. *Frontiers in Medicine*, *11*, 1393123. DOI: 10.3389/fmed.2024.1393123 PMID: 39139784

Parise, G., Parise, L., Allegri, M., De Marco, A., & Anthony, M. A. (2020). Operational resilience of hospital power systems in the digital age. *IEEE Transactions on Industry Applications*, *57*(1), 94–100. DOI: 10.1109/TIA.2020.3032941

Pichan, A., Lazarescu, M., & Soh, S. T. (2018). Towards a practical cloud forensics logging framework. *Journal of Information Security and Applications*, *42*, 18–28. DOI: 10.1016/j.jisa.2018.07.008

Prateek, M., & Rathore, S. P. S. (2025). Clinical validation of AI disease detection Models—An overview of the clinical validation process for AI disease detection models, and how they can be validated for accuracy and effectiveness. *AI in Disease Detection: Advancements and Applications*, 215-237.

Quinn, C. (2025). Generative Ai. In *Clinical Practice: A Physician's Guide To Transforming Medicine*. World Scientific. DOI: 10.1142/9789819822218_0001

Ranjitsingh, L. M., & Rao, T. S. (2025). Establish legal and regulatory standards for the testing and validation of AI systems to ensure their reliability and safety in operational environments. *International Journal of System Assurance Engineering and Management*, *16*(10), 3338–3353. DOI: 10.1007/s13198-025-02865-7

Rao, T. R., Mitra, P., Bhatt, R., & Goswami, A. (2019). The big data system, components, tools, and technologies: A survey. *Knowledge and Information Systems*, *60*(3), 1165–1245. DOI: 10.1007/s10115-018-1248-0

Reddy, S., Fox, J., & Purohit, M. P. (2019). Artificial intelligence-enabled healthcare delivery. *Journal of the Royal Society of Medicine*, *112*(1), 22–28. DOI: 10.1177/0141076818815510 PMID: 30507284

Sahinoglu, M. (2016). *Cyber-risk informatics: Engineering evaluation with data science*. John Wiley & Sons. DOI: 10.1002/9781119087540

Schwarzschild, A., Goldblum, M., Gupta, A., Dickerson, J. P., & Goldstein, T. (2021). Just how toxic is data poisoning? a unified benchmark for backdoor and data poisoning attacks. International Conference on Machine Learning, Shandilya, S. K., Datta, A., Kartik, Y., & Nagar, A. (2024). Navigating the regulatory landscape. In *Digital Resilience: Navigating Disruption and Safeguarding Data Privacy* (pp. 127-240). Springer.

Sharma, P. (2024). Enhancing Cyber Resilience: Development, Challenges, and Strategic Insights in Cyber Security Report Websites using Artificial Inteligence.

Sharma, P., Gounder, M., & Kumar, K. (2024). Mastering Feature Engineering: Unlocking the Art of Data Transformation for Enhanced Predictive Modeling with Neural Networks. International Conference on Data Science and Applications, Sloan, R., & Warner, R. (2017). *Unauthorized access: The crisis in online privacy and security*. Taylor & Francis.

Sobb, T., Moustafa, N., & Turnbull, B. (2025). Responsible resilience in cyber–physical–social systems: A new paradigm for emergent cyber risk modeling. *Future Internet, 17*(7), 282. DOI: 10.3390/fi17070282

Srijayanthi, S., & Sethukarasi, T. (2023). Design of privacy preserving model based on clustering involved anonymization along with feature selection. *Computers & Security, 126*, 103027. DOI: 10.1016/j.cose.2022.103027

Tao, H., Bhuiyan, M. Z. A., Rahman, M. A., Wang, G., Wang, T., Ahmed, M. M., & Li, J. (2019). Economic perspective analysis of protecting big data security and privacy. *Future Generation Computer Systems, 98*, 660–671. DOI: 10.1016/j.future.2019.03.042

Verma, P., Newe, T., O'Mahony, G. D., Brennan, D., & O'Shea, D. (2025). Towards a Unified Understanding of Cyber Resilience: A Comprehensive Review of Concepts, Strategies, and Future Directions. *IEEE Access : Practical Innovations, Open Solutions*. Advance online publication. DOI: 10.1109/ACCESS.2025.3551887

Wang, B., Sun, F., & Luan, Y. (2024). Comparison of the effectiveness of different normalization methods for metagenomic cross-study phenotype prediction under heterogeneity. *Scientific Reports, 14*(1), 7024. DOI: 10.1038/s41598-024-57670-2 PMID: 38528097

Wang, Z., Ma, J., Wang, X., Hu, J., Qin, Z., & Ren, K. (2022). Threats to training: A survey of poisoning attacks and defenses on machine learning systems. *ACM Computing Surveys, 55*(7), 1–36. DOI: 10.1145/3538707

Wasif, N. (2024). *Enhancing Cloud Security with AI-Driven Data Pipelines for Robust Infrastructure Protection: A Guide to Meeting HIPAA*. IAM, and SOX Compliance.

Whig, P., Aggarwal, A., Ganeshan, V., Modhugu, V. R., & Bhatia, A. B. (2024). AI for Secure and Resilient Cyber-Physical Systems. In *Artificial Intelligence Solutions for Cyber-Physical Systems* (pp. 40–63). Auerbach Publications. DOI: 10.1201/9781032694375-2

Williams, C., Watson, T., Bryant, I., Mahrra, J., Miller, W. D., Fonash, P. M., Badillo, B., Abrams, M., Nagarajan, A., & Sood, A. (2012). Resilient cyber ecosystems. *Crosstalk, 25*(5).

Zbrzezny, A. M., & Grzybowski, A. E. (2023). Deceptive tricks in artificial intelligence: Adversarial attacks in ophthalmology. *Journal of Clinical Medicine*, *12*(9), 3266. DOI: 10.3390/jcm12093266 PMID: 37176706

# Chapter 6
# Ransomware Threats in Healthcare Systems:
## Encryption-Based Attacks and Defensive Strategies

**Keshav Sinha**
http://orcid.org/0000-0003-1053-3911
*University of Petroleum and Energy Studies, Dehradun, India*

**Roopa Vuppula**
http://orcid.org/0000-0001-8568-5720
*Woxsen University, India*

## ABSTRACT

*The healthcare systems have become the most common target of ransomware attacks worldwide. The data consists of invaluable patient information, clinical processes and the unrelenting susceptibility of medical systems. It offers an extensive review of ransomware as a healthcare environment threat, its anatomy (starting with initial infection and behavioral development), cryptographic file encryption algorithms, and a deep examination of double extortion models complexity. The chapter analyzes the ransomware infection of healthcare-specific vulnerabilities such as Internet of Medical Things devices, Electronic Health Record systems, PACS imaging archives and HL7 clinical data interfaces. The main contribution is developing a complete defensive approach and Governance, Risk, and Compliance framework mapping ransomware countermeasures within the frameworks of the HIPAA Security Rule, NIST Cybersecurity Framework 2.0, and ISO 27001:2022 standard. The chapter also ends by providing practical suggestions to the cybersecurity teams, compliance officers, and clinical governance stakeholders.*

DOI: 10.4018/979-8-3373-9119-9.ch006

## INTRODUCTION

Ransomware has emerged as the defining cybersecurity threat of the present decade, with disproportionately severe and escalating impact on the healthcare sector. Making the convergence of irreplaceable patient information, life-sensitive operations, disjointed legacy infrastructure, and continued under-investment in cybersecurity uniquely appealing to ransomware attackers interested in both the largest profit margins and the least resistance to financial security requirements has pushed healthcare organizations to the top of the agenda. The magnitude of the issue is quantifiable and frightening. According to ransomware groups, there were more than 5,400 successful attacks worldwide in 2024 (Veriti Research, 2025), and the healthcare sector witnessed a 32% increase in cyberattacks compared to the previous year (CTIIC, 2024). The Sophos State of Ransomware in Healthcare report finds that 2 out of every 3 surveyed healthcare organizations reported being victimized by ransomware in 2024, the highest rate since 2018 (Sophos, 2024). In 2025, the recorded average cost of a healthcare data breach reached USD 7.42 million per incident, the highest across all industries (Jiang et al., 2025). The 100-million-person breach of the secured health data of 100 million people in the February 2024 ransomware attack of Change Healthcare, a subsidiary of UnitedHealth Group in handling around 40 percent of all health insurance claims made in the U.S., caused weeks of disrupted care delivery throughout the country and cost response efforts 2.4 billion dollars, making it the largest healthcare cyber incident on record (Jiang et al., 2025).

When ransomware laterally traverses the clinical network, causing intensive care unit systems to lose network connectivity, the ability to monitor patients is jeopardized. WannaCry Ransomware attack on the National Health Service in England and Wales in 2017 canceled about 19,000 appointments, got ambulances bused out of stricken Emergency Departments, and caused at least 80 NHS trusts to temporarily close down - proving beyond all doubt that a ransomware attack in the healthcare environment is not a data security issue but a patient safety crisis. Although this is a serious threat with an increasing rate, healthcare organizations continue to spend significantly less on cybersecurity than other similar fields. Healthcare normally spends up to four to seven percent of its information technology budgets on cybersecurity, and financial institutions are spending about 15 percent. Such a structural investment gap, exacerbated by a complex layer of legacy clinical infrastructure, complex third-party vendor markets, regulatory compliance overhead, and operational constraints on clinical workflows, creates the preconditions for the ongoing and growing vulnerability.

## Why Healthcare Is Disproportionately Vulnerable

Healthcare organizations are disproportionately appealing targets of ransomware campaigns, influenced by several interrelated structural features. These properties are a condition for developing defenses that are actually tailored to the real threat environment, rather than based on generic cybersecurity frameworks designed for environments with fewer constraints. Healthcare organizations are of extraordinary value on criminal markets as their data can be. Electronic health records containing extensive personal, financial, and medical histories fetch 10–25 times more on dark web marketplaces than credit card credentials (KnowBe4, 2023). This large volume of data facilitates the direct ransom payment role, where the organization would be incentivized to pay in order not to disrupt operations, and the dual extortion role, where the threat of publishing stolen patient records would result in a second, separate coercive force that would require action even after encrypted systems are recovered from a backup. The average ransom demand against healthcare providers reached an estimated USD 7 million in 2025, with the highest recorded single-provider demand reaching USD 100 million (Sophos, 2025). The Internet of Medical Things presents a large, architecturally challenging-to-secure attack surface. Embedded operating systems in medical devices (infusion pumps, patient monitors, ventilators, imaging systems, clinical analyzers, and networked diagnostic devices) typically have longer lifecycles and are not updated as often as the rest of the enterprise information technology infrastructure.

## Motivation and Research Gap

As ransomware attacks against health systems become more frequent, more serious, and more complex, there is a huge gap between the current state of health systems' cybersecurity and their understanding of it, hindering their ability to respond effectively. There are three levels at which this gap works. From a technical perspective, most healthcare security teams today are well equipped with perimeter defense capabilities but lack the validation and knowledge to detect ransomware components, pre-encryption behavioral signatures, and logic specific to healthcare that targets file operations, identifying the most vulnerable and coercive clinical systems as ransomware encryption targets. This type of technical sophistication enables detection systems to be misconfigured, inappropriate alert thresholds to be set, and actions to be taken too late in the attack life cycle or before clinical disruption. In terms of operational processes, there is a lack of understanding of the interplay between the technical processes of ransomware and the clinical operational impacts at the practical level, where clinicians, informaticists, security personnel, and administrators will have to work together to implement and put in place effective defenses. Security measures that do not account for clinical workflow requirements and operational continuity are often circumvented or incompletely enforced, resulting in a disparity between policy on paper and operational practice that ransomware attackers are all too happy to exploit.

## 2. LITERATURE REVIEW

This chapter synthesizes evidence from a structured review of peer-reviewed literature and authoritative grey literature published between 2018 and 2025. Databases searched include IEEE Xplore, PubMed/MEDLINE, Scopus, and ACM Digital Library, supplemented by reports from NIST, HHS Office for Civil Rights, Sophos, Forescout, and the Health-ISAC. Search terms included combinations of: ransomware AND healthcare, ransomware AND hospital, hybrid encryption AND malware, Zero Trust AND healthcare security, HIPAA AND cybersecurity, and IoMT AND ransomware. Inclusion criteria required: (i) peer-reviewed status or recognized authoritative source, (ii) direct relevance to ransomware threats or defenses in healthcare or clinical environments, and (iii) publication after 2018 to reflect the post-double-extortion era. Studies focusing exclusively on non-healthcare sectors without transferable findings were excluded. A total of 38 primary sources met the inclusion criteria and are cited throughout the chapter.

### Human Factors & Clinician Security Behavior

In healthcare settings where clinical needs often take priority over security measures, technical controls alone are insufficient. When patients are at risk of a concerning incident, clinicians routinely ignore security authentication and access controls, as Cresswell et al. (2017) showed, leaving security gaps that ransomware operators fill. Sheikh and Cresswell (2018) also confirmed that the implementation of EHRs causes disruptions in the work process, which leads to social engineering attacks on EHRs because it lowers the cognitive resources of staff responsible for security vigilance. Koppel et al. (2015) noted, however, that workarounds against security controls are commonplace in clinical environments and should be considered a part of the structure of healthcare security posture, not failures.

### Understanding the economics of ransomware and cyber insurance

Dupont (2019) has systematically researched the economic architecture of ransomware as an industry and presented ransomware operations as a rational economic enterprise with cost structures, profit margins, and market dynamics similar to those of legitimate service businesses. According to the Ransomware Task Force (2021), cyber insurance is also a key structural influence on ransom payment behavior, as organizations with cyber insurance coverage are statistically more likely to pay ransoms, as insurers often consider the cost of ransom payments to be cheaper than extended recovery.

## Comparing HIPAA, NIS2, and GDPR compliance

There are significant differences in jurisdictions around the regulatory framework for cybersecurity in healthcare. HIPAA (45 CFR Part 164) regulates covered entities and business associates of the United States, establishing administrative, physical, and technical requirements for safeguarding electronic protected health information, along with requirements to notify of breaches within 60 days of discovery. The EU NIS2 Directive (2022/2555/EU) comes into effect on 24 October 2024. It defines healthcare as a highly critical sector, with a number of obligations, such as incident reporting (within 24 hours of being aware of it), multi-factor authentication requirements, security obligations regarding the supply chain, and personal liability for senior management of an organization that does not comply. If a healthcare organization processes personal data of EU residents, then the General Data Protection Regulation (GDPR, 2016/679/EU) will apply, which mandates that notification be made to supervisory authorities within 72 hours of a breach. In the absence of evidence that it was previously encrypted, a ransomware attack against patient data is a presumption of GDPR violation.

## Detection Evasion Techniques

A comprehensive ransomware detection solution should recognize the level of sophistication ransomware operators are using to evade detection. Polymorphic ransomware variants recompile their binary signatures at every new occurrence, thus evading the signature-based detection of antivirus programs. Living-off-the-land (LotL) techniques are those used by ransomware operators that involve using native Windows administrative tools, including PowerShell, WMI, PsExec, and certutil, instead of custom malware binaries, and are actively designed to bypass endpoint security platforms that attempt to identify unknown executable files.

## Objectives and Contributions

Table 1 presents the distinct contributions to the understanding and practice of ransomware defense in healthcare environments:

*Table 1. Summary of Chapter Contributions to Healthcare Ransomware Defense*

| Contribution | Description |
|---|---|
| **Healthcare-Centric Ransomware Analysis** | A comprehensive and systematic analysis of ransomware taxonomy, vectors of attack, ransomware behavioral kill chain, and clinical impact, along with three influential real-life ransomware attacks in the healthcare sector. |
| **Cryptographic Mechanism Analysis** | An in-depth study of the various hybrid variants of encryption schemes used in the latest generation of ransomware families (ECC, RSA-2048, AES-256, and ChaCha20) and their application in healthcare file systems and clinical data formats. |
| **Multi-Layer Detection Framework** | A structured, operationally deployable detection model using file entropy analysis, network anomaly monitoring, SIEM behavioral correlation, and machine-learning classification, with healthcare-specific calibration guidance for each of the layers. |
| **Healthcare-Specific Defensive Architecture** | A multi-layered security approach that incorporates Zero Trust principles, tailored to the unique security needs and operational needs of EHR systems, PACS servers, IoMT devices, and clinical workflows, while ensuring security without compromising clinical workflow. |
| **Integrated GRC Framework Mapping** | One of the main contributions is that it maps the ransomware defense controls defined in the HIPAA Security Rule, NIST Cybersecurity Framework 2.0, and ISO 27001:2022, allowing healthcare organizations to become compliant with all three while gaining operational security effectiveness. |
| **Ransomware Audit Planning Model** | A practical, evidence-based ransomware audit checklist and readiness assessment methodology to help healthcare organizations assess their control posture, fill in gaps, and show readiness for regulators and auditors. |
| **End-to-End Incident Response Strategy** | A consistent, ransomware-specific incident response lifecycle that incorporates technical containment, forensic investigation, HIPAA breach notification requirements, clinical continuity planning, and recovery government. |

The rest of this chapter has been structured in the following manner. In Section 2, the author analyzes the ransomware anatomy, and Section 3 explores the cryptography used in current ransomware and its focus on healthcare data typologies. Section 4 provides the multi-layer detection model, and Section 5 elaborates on the overall defensive approach and integrated GRC system. In Section 6, the chapter ends by giving a strategic suggestion to the healthcare security leadership.

## 3. RANSOMWARE ANATOMY AND BEHAVIOR

Ransomware is an inclusive and dynamic family of malicious software that denies authorized users access to their systems or data using technical implementation, mainly encryption, and demands payment in exchange for restitution. It is pivotal to understand the taxonomy of the types of ransomware so that defenses can be created that are adjusted to the particular mechanisms used by a particular kind of ransomware. The oldest type of these threats is Locker Malware, which works by denying power to the device or operating system it affects, although files are not always encrypted. It is normally accompanied by a lock message on a full screen pretending to be the law enforcement or system administrators, and requires payment to resume functionality. Although locker ransomware is not as widely used in modern attacks that target hospitals, it still applies to resource-limited IoMT devices whose operating system can be easily hijacked, instead of targeted files being encrypted. The most common new type is crypto ransomware that uses powerful cryptographic algorithms to securely encrypt specified files, file systems, or even whole drives, making the data unusable without the decryption key, which the attacker holds. The new generation of crypto ransomware attacking health care uses hybridized encryption designs - fast symmetric algorithms like AES-256 to encrypt a large volume of medical data, and asymmetric algorithms like RSA-2048 or ECC to protect the symmetric encryption key. This construction is computationally efficient (scalable to large data volumes) and cryptographic (recovery without the attacker's private key is impossible). Hybrid ransomware, also viewed through the prism of the double extortion model, is a combination of file encryption and data exfiltration. The ransomware transports out a section of high-value data quietly, before executing the encryption payload, to an attacker-controlled infrastructure. The victim is then exposed to two threats at the same time: (i) inaccessibility of encrypted information and (ii) publicity or sale of stolen sensitive records. This paradigm, pioneered by the Maze group in 2019 and now standard practice among major ransomware operators including LockBit, RansomHub, and ALPHV/BlackCat (Alraizza & Algarni, 2023), has essentially cannibalized the principal protective utility of offline backups. An organization that has great backup hygiene is able to bring up encrypted systems; however, it is not able to bring back the exposure of stolen patient records.

Ransomware-as-a-Service is a business model for the majority of modern-day healthcare ransomware deployed. The ransomware platform, including the encryption engine, command and control infrastructure, payment portal, and negotiation interface, is the core development team (e.g., the Wizard Spider group involved in the Conti toolkit). Affiliate operators make a subscription payment or revenue share to deploy the platform within the targets of their choice. This paradigm has significantly reduced the technical cost of engaging in advanced ransomware attacks, allowing attackers with fewer technical skills to use enterprise-quality malware to target hospitals and healthcare systems. Figure 1 presents the ransomware taxonomy in Healthcare Environments, showing four main categories: Locker, Crypto, Hybrid, and Ransomware-as-a-Service with sub-types, encryption methods, and primary healthcare target systems.

*Figure 1. Ransomware Taxonomy in Healthcare Environments*

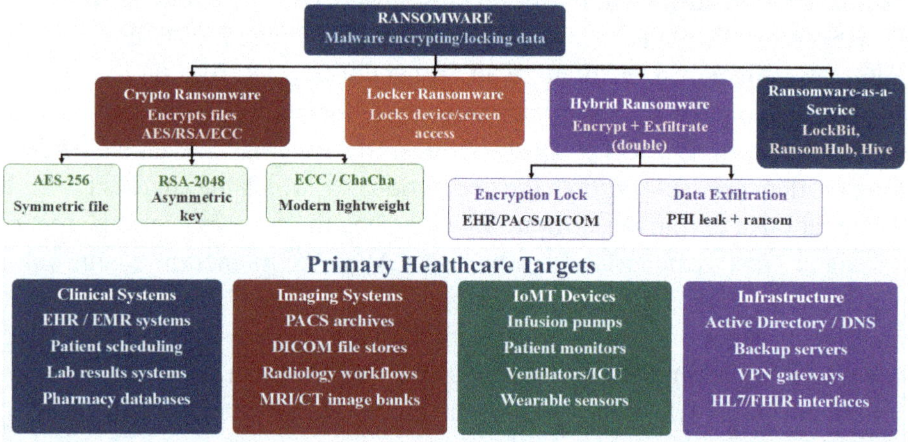


## Infection Vectors in Healthcare

To design effective controls to prevent ransomware, it is necessary to understand how ransomware gets into healthcare settings. The area of attack is wide and conditioned by the nature of work in clinical settings. The most common initial access method is phishing email, accounting for approximately 34 percent of confirmed healthcare ransomware incidents (Sophos, 2024).

The second most notable number is that of remote desktop Protocol exploitation, which caused approximately 28 percent of healthcare ransomware incidents (Sophos, 2024). Remote clinical, medical device management, and vendor support connections often have RDP propagated on public-facing interfaces in healthcare organizations. Attackers' brute-force RDP endpoints to use exposed credentials and buy stolen credentials in the initial access brokers within underground marketplaces. In 2021, the Health Service Executive (HSE) Ireland Conti attack the largest recorded ransomware attack on a national health service, which was initiated via a compromised RDP connection by the Wizard Spider group (Health Service Executive, 2021).

Exploits such as vulnerabilities, especially against VPN gateways, remote access infrastructure, and unpatched clinical application servers, have been on the increase as a vehicle. In a Sophos analysis of vulnerabilities exploited in 2025, vulnerability and credential-based attacks were identified as the primary technical root cause of healthcare incidents, accounting for 33 percent (Sophos, 2025). The high rate of unpatched legacy systems in healthcare, caused by the risk of disruption of operational operations of clinical systems by patching them and vendor restrictions on certified medical device software, forms a continuous vulnerability list that ransomware operators actively scan and exploit. Figure 2 presents the primary ransomware infection vectors in Healthcare Systems. Six entry paths converge on the hospital network, with phishing (34%), RDP exploitation (28%), and vulnerability exploitation (33%) as leading vectors in 2024-2025.

*Figure 2. Primary Ransomware Infection Vectors in Healthcare Systems*

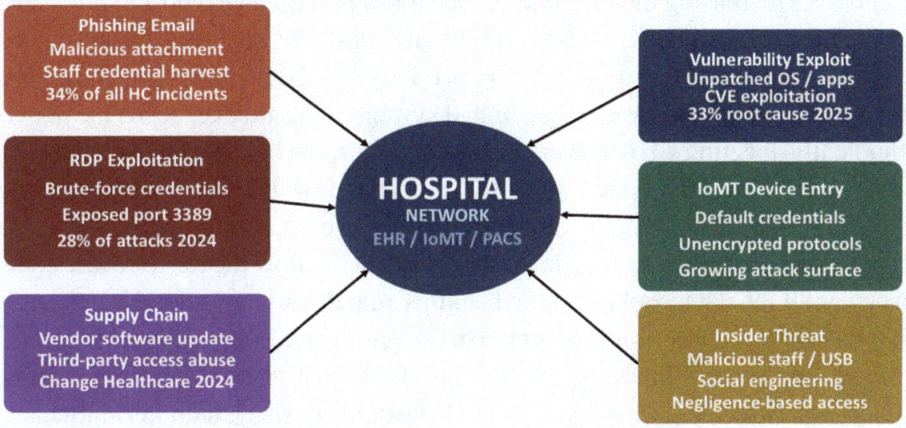


## Ransomware Kill Chain in Healthcare

Instead, ransomware attacks on healthcare organizations are not one-punch operations but a well-organized campaign that often takes days or weeks before the ransomware encrypts its payload. The knowledge of the kill chain allows the defenders to determine areas to interfere at any stage. The reconnaissance phase entails a systematic intelligence collection on the target organization. Open-source intelligence used by attackers to determine technology vendors, software versions, network topology, exposed services, and email addresses of staff members includes healthcare provider directories, LinkedIn profiles, vendor announcements, and publicly accessible medical devices network scans. Targets are considered based on their financial ability to pay ransom, their reliance on computer systems to carry out their operations, and the fullness of their backup systems. The attacker gains access to a single host in the healthcare system - either a clinical workstation, an administrative PC, or an exposed server. At this point, the concession is often not visible to the security team of an organization.

Persistence makes sure that the attacker's access remains intact despite a reboot, credential rotation, and even regular security scans. Some of the mechanisms of persistence are registry-based startup entries, scheduled jobs, service installation, and deployment of commercial remote access tools like Cobalt Strike beacons, which can be configured to combine legitimate patterns of administrative traffic and attacker command and control traffic. The HSE Ireland attack involved approximately eight weeks of undetected persistence (Health Service Executive, 2021), which depicts the dwell time element of professional ransomware campaigns. Lateral movement encompasses increasing the foothold of the attacker on their first host to other structures in the healthcare network. Methods involve pass-the-hash attacks on Windows authentication, abuse of Active Directory privileges, SMB relay attacks, and entering into trust relationships between the clinical systems. The attacker scans the network methodically, locating EHR servers, PACS archives, the backup infrastructure, and domain controllers - the systems that the encryption of the encryption will impact the organization in the most useful way. Privilege escalation aims at the domain administrator account or system-level access that will allow the ransomware code to overpower all the data available, stop backups, and destroy volume shadow copies, which will otherwise permit recovery. This stage is usually characterized by taking advantage of Active Directory configurations, kernel abuse, or theft of service account credentials. Figure 3 presents the Ransomware Kill Chain in Healthcare. It consists of a 7 Stage Attack Progression from Reconnaissance through Extortion, with healthcare-specific impact at each phase, including EHR encryption, PACS disruption, and clinical emergency conditions.

*Figure 3. Ransomware Kill Chain in Healthcare*

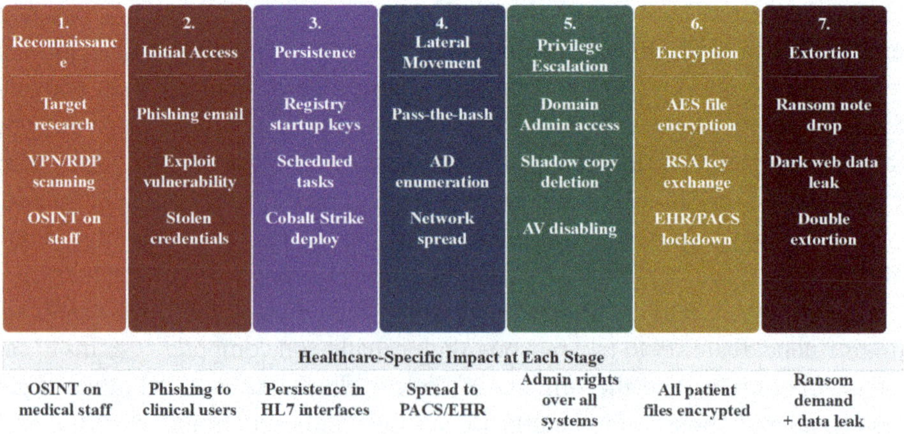

## Notable Healthcare Ransomware Incidents

Three historic events demonstrate how the nature of healthcare ransom has taken a new course and its practical clinical implications. The May 2017 WannaCry attack took advantage of the EternalBlue vulnerability of the Windows SMB protocol to spread automatically across unpatched systems. The underlying vulnerability was identified and reported in 2014, and Microsoft had provided a patch two months prior, but it was still unpatched at the time of the attack. In England and Wales, over 80 NHS trusts were impacted in less than an hour, 603 primary care organizations and 595 GP practices suffered, and around 19,000 appointments were postponed or rerouted. Some of the emergency departments were shut down, ambulances were diverted, and important diagnostic equipment was unavailable. The total estimated cost for the NHS was GBP 92 million (Forescout Technologies, 2024). The event demonstrated that there was a systemic neglect of implementing available security patches to clinical infrastructure and brought into focus the ultimate impacts of ransomware on patient safety in a population-scale health system. A qualitative escalation was achieved with the Conti ransomware attack on the Irish Health Service Executive in May 2021. The HSE attack, in contrast to the automatic self-propagation of the WannaCry, was a carefully thought-out human-alleged campaign. It was first accessed by a malicious Microsoft Excel attachment in a phishing email on 18 March 2021. The attackers estimated between eight weeks to gain persistence, map the HSE network, exfiltrate data, and prepare the encryption payload, and delivered it on 14 May 2021. Approximately 80,000 devices across the national health system were compromised (Health Service Executive, 2021).

Screening for cancer was halted, services to the maternity were marred, radiology activities were thrown into limbo, and the hospital management information system collapsed. To compensate, remediation costs exceeded EUR 100 million, with a further EUR 650 million required to upgrade and strengthen the HSE's information technology infrastructure (Health Service Executive, 2021). After the February 2024 attack on Change Healthcare, the systemic danger of monopolistic healthcare technology intermediaries became apparent. UnitedHealth Group subsidiary Change Healthcare handles about 40 percent of all health insurance claims in the U.S. The ALPHV/BlackCat ransomware group gained initial access using stolen credentials on a Citrix remote access portal that lacked multi-factor authentication enforcement (Jiang et al., 2025). Arguably, this interruption caused the subsequent failure of pharmacies to take prescription orders, interfered with hospitals' filing claims, and disrupted the workflow of the thousands of provider organizations at once. The attack compromised the secured health data of 100 million people and cost 2.4 billion dollars in response efforts - setting a new standard in the number of victims of ransomware in the healthcare industry.

## 4. Encryption Designs And Lifecycle Of Healthcare Attacks

The success of the ransomware as an extortion instrument is entirely hinged upon the effectiveness and appropriateness of its cryptographic application. The ransomware families today have developed advanced hybridized cryptography designs that integrate both the computing power of symmetric cryptography and the key management features of asymmetric cryptography, generating encryption systems that are essentially unbreakable in the absence of the private key of an attacker. The foundational cryptographic architecture employed by LockBit, Conti, ALPHV/BlackCat, and the majority of active healthcare-targeting ransomware families follows a two-layer hybrid design (Li et al., 2025; MITRE Corporation, 2024). The command and control system of an attacker is used to generate a key pair based on either RSA-2048 or elliptic curve cryptography (ECC). The ransomware binary is sent to the victim system, which contains the public key. The ransomware code creates a distinct symmetric key, which is usually a 256-bit AES key, per target or unique file, based on the implementation. The contents of the file are encrypted, either with AES-256 in cipher block chaining or Galois/Counter Mode, which offers confidentiality and, in the latter, authenticated encryption. Encryption of the AES session key is then performed with the RSA public key of the attacker, and the encrypted key material is stored or embedded in the encrypted file along with it. The original AES key is then wiped off the records.

Some modern ransomware families are using variants of elliptic curve cryptography, especially the Curve25519 algorithm, instead of or in addition to the RSA-2048. ECC has the same level of security, however, with significantly reduced keys - a 256-bit ECC key offers about the same level of security as a key with 3072 bits of RSA key - it is easier to generate, quicker to use, and more challenging to factor. LockBit 3.0, responsible for the sophisticated breach of NHS-affiliated systems, employed ECC to encrypt symmetric session keys (Li et al., 2025) that provided an additional layer of security that severely hampered the recovery of the technical files. The Hive ransomware family, active during 2022–2023 and targeting hospitals and government agencies, also implemented ECC (Alraizza & Algarni, 2023) to create an encryption difficulty that is practically irreversible by investigators without the cooperation of the attacker.

*Figure 4. Hybrid Encryption Flow in Modern Ransomware (AES-256 + RSA-2048)*

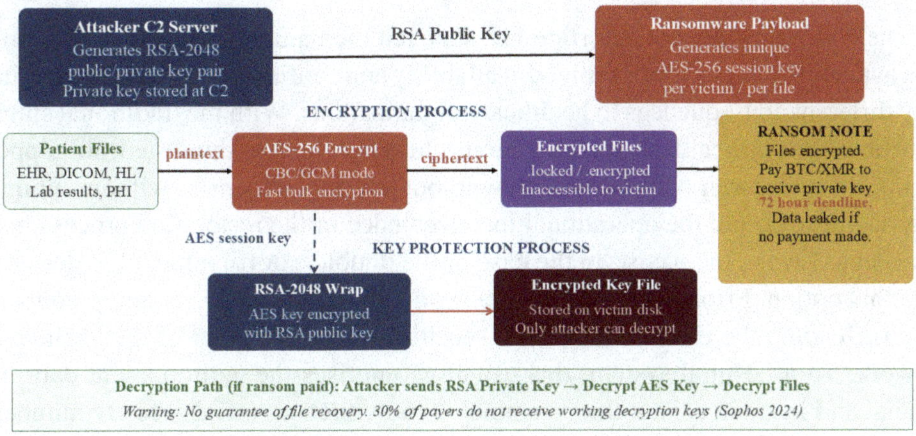


## Healthcare-Specific File Targeting

Hackers of healthcare have developed file-targeting logic to focus on the most disruptive and pressureful operations with maximum impact by focusing on the types of data most vital to clinical functions and least accessible through data backup. The main target is EHR systems. EHR databases are the formatted clinical information that clinicians rely on to provide safe patient care–the demographics, diagnoses, medications, allergies, clinical notes, and treatment histories of patients. EHR-based ransomware attacks are often characterized by the encryption of a database coupled with the deletion or encryption of application configuration files, credential stores, and connection strings to such a degree that the underlying database can be recovered, but the clinical application layer cannot instantly reconnect to it. PACS and DICOM imaging archives are urgently needed targets due to vast amounts of data and the clinical urgency of imaging data in diagnostic and surgical planning. A PACS archive found in a typical hospital is terabytes of DICOM-formatted imaging studies accrued over the years or decades. The replication of these studies in off-site backup is not often completely replicated due to the cost and bandwidth of replicating large volumes of imaging. The deletion of imaging archives is thus specifically coercive, as restorations, including backups, can be either incomplete or take months. Both direct encryptions and disruption multipliers are represented by HL7 and FHIR interfaces, the clinical messaging standard under which various healthcare systems exchange patient data.

## Double Extortion In Healthcare

The concept of double extortion has changed the nature of ransomware from a data availability attack to a combined availability and confidentiality attack, carrying very different consequences to healthcare organizations. With the traditional single extortion model, a healthcare organization, which has trustworthy, tested, air-gapped backups, may recover operations, even without interface expenses, without submitting the ransom, and the operational inconvenience of the restoration process may be accepted as the main cost. In the case of the double extortion model, it does not give this option. Prior to placing the encryption payload, attackers enjoy hours or days offloading the most valuable and sensitive data quietly out of the healthcare network. To a hospital system, this usually comprises the entire patient data, financial and insurance data, the personnel records such as social security numbers and credential files, as well as any proprietary research data and pharmaceutical information possessed by academic medical centers. The stolen data is uploaded to the infrastructure under the control of the attackers. After the deployment of the encryption payload, the ransom sum is complemented with evidence of the exfiltration they have performed, which is usually posted as sample files to a dedicated dark web leak site, and failure to pay will lead to the full publication of the entire stolen data.

*Figure 5. Healthcare-Specific Ransomware Attack Lifecycle*

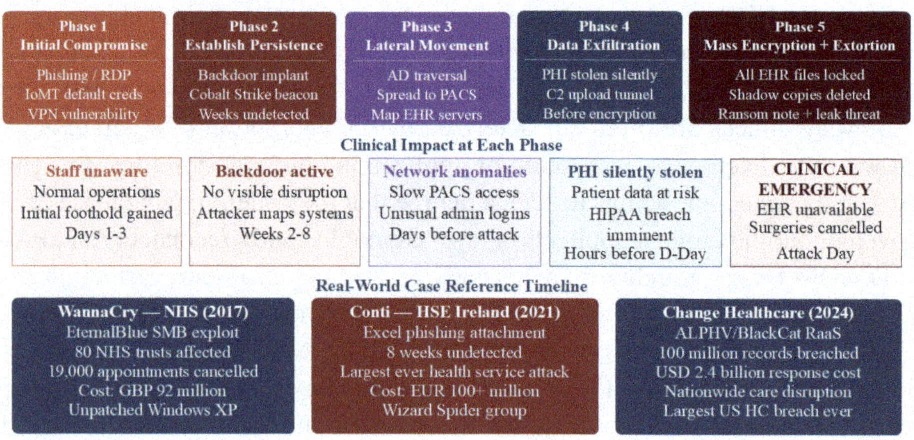

## 5. DETECTION AND IDENTIFICATION STRATEGIES

Temporal is the main problem of ransomware detection in healthcare: by the time the encryption payload has executed, releasing its operational disruption into the limelight, the attack has already achieved its initial goal. The financial and clinical impact of ransomware is not defined by whether or not the encryption will be overturned, but rather by a prolonged period of unavailability of clinical systems and data leaks. Successful detection should thus look at targeting the pre-encryption steps of the kill chain - reconnaissance, persistence, lateral movement, and privilege escalation at stages where the intervention can actually ensure that the encryption event does not even take place.

### File Entropy Analysis

Shannon entropy is used to have a quantitative measure of information density in data. Ideally, encrypted data would have the entropy of the output of the encryption (measured in bits per byte) equal to 8.0 bits, illustrating the limitation of such data to be statistically identical to random noise. Entropy values of unencrypted files containing natural language text, structured database records, or formatted documents typically fall between 3.0 and 5.5 bits per byte (Schmidt et al., 2023; Razavi et al., 2023). Baseline entropy in DICOM medical imaging and compressed medical data can be larger, although it is usually less than 7.0 bits per byte. Ransomware encryption leaves an entropy signature - the malware will increase its entropy very fast as it reads files by first adjusting their entropy to a threshold, then soaring to a near 7.8 to 8.0 bits per byte.

### SIEM, EDR, and Machine Learning Detection

Security Information and Event Management platforms deliver the correlation layer that converts single security events across different sources, endpoint agents, network monitors, authentication logs, application logs, and threat intelligence feeds into subsequent incident alerts that capture the multi-stage reality of ransomware campaigns. Building a SIEM to detect ransomware in healthcare will need an effective SIEM configuration that enables it to identify kill chain correlation rules instead of identifying the isolated occurrence of each event incident. An attempt to log in once is not an issue. A brute force indicator is the number of failed authentication attempts (one source against many targets in 10 minutes). Authentication attempts that failed, and then successful authentication, followed by a new scheduled task, followed by SMB scanning on the authenticated host, are indicators of a high-confidence kill chain that should be immediately investigated and responded to automatically. User and Entity Behavior Analytics normalizes the typical behavior of individual users, service accounts, and devices, and notifies when observed behavior is significantly different than the baselines. Recent studies have demonstrated that ensemble approaches combining random forest classifiers, gradient-boosted trees, and LSTM sequence models processing behavioral feature vectors, including file access rates, API call sequences, network connection patterns, and registry modification activity, achieve ransomware detection accuracy exceeding 99 percent across diverse ransomware family samples (Lee et al., 2025; Ferdous et al., 2025; Ispahany et al., 2024). The central issue of operation is how to cope with false positive rates in clinical settings where valid clinical processes can be met with behavioral patterns of superficial similarity to ransomware - bulk file processing, scheduled database export separations, and medical imaging compression operations all create patterns of file system activity that naive classifiers would misclassify. Figure 6 presents the Multi-Layer Ransomware Detection Framework for Healthcare, combining file entropy analysis (Layer 1), network anomaly detection (Layer 2), and SIEM/EDR/ML behavioral detection (Layer 3), with specific indicators of compromise for each layer.

*Figure 6. Multi-Layer Ransomware Detection Framework for Healthcare*

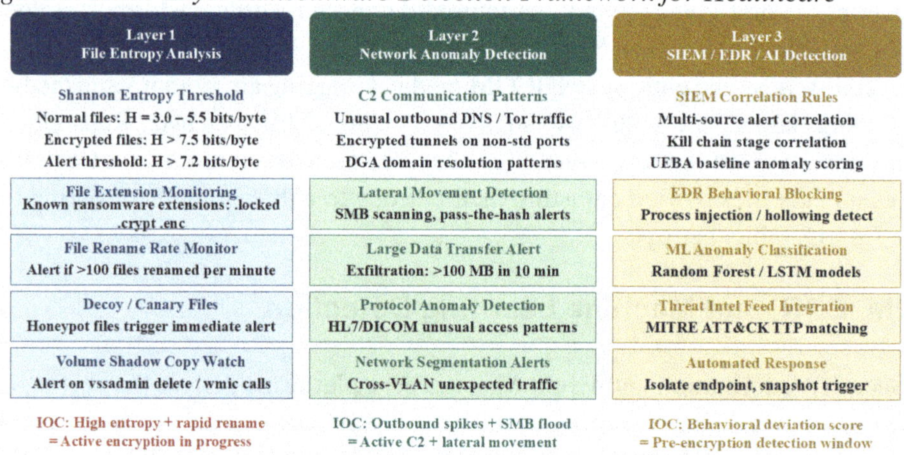


## 6. AUDIT PLANNING, STRATEGIES TO ADDRESS DEFENSE, AND GRC FRAMEWORK

The architectural principles of healthcare ransomware protection are the layered security model. The controlled use of security controls stands distant from the technology stack, such that a hacker can never have unlimited access to clinical data or operational systems. It is coupled with well-known concepts of Zero Trust, namely, the policy, according to which no user, device, or network segment should be trusted by default, regardless of its network presence. Layered defense may provide a space in which the lateral movement and privilege escalation patterns characteristic of ransomware are always identified, contested, and prevented. Next-generation firewall rules ought to heavily restrict outbound and inbound traffic at the perimeter layer, explicitly denying by default and explicitly authorizing explicitly defined allow rules of documented clinical data flows. Before deliveries to clinical staff, email security gateways are recommended to examine all incoming email to identify malicious and phishing attachments and indicators. All connections to VPN and remote access infrastructure must be multi-factor authentication-enabled, as demonstrated by the Change Healthcare breach, in which the absence of MFA on the Citrix remote access portal directly enabled initial access (Jiang et al., 2025). The Network boundaries should be fitted with an Intrusion Prevention System and set to a predefined set of healthcare-specific rules addressing the patterns of clinical protocol exploitation. Figure 7 presents the Layered Defense Architecture for Healthcare Ransomware Protection. Five concentric defense layers from the data core through perimeter implement Zero Trust principles, with specific controls for EHR systems, PACS archives, and IoMT devices at the core.

*Figure 7. Layered Defense Architecture for Healthcare Ransomware Protection*

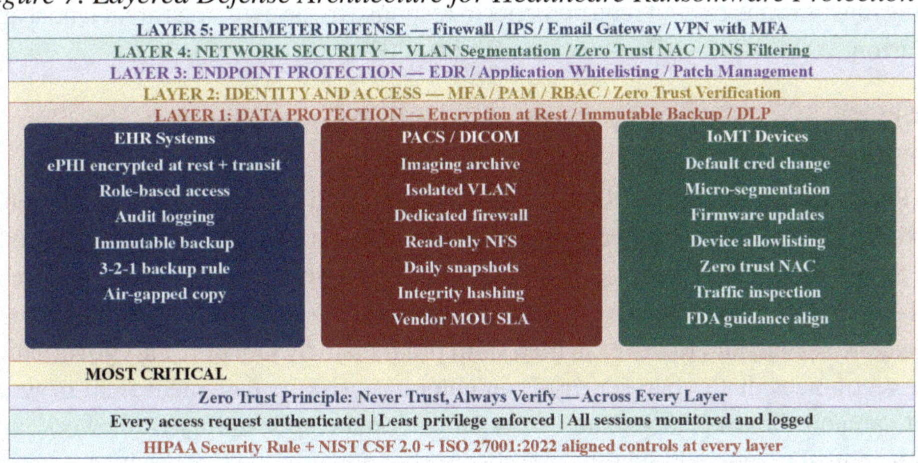

## Backup and Recovery Strategy

Healthcare organizations need to have installed backup architectures, specially built to survive the intended destruction manifested by ransomware operators prior to them introducing their encryption payload. The 3-2-1 backup rule is the starting point, which is to have three copies of data in two forms of storage media, and one off-site. In the case of healthcare settings, two more requirements need to be added to this baseline immutability and offline isolation. To validate the full recovery of representative datasets in all levels of backups, such as daily incremental or weekly full and offline archive copies, healthcare organizations ought to provide quarterly tests of restores, which verify that the actual recovery time goal has been met as compared to the scheduled Recovery Time Objective (RTO). These tests have to be documented, and their results reviewed by clinical governance and information security leadership.

## GRC Framework: HIPAA Security Rule

The HIPAA Security Rule, which is codified in 45 CFR part 164, provides the minimum administrative, physical, and technical safeguard requirements to the covered entities and business associates that use electronic protected health information. On 20 December 2024, the Department of Health and Human Services proposed significant amendments to the HIPAA Security Rule explicitly strengthening ransomware-related requirements in response to the evolving threat landscape (Marron, 2024; HHS Office for Civil Rights, 2024).

## GRC Framework: NIST Cybersecurity Framework 2.0

Published in February 2024, NIST Cybersecurity Framework 2.0 (National Institute of Standards and Technology, 2024) represents the first major revision to the foundational NIST cybersecurity guidance framework since its initial release in 2014. CSF 2.0 broadens the five original pillars of functions, namely Identify, Protect, Detect, Respond, and Recover, with a sixth pillar, namely Govern. This governance role recognizes that cybersecurity is an enterprise risk management field of work that demands board presence and an organizational responsibility framework, and not technical practice. In healthcare ransomware defense, the Governance function aligns with building a cybersecurity governance structure with established roles, responsibilities, and accountability to manage the ransomware risk. This consists of an executive-approved cybersecurity risk management plan, periodic board-level reporting on cybersecurity risk posture, and incorporation of cybersecurity goals into organizational strategic plans. The Governance component of the supply chain risk management is especially applicable to healthcare since it has been proven that ransomware has concentrated on getting into the healthcare system through vendor relationships, as in the case of Change Healthcare. Identifying function is equated with the upkeep of technology asset inventory and network map, as mandated by the new HIPAA Security Rule, which entails annual risk assessment, including ransomware as a candidly considered vulnerability, and situational awareness of the threat landscape through threat intelligence subscriptions and involvement with the Health-ISAC information sharing community. The Protect function is equated to the access control, encryption, backup, patch management, and endpoint protection controls as in Sections 5.1 to 5.3. The Detect function corresponds to the detection framework outlined in Section 4, such as continuous monitoring, the ability to detect anomalies, and the ability to hunt threats. The Respond and Recover functions are aligned to the incident response planning, forensic investigation procedures, communication plans, and recovery capabilities provided in Section 5.7. The focus of CSF 2.0 on constant improvement - learning by internal incident as well as utilizing threat intelligence on incidents affecting comparable organizations should be allocated to habitual incident response workouts, post-incident audits, and updates to the control structure according to lessons learned.

## GRC Framework: ISO 27001:2022

ISO 27001:2022 is an internationally recognized information security management standard against which healthcare organizations can certify their security governance programs, and this guarantees they develop a high degree of security governance as externally established. In the 2022 revision of the standard, Annex A to 93 controls have been reorganized and revised, and are grouped into four themes: organizational controls, people control, physical controls, and technological controls. A number of Annex A controls are ransomware relevant. Information backup Control A.8.13 states that a backup policy needs to be documented, tested, and periodically reviewed as per the 3-2-1 and immutability principle presented in Section 5.2. The control A.8.24 on cryptography usage needs a written cryptographic policy (encryption of data at rest/in transit, key management, and using approved cryptographic algorithms) - a direct support of the protection of exposure of ePHI to exfiltration. Control A.8.2 on the topic of privileged access rights handles the access management controls that ransomware operators cannot access in order to accomplish their attacks, which is by gaining the domain administrator privileges. Controls A.5.24-A.5.27 deal with incident management on a holistic scale: planning and preparation, assessment and decision-making, response to information security incidents, and incident learning. These controls are the framework for the incident response planning guidance in Section 5.7. In particular, control A.5.25 includes the condition that organizations must analyze whether the information security incident reported should be considered a data security incident - the assessment that the condition applies to the ransomware attacks, which additionally involves the analysis of whether ePHI was accessed or exfiltrated prior to encryption. Figure 8 presents GRC Framework Mapping across HIPAA Security Rule, NIST CSF 2.0, and ISO 27001:2022 for five ransomware control domains: Governance and Risk, Access Control, Encryption and Data Protection, Detection and Monitoring, and Incident Response.

*Figure 8. GRC Framework Mapping across HIPAA Security Rule, NIST CSF 2.0, and ISO 27001:2022*

| Control Domain Ransomware Focus | HIPAA Security Rule 45 CFR Part 164 2025 | NIST CSF 2.0 6 Core Functions Feb 2024 | ISO 27001:2022 Annex A 93 controls |
|---|---|---|---|
| Governance and Risk | **164.308(a)(1) Annual risk** assessment required Risk register mandatory Board-level oversight | **GV.OC and GV.RM** Governance strategy Risk management Supply chain risk | **A.5 IS Policies** A.6 Organisation IS Risk treatment plan SoA documentation |
| Access Control | **164.312(a)(1)** Unique user IDs Emergency access proc Automatic logoff req | **PR.AA Access Control** Identity management MFA enforcement Least privilege | **A.8.2 Privileged access** A.8.3 Info access A.8.5 Secure authn A.8.6 Capacity mgmt |
| Encryption and Data | **164.312(a)(2)(iv)** Encrypt ePHI at rest Encrypt in transit 72hr restore plan | **PR.DS Data Security** Data at rest protect TLS in transit Backup recovery | **A.8.24 Cryptography** A.8.13 Info backup A.8.14 Redundancy A.8.15 Logging |
| Detection and Monitoring | **164.312(b) Audit** HW/SW audit controls Activity monitoring Audit trail integrity | **DE.CM Monitoring** Continuous monitoring Anomaly detection SIEM analysis | **A.8.15 Log monitoring** A.8.16 Activities A.8.17 Clock sync A.5.25 IS events |
| Incident Response | **164.308(a)(6) IR plan** 60-day breach notify Forensics preserve Documented procedures | **RS.MA and RC.RP** Incident management Recovery planning Comm plan | **A.5.24 IR planning** A.5.25 Assessment A.5.26 Response A.5.27 Learn from inc |

## Ransomware Readiness Audit Planning

In Ransomware audit planning, the strategic framework outlined in Sections 5.4 through 5.6 is converted into an organized, evidence-based ransomware readiness assessment. Ransomware audit is different compared to a general information security audit in that it requires a very specific focus on the controls based on which an organization can prevent, detect, contain, and recover after a ransomware attack with satisfactory patient safety and data protection results. The essential ransomware audit checklist of healthcare organizations includes the following types of controls, as presented in Table 2.

*Table 2. Ransomware Audit Controls Checklist*

| Control Domain | Audit Test Procedure | Evidence Required | Framework Ref. |
|---|---|---|---|
| Asset Inventory | Verify a complete inventory of all IT and IoMT assets. Confirm network diagram accuracy. | Asset register + network diagram | HIPAA 164.308 / NIST GV |
| MFA on all remote access | Test all VPN, RDP, Citrix, and cloud portals for MFA enforcement without exception. | Authentication logs + config screenshots | HIPAA 164.312 / NIST PR.AA |
| Patch management SLAs | Review patch records for critical CVEs. Verify 30-day remediation for internet-facing systems. | Patch tickets + vulnerability scan reports | HIPAA 164.308 / NIST PR.MA |
| Backup completeness | Verify 3-2-1 backup compliance. Tests restore from each backup tier. Verify immutability config. | Restore test records + backup policy | HIPAA 164.308 / NIST RC.RP |
| Network segmentation | Verify IoMT, PACS, and EHR in separate VLANs. Test inter-VLAN access controls. | Firewall rulesets + network diagram | NIST PR.IR / ISO A.8.22 |
| Shadow copy protection | Verify VSS deletion commands are detected and blocked by endpoint security. | EDR policy config + test logs | NIST DE.CM / ISO A.8.15 |
| Incident response plan | Review the IR plan for ransomware-specific procedures. Verify tabletop exercise records. | IR plan document + exercise records | HIPAA 164.308 / ISO A.5.24 |
| Staff awareness training | Verify phishing simulation results and security awareness training completion rates. | Training records + simulation reports | HIPAA 164.308 / ISO A.6.3 |
| Vendor access management | Review third-party access controls. Verify MFA and least-privilege for all vendors. | Vendor access register + audit logs | HIPAA 164.308 / NIST GV.SC |
| Breach notification readiness | Verify documented procedures for 60-day HIPAA breach notification. Review past notification history. | Notification procedures + test records | HIPAA 164.404 / ISO A.5.26 |

To mitigate the effects of the ransomware, healthcare organizations need to establish response procedures specific to ransomware that combine technical forensics and recovery-based information security response with the clinical operations continuity planning of the business continuity management.

## Ransomware Negotiation and Payment Decision Framework

Once ransomware encryption has been used and clinical systems are down, the healthcare leader has to make a choice and pay the ransom or try to resist it. This decision must be taken in real-time with incomplete information and with information from the IT security team, legal team, clinical leadership, executive management, and cyber insurance carriers. A well-designed decision framework minimizes the likelihood of decisions being made reactively that can exacerbate outcomes. Backup viability: (i) Is it possible to get clinical systems back online within an acceptable amount of time using existing unencrypted backups? The longer it takes to recover from backups, the stronger the case for payment becomes if the time is greater than clinical safety limits. (ii) Confirmed exfiltration: Has there been any forensic analysis or proof that a data exfiltration occurred by an attacker? If ePHI is exfiltrated, there is no requirement for payment to trigger the notification requirements, and the additional value of paying for the disclosure must be balanced against the risk of it. (iii) Threat actor credibility: Does the ransomware group have a history of delivering working decryption tools when ransom is paid? The former groups that create Ransomware-as-a-Service (RaaS) with a reputational incentive for honoring payments are not the same as the opportunists who accept payment but are not capable of providing decryption. Regulatory/legal position: payments to sanctioned threat actors could be in violation of OFAC regulations. Any legal counsel needs first to verify that the identified threat actor is not on the sanctions lists before approving payment. (v) Insurance coverage: The policy terms of cyber insurance policies should be reviewed—many policies have conditions that require the insurer's approval of ransom payments in order to maintain coverage. Healthcare organizations should create a pre-incident Ransomware Response Committee (RRC) that includes a CISO, General Counsel, Chief Medical Officer, CFO, and a Public Affairs officer, all with agreed governance and escalation, to ensure that governance is not improvised during the incident.

## Crisis Communication and Patient Notification Strategy

Healthcare ransomware incidents have multiple concurrent and legally defined communication requirements that need to be managed simultaneously with multiple audiences. A lack of proper communication can heighten regulatory risk, erode patient trust, and cause more secondary reputational harm than the cost of the attack itself.

HIPAA mandates that covered entities inform people that their personal health information has been compromised within an "undue delay" of 60 calendar days after a breach with unsecured ePHI has been discovered. If there is a breach involving 500 or more individuals in a state or jurisdiction, individual notification is in addition to a prominent media notice. The same 60 days must be given to the HHS Office for Civil Rights. Where an investigation finds that, before encryption, access, or exfiltration of ePHI occurred, notification requirements are triggered even if ransom was paid or systems were recovered from backups. Internal communication should ensure that clinical teams are aware of any problems with the system and what to do in the event of downtime to ensure continuity of care. All external communications with the public, media, and partner organizations must be handled through a designated spokesperson and, with legal counsel input, with a view to avoiding additional regulatory or litigation exposure. Pre-wrote letters to be sent to patients, regulators, and media for ransomware-type incidents should be included with incident response planning and reviewed every year.

## Healthcare-Specific Tabletop Exercise Design

Tabletop exercises are the main way healthcare organizations can test their ransomware incident response capabilities without putting their systems at risk. A successful healthcare ransomware tabletop exercise should simulate the reality of a multi-domain attack and involve the same type of decision-making that happens during an actual incident—both across clinical operations and IT security, as well as legal, communications, and executive decisions. A suggested outline of the flow of a healthcare ransomware tabletop exercise is as follows. Phase 1 (Initial Discovery): IT staff says that several clinical workstations are showing ransom notes and that they cannot access the EHR. Participants should be able to: Run the Incident Response plan, determine the extent of the impacted systems, engage clinical Downtime procedures, and alert executive leadership. Phase 2 (Scope Expansion): After doing a forensic analysis, it is discovered that the PACS archive and backup servers on the network are also encrypted. The attacker calls the organization with a ransom demand and sends samples of the stolen patient information. Participants should be able to: Evaluate Payment decision criteria, involve a cyber insurance carrier, Identify HIPAA breach notification requirements, and start an external forensic investigation. Phase 3 (Recovery and Communication): Backup restoration is in progress from copies in an air-gap, but may take 72 hours. Media inquiries are taken. The participant(s) are responsible for: Phased System Recovery Priority Plan, Coordinate Patient Notification, and Manage Public Communications. A structured after-action review should be conducted after the exercise to capture lessons learned, gaps identified, and controls that need to be improved, with a remediation tracking system to ensure that findings are addressed prior to the next exercise cycle.

## Post-Quantum Cryptography on healthcare data retention

Given the rise of cryptographically valuable quantum computers in the next decade, current security planning must already take into account the impact on healthcare data. There are longer retention periods for healthcare records, especially as mandated by state and federal legislation, which typically mandates that medical records be kept for 7 to 10 years and sometimes longer for pediatric records. The future power of a quantum computer means that data that could be encrypted today with RSA-2048 or ECC-based cryptography may be decrypted in the future, something ransomware operators may be exploiting right now: harvest now, decrypt later. In 2024, NIST finalized its standardization process for PQC and published

FIPS 203 (ML-KEM, based on CRYSTALS-Kyber), FIPS 204 (ML-DSA, based on CRYSTALS-Dilithium), and FIPS 205 (SLH-DSA, based on SPHINCS+). Healthcare organizations should start planning a cryptographic migration plan that accounts for any systems running EHRs with long retention periods, prioritizes migration to post-quantum cryptographic algorithms for data at rest and in transit, and provides for the cryptographic agility of medical imaging archives and EHR platforms. The planning for this should start now, with the transition of cryptographic infrastructure in complex healthcare environments being a multi-year process.

## SIEM Correlation Rule Example for Healthcare Ransomware Detection

To operationalise the detection framework described in Section 4, the following pseudo-code illustrates a healthcare-specific SIEM correlation rule targeting the pre-encryption kill chain activity characteristic of human-operated ransomware campaigns:

```
RULE: Healthcare_Ransomware_PreEncryption_KillChain
CONDITION: WITHIN 30_MINUTES:
[Event A] auth_failures >= 5 FROM single_source_ip TARGETING
healthcare_domain_controllers
AND [Event B] successful_auth FROM same_source_ip WITHIN 5_
MINUTES OF Event_A
AND [Event C] new_scheduled_task OR new_service_created ON
authenticated_host
AND [Event D] smb_lateral_scan FROM authenticated_host TO
>10 internal_hosts
AND [Event E] vssadmin_delete OR wmic_shadowcopy_delete DE-
TECTED ON any_host
ALERT: CRITICAL – Ransomware Kill Chain Indicator
RESPONSE: isolate_host(Event_B.host), notify_soc_oncall,
open_incident_ticket
```

Tuning guidance: In healthcare environments, Event D thresholds must be calibrated to exclude legitimate scheduled EHR database export processes, which generate high-volume internal file access. Baseline profiling of clinical application service accounts should be completed before deploying this rule to minimize false positive volume during business hours.

## Zero Trust Implementation Guidance for Small Rural Hospitals

Small rural hospitals that have lower IT staff resources are especially challenged with implementing Zero Trust architecture. Prioritized guidance for implementation is provided below, starting with the highest priority guidance for reduced risks per unit of implementation effort, and continuing with lower priority guidance for reduced risks. Priority 1 — Multi-Factor Authentication (Immediate, Low Cost): Implement MFA on all remote access portals, VPN concentrators, and cloud-based EHR access. Implementing free-tier MFA (Microsoft Authenticator, Google Authenticator) solutions is relatively inexpensive and can be integrated with most existing remote access infrastructure. This one control alone would have stopped the Change Healthcare breach and is the most effective control that resource-constrained organizations can implement. Priority 2 — Privileged Access Segmentation (Short Term): Implementing a separate administrative user account for members of the IT staff from their normal clinical user accounts. The authentication level of administrative functions should be elevated and require a different logon. This reduces the scope of credential spoofing. Priority 3: Immutable Cloud Backup (Short Term, Subscription Cost): Store critical EHR data in an immutable cloud backup system (short term, subscription cost). Ransomware-resistant backup is available at subscription tier costs for small organizations with AWS S3 Object Lock, Azure Immutable Blob Storage, and similar. Priority 4 — Basic Network Segmentation (Medium Term): VLAN Segmentation of IoMT devices from clinical workstations and administrative systems. The vast majority of managed switches, which are used in most rural hospitals, will allow VLAN configuration at no extra expense. This helps to stop IoMT devices from acting as lateral movement routes to the EHR infrastructure. Priority 5 — Endpoint Detection and Response (Medium Term, Subscription Cost): Implement a cloud-based EDR solution in clinical workstations. There are a number of EDR vendors that provide pricing and managed detection solution options suitable for organizations that have no dedicated security operations personnel.

## Pure Exfiltration Ransomware: Detection and Defence Implications

An emerging variant of the ransomware threat model involves groups that exfiltrate sensitive data without deploying encryption payloads, relying exclusively on the threat of data publication to coerce payment. This pure extortion model, observed in operations by groups including Clop and certain RansomHub affiliates, eliminates the operational disruption that traditionally triggers rapid incident detection, allowing attackers extended dwell time and avoiding the triggering of backup-monitoring and file-encryption detection controls.

The detection and defense implications differ significantly from encryption-based ransomware. File entropy analysis (Section 4.1) and volume shadow copy deletion monitoring are ineffective, as no encryption occurs. Detection must shift to data exfiltration indicators: anomalous outbound data volumes, connections to cloud storage services not in the approved baseline (Mega.nz, Dropbox, OneDrive from non-standard applications), large-scale staging of data in temporary directories, and compression of clinical data volumes in unusual locations. DLP (Data Loss Prevention) controls monitoring outbound data flows from EHR export directories and PACS archives, which become primary detection mechanisms. HIPAA breach notification obligations are triggered at the moment of confirmed exfiltration, regardless of whether encryption or ransom demand follows. Healthcare organizations should extend their incident response procedures and tabletop exercise scenarios to explicitly include the pure exfiltration threat model, ensuring that detection playbooks and communication protocols address incidents in which no encryption occurs.

## 7. CONCLUSION

In withering operational disruption attacks (availability attacks) with regulatory and reputational impact of data breach, ransomware has become the hallmark cybersecurity threat to the healthcare system in the present decade, which exploits the potential of the legacy of malicious actors to infiltrate IT systems and the associated financial and reputational impacts of uncoordinated IT operations (extortion and extortion). The threat will not stand still: ransomware actors are constantly upgrading their tooling, approaches to targets, and the mechanisms of extortion, responding to the defensive strengthening, regulative actions, and the activity of law enforcement. Healthcare organizations that consider solving the ransomware defense to be a matter of the past may be easily surpassed by a threat that has already shown its ability to constantly evolve. The chapter has presented a clear analysis of the ransomware menace in terms of its cryptographic basis up to its clinical implications and has devised a holistic defensive infrastructure that deals with the technical and legislative aspects of successful defense. The insight that is chief to the defensive approach is that the ransomware is not a one-time event that needs a one-time control, but a multi-phase initiative that needs associative defenses taking place throughout the kill chain: Prevention: controls that eradicate initial access vectors Pre-encryption: Observation capabilities that identify the kill chain activity before it implements encryption Containment: Lateral movement controls and backup destruction is needed Multi-stage destruction Recovery. The GRC framework, created in Section 5 ransomware defense mapping between HIPAA, NIST CSF 2.0, and ISO 27001:2022, offers healthcare organizations a compliance architecture that both meets the requirements of the regulations and is operationally effective in security controls. This framework is transformed into verifiable and evidence-based evaluations that can be used both in internal governance and in external certification needs, as guided by the audit planning guidance. The healthcare organizations, which have the controls that were presented in this chapter, performing their implementation by regular exercises and audits, and continuously updating their posture according to the changes in the threat landscape, will be much better prepared to defend their patients, their data, and their clinical operations against the ransomware threat. Future research and practice directions involve applying artificial intelligence to real-time ransomware watchful measures in medical settings, building healthcare-specific threat intelligence disseminations to allow attack indicators to spread swiftly across the industry, the security implications of cloud-based EHR platforms to ransomware risks and recovery, and the future post-quantum cryptographic evolution of ransomware weaponry and its impact on existing encryption-based defenses. The long-term viability of the digital conversion of healthcare systems will be anchored on the long-term implementation of the defensive principles, governance structures, and working disciplines outlined in this chapter with respect to security, resilience, and patient safety.

## CONFLICTS OF INTEREST

The author(s) declare no conflicts of interest with respect to the research, authorship, or publication of this chapter.

## ACKNOWLEDGMENTS

The author(s) wish to acknowledge the support of the School of Computer Science, UPES Dehradun, in facilitating this research. No external funding was received for this work.

## REFERENCES

Alraizza, A., & Algarni, A. (2023). Ransomware Detection Using Machine Learning: A Survey. *Big Data and Cognitive Computing*, *7*(3), 143. DOI: 10.3390/bdcc7030143

Cresswell, K., & Sheikh, A. (2017). Organizational issues in the implementation and adoption of health information technology innovations: An interpretative review. *International Journal of Medical Informatics*, *86*, 1–14. DOI: 10.1016/j.ijmedinf.2015.09.012 PMID: 23146626

CTIIC / Office of the Director of National Intelligence. (2024). Ransomware attacks surge in 2023; attacks on the healthcare sector nearly double. https://www.dni.gov/files/CTIIC/documents/products/Ransomware_Attacks_Surge_in_2023.pdf

Department of Health and Human Services, Office for Civil Rights. (2024). Cybersecurity resources for HIPAA-regulated entities. https://csrc.nist.gov/files/pubs/sp/800/66/r2/final/docs/sp800-66r2-cybersecurity-resources.pdf

Dupont, B., Côté, A.-M., Savine, C., & Décary-Hétu, D. (2019). The ecology of trust among hackers. *Global Crime*, *17*(2), 129–151. DOI: 10.1080/17440572.2016.1157480

European Parliament and Council. (2016). *Regulation (EU) 2016/679 (General Data Protection Regulation)*. Official Journal of the European Union.

European Parliament and Council. (2022). *Directive (EU) 2022/2555 on measures for a high common level of cybersecurity across the Union (NIS2 Directive)*. Official Journal of the European Union.

Ferdous, J., Islam, R., Mahboubi, A., & Islam, M. Z. (2025). A novel technique for ransomware detection using image based dynamic features and transfer learning to address dataset limitations. *Scientific Reports*, *15*(1), 32342. Advance online publication. DOI: 10.1038/s41598-025-17647-1 PMID: 40897752

Forescout Technologies. (2024). Ransomware in healthcare: The NHS example and what the future holds. https://www.forescout.com/blog/ransomware-in-healthcare-the-nhs-example-and-what-the-future-holds/

Health Service Executive (2021). Conti cyber attack on the HSE: A report by PricewaterhouseCoopers. Published December 2021.

Ispahany, J., Islam, M., Islam, M. Z., & Khan, M. A. (2024). Ransomware Detection Using Machine Learning: A Review, Research Limitations and Future Directions. *IEEE Access : Practical Innovations, Open Solutions*, *12*, 68785–68813. DOI: 10.1109/ACCESS.2024.3397921

Jiang, J. X., Ross, J. S., & Bai, G. (2025). Ransomware Attacks and Data Breaches in U.S. Health Care Systems. *JAMA Network Open*, *8*(5), e2510180. DOI: 10.1001/jamanetworkopen.2025.10180 PMID: 40366661

KnowBe4 (2023). Hacked healthcare: A global crisis in cybersecurity. https://www.knowbe4.com/hubfs/Global-Healthcare-Report-and-Timeline-EN_US.pdf

Koppel, R., Smith, S., Blythe, J., & Kothari, V. (2015). Workarounds to computer access in healthcare settings. *Studies in Health Technology and Informatics*, *208*, 287–291.

Lee, J., Kim, J., Jeong, H., & Lee, K. (2025). A Machine Learning-Based Ransomware Detection Method for Attackers' Neutralization Techniques Using Format-Preserving Encryption. *Sensors (Basel)*, *25*(8), 2406. DOI: 10.3390/s25082406 PMID: 40285096

Li, J.. (2025). Analysis of LockBit 3.0 and its infiltration into Advanced's infrastructure crippling NHS services. arXiv:2308.05565.

Marron, J. A. (2024). *Implementing the health insurance portability and accountability act (HIPAA) security rule*. National Institute of Standards and Technology., DOI: 10.6028/NIST.SP.800-66r2

MITRE Corporation. (2024). MITRE ATT&CK framework v14: Enterprise matrix ransomware techniques. https://attack.mitre.org/

National Institute of Standards and Technology. (2024). Cybersecurity Framework 2.0. *NIST CSWP*, *29*. Advance online publication. DOI: 10.6028/NIST.CSWP.29

National Institute of Standards and Technology. (2024). Post-quantum cryptography standards: FIPS 203, FIPS 204, FIPS 205. https://csrc.nist.gov/projects/post-quantum-cryptography

Ransomware Task Force. (2021). Combating ransomware: A comprehensive framework for action. Institute for Security and Technology. https://securityandtechnology.org/ransomwaretaskforce/

Razavi, H., . . .. (2023). Entropy sharing in ransomware: bypassing entropy-based detection of cryptographic operations. Sensors. https://pmc.ncbi.nlm.nih.gov/articles/PMC10934942/

Schmidt, A.. (2023). Effective ransomware detection using entropy estimation of files for cloud services. *Sensors (Basel)*, *23*(6), 3023. DOI: 10.3390/s23063023 PMID: 36991730

Sheikh, A., & Cresswell, K. (2018). Addressing the human aspects of EHR-enabled health system change. *Journal of the American Medical Informatics Association : JAMIA*, *25*(3), 225–226. DOI: 10.1093/jamia/ocx152

Sophos. (2024). The state of ransomware in healthcare 2024. Sophos Research Report.

Sophos. (2025). The state of ransomware in healthcare 2025. Sophos Research Report.

Sudheer, S. (2024). Ransomware Attacks and Their Evolving Strategies: A Systematic Review of Recent Incidents. *Journal of Technology and Systems*, *6*(7), 32–59. DOI: 10.47941/jts.2399

UcedaVelez. T., & Morana, M. M. (2015). Risk centric threat modeling: Process for attack simulation and threat analysis. Wiley.

United Kingdom NHS. (2017). WannaCry ransomware attack spreads worldwide. BMJ / PMC. https://pmc.ncbi.nlm.nih.gov/articles/PMC5461132/

Veriti Research. (2025). Healthcare ransomware statistics 2025. Cobalt / Veriti Analysis. https://www.cobalt.io/blog/healthcare-data-breach-statistics

## KEY TERMS AND DEFINITIONS

**Double Extortion:** Ransomware attack variant where the attacker steals sensitive data without making a noise and drops the encryption payload before threatening to leak or sell the stolen information or data unless a ransom is exchanged.

**Electronic Health Record (EHR):** An electronic system that stores all health records of patients, including diagnoses, medications, treatment history, lab results, and clinical notes.

**Governance, Risk, and Compliance (GRC):** A united mode of governance within an organization that orchestrates information security controls with regulatory, risk management, and business operational goals.

**Hybrid Encryption:** This type of cryptography is a ransomware attack that is implemented using a cryptographic design in which the bulk data is encrypted by symmetric encryption, typically AES-256 in CBC or GCM mode.

**Immutable Backup:** A backup storage setup where once written data cannot be encrypted, modified, or deleted by any account, not even accounts of domain administrators that have been compromised by ransomware.

**Indicators of Compromise (IOCs):** The visible traces or patterns of actions that will provide great certainty that a system has been or is being affected by ransomware.

**Internet of Medical Things (IoMT):** The system of interconnected medical equipment, clinical monitoring devices, and healthcare information systems communicating through the IP networks in a clinical setting.

**NIST Cybersecurity Framework (CSF 2.0):** A voluntary framework released by the National Institute of Standards and Technology that assists organizations in controlling and mitigating the risk of cybersecurity.

**Ransomware:** This is a type of malicious software that blocks legitimate users from accessing their data or computer system, usually with powerful encryption, and requires a ransom to be paid to repair it.

**Shannon Entropy:** A measure of the information density or randomness of data, in bits per byte. With an encrypted file, the theoretical maximum entropy is 8.0 bits per byte, and detection systems based on entropy can identify files that have been encrypted by ransomware by detecting an increase in entropy beyond a fixed limit when interacting with the file system.

**Zero Trust Architecture:** It is a security architecture model that is founded upon the idea of consulting no users, devices, or network segments at all, irrespective of where they are located in the network.

Chapter 7

# Benefits, Difficulties, and Healthcare 4.0:
## Effects of Blockchain Technology in Medicine

**Togonova Shoxida**
*Urgench State Pedagogical Institute, Uzbekistan*

**Zarifa Mamadieva**
*Termez University of Economics and Service, Uzbekistan*

**Seitnazarov Kuanishbay Kenesbaevich**
*Nukus State Pedagogical Institute, Uzbekistan*

**Anorgul Ashirova**
http://orcid.org/0009-0006-7271-3634
*Mamun University, Uzbekistan*

**Sabyasachi Pramanik**
http://orcid.org/0000-0002-9431-8751
*Haldia Institute of Technology, India*

**Valisher Sapayev**
http://orcid.org/0000-0002-6751-5864
*Mamun University, Uzbekistan*

**Abdullayev Abdulla Fayzulla Ugli**
*Tashkent State University of Economy, Uzbekistan*

## ABSTRACT

*Machine optimization for a variety of industrial applications is now possible because to the development of AI methods and their translation into intelligent automated processes using the Internet of Things (IoT). One noteworthy development that occurred was the healthcare industry's tremendous advancement, which paved the way for the development of Health 4.0. The IoT, Internet of Services (IoS), Medical Cyber-Physical Systems (CPS), Health Cloud, Health Fog, and other cutting-edge technologies are all part of this new age. Securing all medical devices with internet connections is the biggest obstacle to electronic healthcare. Due to its efficiency*

DOI: 10.4018/979-8-3373-9119-9.ch007

*and dependability, blockchain—a distributed, immutable ledger or database—is having more popularity in a number of industries, like medical applications. Its benefits include immutability, better security, and decentralization. This chapter provides a realistic assessment of blockchain's advancement in healthcare with the goal of examining the advantages and difficulties of adopting blockchain technology in medicine 4.0.*

## 1. INTRODUCTION

Technology has made it easier for entities in the actual world to communicate with one another. To develop safe transactions, however, the data that is transmitted between two organizations must be kept private. Tokenization, robust authentication and authorization procedures, fraud monitoring, encryption methods, and the use of cyber security techniques may all be used to safeguard transactions. As per the discussion of (Mukherjee, P., et al. 2020), it is needed to include physical security, encryption security, emission security, and transaction security factors in order to build a secure communication and transactions. Protecting the authorization and authentication procedures used by different organizations to access data is part of encryption security. Emission security talks about the steps that need to be performed to convince an organization to grant or refuse permission in order to stop assaults. The purpose of transaction security is to ensure the security of sensitive data when going for business across a network that includes many parties. The transaction security is the most important of all these security measures as it might result in significant losses in digital transactions. Transparency preservation is the superior strategy for preserving transaction security. Traditional centralized networks are opaque when it comes to exchanging data with other parties, have immutable data, struggle with network latency, have less redundant data, and are more open to attack. A primary disadvantage of a consolidated framework is the possibility of a lone point of failure, which may result in data loss. Its narrow data transfer scope is accompanied by concerns related to scalability and security. By using a decentralized approach, the centralized system's shortcomings were addressed. Every node in a decentralized system has the ability to make decisions; the aggregate of all the nodes determines which node gets the request and answer first. Bitcoin is among the greatest examples. The benefits of a decentralized system include the capacity to scale vertically, which improves the scalability structure described by (Mahajan, H.B. et al. 2022). Decentralized framework also discards the prospect of a lone point failure. Even yet, there may still be decentralization constraints, such as which nodes succeeded or failed. Blockchain technology (BCT) is among the greatest examples of a decentralized system. Implementations for BCT are established in the areas of cryptocurrency, medicine, multimedia, banking, insurance, energy, and society. BCT has applications in healthcare that include patient monitoring, record-keeping, enhanced transparency, and privacy protection. BC uses the hashing algorithm on many nodes in a network to store digital data in a secure manner. One BC protocol example that confirms the legality of drugs and medications via the pharma supply chain management system is MediLedger. By offering immutable records and data management with tampering, the BC also contributes to a decrease in mistakes and frauds in clinical trials. This is achieved by hashing a new block and adding a time stamp. By capturing data via sensors built in wearable devices, BC extends its reach into the IoMTs. Depending on the authentication from the stack holders, the IoMT devices carefully monitor the victim's body, and the produced data will be safely saved as blocks in cloud storage utilizing the BC method. Therefore, BC has a good effect on how the medical sector is managed, facilitating enhanced security, transparency, and patient information privacy protection. The chapter's remaining parts are arranged as shown here: Section 2 covers the overview on BC technology, and Section 3 covers the review process methodology, while Sections 5 and 6 discussed the implications and implementations of BCT in the medicine. Section 4 offered an examination of the current condition of the industry. Real-time solutions and their implications are covered in Sections 7 and 8, and the performance and loopholes of utilizing BCT in the medical arena are covered in Section 9. In Section 10, we looked at commercial strategies to advance BCT in healthcare 4.0. Recommendations for further development were provided at the conclusion of Section 11.

## Literature Review

Numerous studies have already shown BC's potential to facilitate medical data interchange and assist a range of additional diagnostic applications. For example, tracking and storing confidential healthcare data on a private BC is one of possible illustrations of the Healthcare Data Gateway technique, which was first presented by (Orabi, M.M., et. al. 2025). Patients using this personalized healthcare approach are free to see, track, and control their own medical data and clinical records that are kept on a privatized BC (a centralized database framework having restricted access control granted to authorized or particular users). In a different research, utilized a private BC constructed on the Ethereum protocol to remove the security matters connected to a distant patient tracking framework and enable the secured usage of healthcare sensors. In addition to keeping a safe, secure, and current patient history, their BC-based approach may enable secured real-time distant tracking, enabling doctors to follow the medical condition of their victims from remote places. By using a public BC—a decentralized database framework with open access command to everybody linked to the network—in encrypted data, (Raj, A., et al. 2024) also illustrated a technique in storing healthcare data securely. Using this technique, a BC-based personal health record is created by publicly depositing the encrypted medical data. Patients now have enhanced control to their clinical data according to their proposed method that permits them to smoothly monitor and access their data and append to it and connect it with any allied care giving organization. According to a different survey (Cihan, S., et al. 2025) proposed a system for controlling and sharing victim's private healthcare data that combined BCT with cloud storage. The suggested plan may be used to accomplish the secured sharing and repository of private victim's health information. The proposed method is distinct in that it eliminates the need for outside parties by providing victims having total control over their private healthcare information.

For assessing the healthcare condition of victim diseases, (Ibrahim, A.M., et al. 2025) has suggested BC architecture depending on simultaneous execution and artificial medical technologies. In order to make clinical decisions, the suggested approach finds the victim's general health, disease detection, and course of healing. It also analyses the related therapeutic processes using computer trials and parallel executions. To find the capability of disease detection and benefit of therapy, the suggested technique has been tested on both fake and actual healthcare frameworks.

BloCHIE is a novel BC-dependent platform for exchanging healthcare data which was constructed by (Akhai, S., et al. 2025). The proposed system evaluates the requirements for medical data exchange, mainly for electronic health records. It also handles various categories of data by combining blockhains across several origins. They paired the platform having on-chain and off-chain verification procedures to confirm the satisfied needs of both authenticity and security.

Doctors and hospitals can significantly intensify healthcare data interchange, and security by using BC technology. Utilizing a related technique (Hammad, M., et al. 2026) put forward a methodical and creative BC-based architecture that can safeguard private patient information, handle important data privacy concerns, and integrate a BC framework across a healthcare framework.

Additionally, BCT has displayed plenty of courage in the healthcare and biological study fields. Prior to initiating a healthcare trial or scrutiny, various healthcare agreements, schemes, and methods may be stored on a BC and credit to the feasible usage of BC technology. This would make the private information pertaining to clinical studies more contemporary, safer and open to the public. Alternately, if correctly executed and verified, smart contracts may also be utilized to assure clarity at various steps of a healthcare research. Researchers introduced a BC-dependent tele-monitoring clinical platform in (Khan, A.A., et al. 2025) in finding and treating harmful tumors in distant patients.

In order to guarantee the accuracy and privacy of patient data in specific medical facilities and in patient residence, the suggested approach creates usage of smart contracts and BCs. DermoNet, a BC-dependent approach in helping dermatology patients through an online skin-related meeting using a tele-skin-related tracking framework, was proposed by (Kumari, M., et al. 2021) in another research. On the contrary, ProActive Ageing is a BC-dependent system which assists aged persons' energetic habits. It must be noted that BCT may be an excellent match for prolonged healthcare remedy procedures including ageing, surgical procedure, and persistent sicknesses like cancer. Additionally, using DNA data saved on BCs, pharmaceutical companies, medication makers, and biomedical researchers may be able to carry out sophisticated international genomic research.

BC has triggered a worldwide analysis expansion due to the prevalent usage of bitcoin and the rapid growth of decentralized stages in both financial and non-fiscal implementations. BC puts it simpler for end users and medical architectures to allot EHRs without interfering with communication. These services are offered via distributed ledger technology interoperability certification and trust lines. With the aim of avoiding unidentified and unapproved access by unlicensed users, present-day medical applications prioritize the security of combined data. Therefore, the primary prerequisites for exchanging EHRs across many users are trust, authentication, and privacy (Kashyap et. al., 2025).

At every level of the BC, security threats are mostly caused by flaws in mechanisms, attack strategies, and security solutions. Although it offers security assurances for a trustless environment, it also encounters a number of privacy and security issues. Numerous governments and organizations have shifted their research attention to BC security (Ben Fekih, R., et al. 2020). In order to contrast and evaluate the current privacy procedures and create a more robust secured protocol in the BC settings, this chapter concentrates on the privacy concerns with BCT and its implementations in the medicine industry. It does this by classifying the privacy threats at the technical level using 6-layer designs. For BC security research, the theoretical architecture of parallel privacy offers helpful theoretical and technological security assistance. In order to provide correct forecast and supervision of illness identification and remedy via parallel implementation, a system dependent on a parallel medical framework is developed to design and depict the victim's state, identification, and therapy technique. The fundamental security objective of BC framework building is to utilize encryption, computer security and various technological methods for safeguarding every tier of BC security systems in accordance with the network system's privacy needs. Data privacy is intimately tied to security goals including content security and privacy.

Speedier and more sophisticated BC remedies and opportunities in improving BC security and achievement will be made possible by quantum technology developed from digital and networked resources. In a quantum cryptosystem, Kashyap talks about how to combine BCT with quantum cryptography. Network technology development and security are closely related, and BCT may effectively mitigate the privacy concerns and security flaws in IoT systems. IoT implementations in hospitals reduce the barriers to communicate between physicians and victims by enabling remote diagnosis in emergency situations via smart devices and sensors. Because BCT decentralizes immutability, security, privacy, and transparency, it is mostly used in the healthcare industry. BC, IoT, and healthcare systems share dependable resources and are interconnected. (Amin, M.S., et al. 2025) carried out a new paradigm research on the security threats and difficulties throughout the technological integration procedure. Monrat examined the difficulties and offered a comparative analysis of the various consensus methods in his work.

### Research Objective

The advantages and risks of BCT in the medical field are not well understood. Therefore, this scoping review's goal is to examine and compile the primary advantages and risks of BCT in the healthcare industry as documented in the literature.

## 2. AN OVERVIEW OF BLOCKCHAIN

This unit covers the foundations of BC technology, including its kinds, salient characteristics, and use in the medical industry.

### 2.1 BC

BC is a separated, immutable database which uses encryption and hashing algorithms to securely record transactions. A hash key from the previous block, a timestamp, a Merkle tree, gas use, and encrypted sender and recipient identities are all included in each block. To make sure that immutable blocks are connected in a chain, the timestamp keeps track of changes made to the data. Every transaction on the BC is protected because it is irreversible.

### 2.2 BC Categories

The 4 categories of BC are public, private, hybrid & consortium, depending on the different use cases (Mackey, T.K., et al. 2019). (i) Anyone with the necessary credentials may view the public BC and its contents. The user will be validated before being added to the ledger and has the ability to see records and perform transactions. As a result, it makes it possible for everyone to check transactions and address flaws since it is open source.

Benefits of open BC: Since public BCs are independent of organizations and operate without authorization, network transparency is preserved. However, users' adherence to security guidelines and standards is ultimately what keeps the BC secure. Drawbacks of a public BC and its scaling problems, network latency, and unfettered access lead to public data heft. As a result, certain non-governmental organizations and social assistance groups may make use of the public BC. (ii) Private BC operates inside a certain organization's restricted environment. A BC of this kind that has appropriate access controls guaranteeing security, authorization, and accessibility will function on a smaller scale. Depending on the dependencies, the organization is free to change the rules and access control over the resources over time. A few private businesses use BC technology, including SCM and voting frameworks. The ideal speed of network transactions is ensured with more control thanks to proper access control and size limitations. The consensus process and transaction validation should only be anticipated in by authorized parties. Drawbacks to private BC Security problems may arise from a lack of openness and the inability for the user to verify the data. (iii) Hybrid BC: This setup combines public and private BCs, allowing the public BC to gather data while the organization maintains access to its features. This is made feasible by the smart contract mechanism, which verifies private entity-verified sensitive information before placing it in blocks with unaltered transactions. The finest example of a hybrid BC is a medical ledger. Advantages of BC hybrids are: There might be limits on the quantity of data hacked because of the closed system permits contact with other parties improving scalability and speeding up transactions. Cons of BC hybrids: This variant of BC is not entirely transparent as the data is shielded from organizational rules. There are fewer incentives to engage in and contribute to the network when the smart contract technique is used with fewer partners. (iv) BC consortium: With restricted access to a certain group, it is referred to as a federated BC. The reconfigured nodes fail to evade the validation process and preserve the consensus processes. This includes a hierarchy of functionality to a single data, such consensus, cooperation, and teamwork. The Proof of Authority, Proof of Significance, Proof of Work, Proof of Stake, Proof of Weight, and Proof of Capacity are all included in this. This BC is used for tracking systems and banking transactions.

**Benefits of BC consortium:** It provides access restrictions in addition to being more scalable and secure.

**Cons of BC consortiums:** more intricately configured than other BCs with several organizations.

## 2.3 Important BC characteristics for the healthcare industry as opposed to other industries

When the health sector employs a standard data management system, patient medical data is integrated, analyzed, and insights are extracted to improve patient outcomes while protecting patient privacy. However, since it is centralized and has a lone point of failure, the data might be compromised. Compared to conventional data administration in the medical sector, BCT provides a quantity of advantages, like secure transactions for medical information and traceability in managing the medicine supply chain. The salient characteristics of BC in the medical sector are shown.

- Safety: Because the BC discards lone points of failure, its decentralized structure significantly lowers the risk of patient record data loss.
- Transparency: By using encryption methods, patients may read and access their e-health data in a transparent manner, which enhances privacy preservation.
- Smart contracts: Smart contracts (Kamel Boulos, M.N., et al. 2018) automatic tasks like insurance claims and patient treatment analysis by enabling safe data exchange among third parties globally and guaranteeing the fulfillment of predetermined agreements.
- Distributed Ledger: a more reliable and transparent solution is offered by enhanced interoperability and data encryption to protect privacy.

## 2.4 Current BC applications in the medical field

This section covers the open-source BC systems now in use in the healthcare industry. These systems serve as a useful tool for efficient on-chain data management, offering improved storage options and enhancing interoperability across medical information. A few of the platforms are mentioned as follows:

- Ethereum: Ethereum (Dhingra, S., et al. 2025) provides interoperability and smart contract applications which have the possibility to fundamentally alter the medical industry. It facilitates data privacy, approval control, and the monitoring of medical devices and products, among other BC use cases. It codes the transactions using Solidity Language.
- IBM BC: This monitors a plethora of aspects of the healthcare sector, including orders, payments, manufacturing, financing, and more. Hyperledger Fabric provides a distributed, secure environment for healthcare systems, which satisfies all of these requirements. While there are several healthcare

applications for Hyperledger Fabric, this presentation will focus on patient medical record management.

- R3 Corda: Pluggable consensus, a consensus method used by Corda, gives users the option to choose the consensus algorithm that best fits their organization.
- Tezos: Tezos is an open-source BCT which may be used to execute smart contracts and conduct peer-to-peer exchanges. XTZ (ISO 4217) is the native currency of the Tezos network. Proof-of-stake is used in the Tezos network to achieve agreement in the medical field.
- EOSIO: The recommended bridge health monitoring technique uses the EOSIO BC (Onur, D., et al. 2025) integration to control the secured repository of real-time IoT data and accomplish pre-programmed logic for data analysis via smart contracts.
- Stellar: Stellar BCT will be used to create an innovative medical platform. Scalability and fast implementation are two of its advantages. BC-dependent health remedies facilitate patient data handling and supply chain administration. The following highlights the chapter's primary contribution:
- A detailed survey of the developments of BCT in the medical sector was conducted.
- There was discussion of the implications and implementations of BC for data security, data monitoring, and privacy protection, data protection from assaults, consensus, and trustworthiness.
- Emphasis is placed on potential solutions and their consequences in the current form.
- The shortcomings and effectiveness of using BCT to the healthcare sector were emphasized.
- Emphasis was placed on business plans to further BC technology's use in healthcare 4.0.

## 3. REVIEW METHODOLOGY

A PRISM technique was used to the review process. To find the study avenues made possible by the BC in the medical industry, the research questions were formulated and a search was conducted in journal databases.

### *3.1 Formulating Research Issues*

Two study questions have been developed to find the importance of BC in the hospitals:

**Q1:** What BC-based remedies may be used in the current medical system?
**Q2:** What Business plans to advance BC use in healthcare 4.0?

## 3.2 The process of searching for documents

The survey focuses on BCT in the medicine domain. The search phrase is utilized to do a global search on the three most popular search engines, like WoS, IEEE Explorer & Scopus. The buzzwords include "smart contracts" (Esmaeilzadeh, P. et al. 2022), "blockchain technology, "healthcare" or "security issues in healthcare", as well as "solutions of BC in healthcare". Figs. 2 and 3 provide the biblometric (Yuman, Y., et al. 2025) analysis of the search technique. The advancements in BCT have resulted in restricted or filtered search results in recent years on 3682 publications were submitted to us on this subject. In order to determine if each work was crucial, we carefully considered its originality, significance, and relevance, paying particular weight to the first research on the BC mechanism. Books, book chapters, conference proceedings, conference reviews, editorials, and survey articles are among the publications. The flow chart for the search procedure is depicted in Fig. 1. The selection criteria for the publications that received the highest ratings for more research are shown in Table 1. The PRISM review process for the BC in the medical industry is described in Figure 1.

*Table 1. The Database Search Process*

| *Publications* | *Count* |
|---|---|
| Articles | 1518 |
| Books | 10 |
| Book chapter | 337 |
| Conference Paper | 1551 |
| Conference review | 2 |
| Editorial | 8 |
| Review | 256 |
| **Total** | **3682** |

## 3.3 Bibliometric analysis

This analysis was carried out to track the author research output for a period using the visualization network. The following viewpoints were examined and the directions of BCT in healthcare were identified using bibliometric analysis: the most significant publications and highly cited authors were found by citation and co-citation analyses, content analysis of the papers, authors, and paper sources. Bibliometric networks were analyzed, visualized, and publications were grouped into several time periods using VoSViewer (Dlamini, Z., et al. 2023). VoS viewer tools are useful for information visualization and may be accessed for free online. They were employed for general visualization as well as the creation of co-authorship and co-citation networks (Khan, A.A., et al. 2025). The year wise publication list was given in Figure 2. Figure 3 gives the bibliometric analysis of the keywords involved.

To increase the announcement of structured evaluation, the PRISMA (Preferred Reporting Items for Systematic reviews and Meta-Analyses) standard was formed. PRISMA gives writers instructions and instances to operate to fully reveal the reasons for a systematic review, the techniques utilized, and the findings. PRISMA 2020, the major PRISMA describing hints, mostly provides orders for publishing methodical evaluation that assess the result of treatments. A quantity of PRISMA extensions help PRISMA 2020, including instructions for announcing particular features or types of organized analysis and other types of proof combinations (like Scoping evaluation).

*Figure 1. PRISMA Methodology review process*

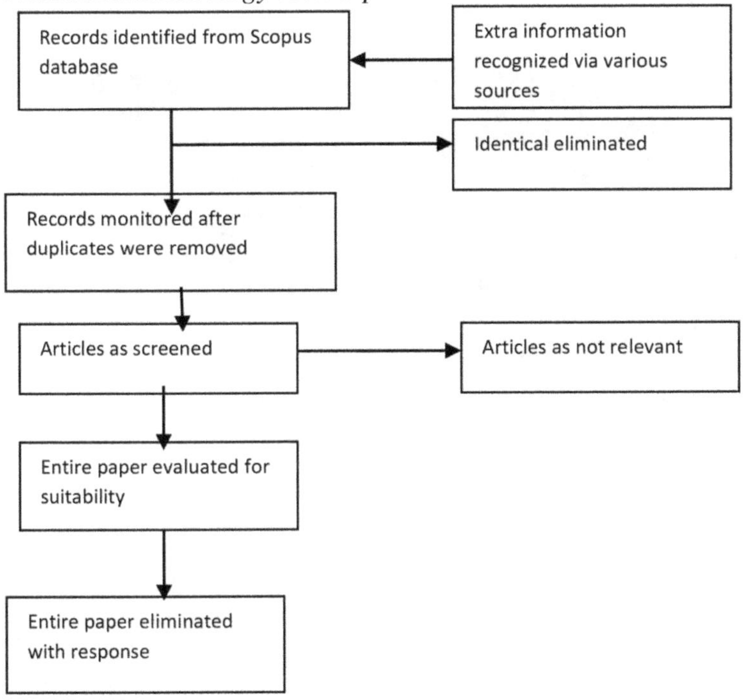

Figure 2. Year Wise Publication list for blockchain in Healthcare sector

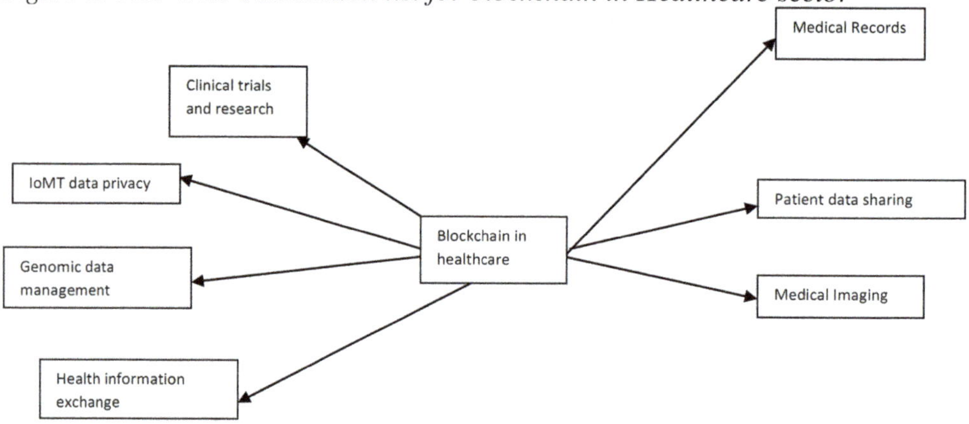


Figure 3. Bibliometric analysis using VoS viewer

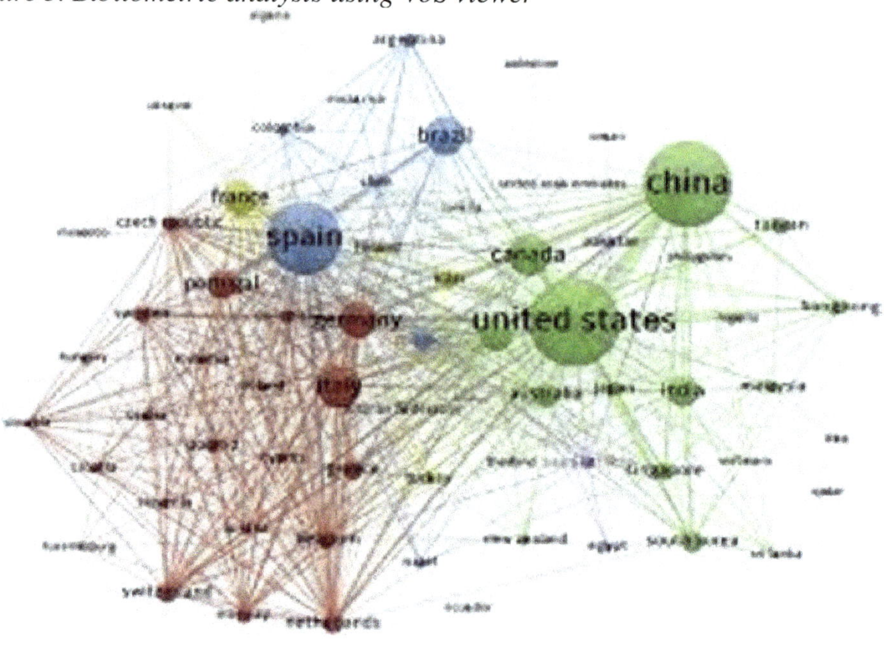

## Framework for IoMT Based on Fog and Blockchain

Figure 4 depicts the framework for fog and blockchain-dependent IoMT systems. Utilizing a fog node between the cloud and Internet of Medical Things device layer seems to have benefits such as support for heterogeneity and interoperability, low latency, and low energy usage. Additionally, this structure promotes flexibility and scalability, allowing for the integration of new applications without interfering with the whole medical framework. The victim's movement is moreover intensified by this kind of setup. For medical records and communications, the Blockchain (BC) layer offers a distributed, private, and secure architecture. Beneath is an clarification of the tiered framework and the roles implemented at every layer. The perception or sensor layer is made up of all the hardware, sensors, and various tracking tools which collect data from victims and, sometimes, the outside world before sending it to the fog layer for future communication.

Fog layer: The communication delay may often be fatal and lead to subpar medical treatment and assistance, which is typically achievable in a cloud-based or centralized design. Additionally facilitating fast answers, the fog layer attempts to reduce the encryption load on IoMT sensors that have restricted processing capability. Information collected through the fog layer is aggregated and sent to the cloud repository layer via the data communication layer, which behaves as a network layer. Since it manages every data flow from the fog layer to the repository layer, this layer is ultimately susceptible.

BC layer: With the aid of the fog layer, the BC layer is in charge of confirming the IoMT gadgets and supporting the end users prior to granting access to the repository layer. This ensures a higher level of data security with lesser delay and lesser load on physically limited devices. By preventing any document alteration without the required consent and verification, it moreover upholds the immutability of information. Interoperability and HIPAA compliance will be further supported by the addition of a BC.

Cloud layer or data repository: This layer houses every record and is in charge of offering facilities and data analytics to assist medical potentials for users of the framework. People see the repository as a lone entity. Nevertheless, it is often a decentralized structure of many repository gadgets that are managed by the BC layer that comes prior to it and thereby preserving security and anonymity.

Utilizing bio-sensors like blood sugar monitors, ECG signals, and blood pressure monitors, the proposed system can detect the victim's details and send the data to the fog node that can be a mobile phone or any nearby device. The data transit layer operates and sends the information after acquiring them from the fog node. The information are ultimately operated and deposited irrevocably with BC combination in the cloud computing layer, addressing the trust concerns associated with IoMT devices and thwarting eavesdropping and unauthorized change. This suggested structure would eliminate latency and time delays, and the BC layer can convey any possible privacy threats.

*Figure 4. IoMT fog platform in medicine*

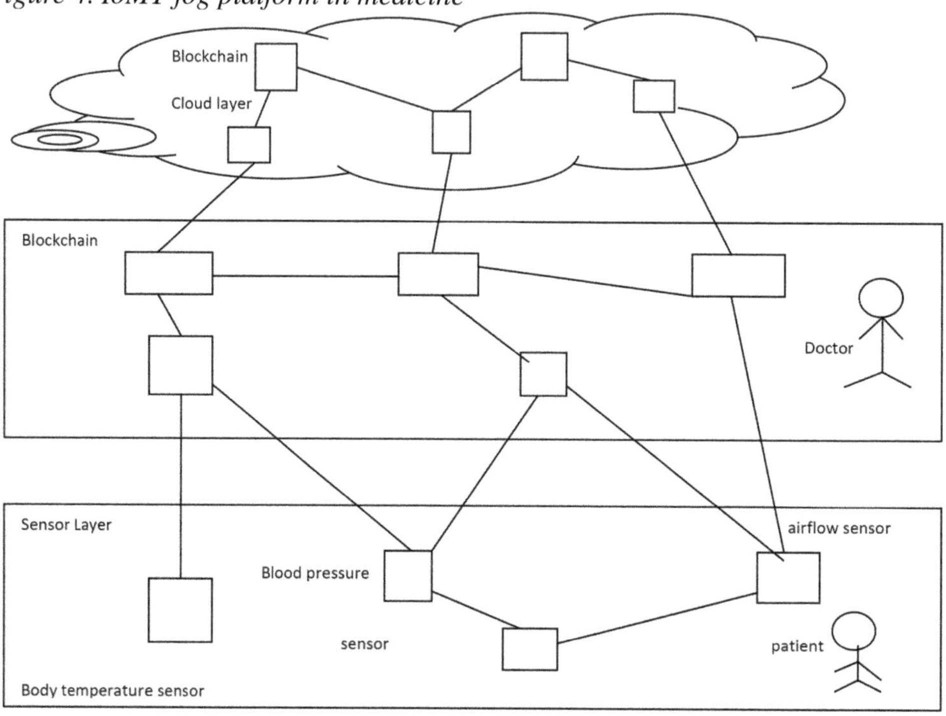


## 4. ANALYSIS OF THE CURRENT STAGE OF HEALTHCARE 4.0

The data management of healthcare sector was carried out from medical records, real-time data access, and contribution of patient engagements, sharing of confident information among the healthcare stake holders, privacy of victim's information with the third party resources, insight of public towards the data management in healthcare sector

(i) Medical records: Medical record is a document that provides detailed information about the patient's history, clinical findings, lab results of the diagnosis, treatment care chart with pre and post operations, progress of the patients and the medication details. These documents need to be protected and should be kept confidential while entering the data in digitalization. Authentication and authorization need to be established properly for the data to be stored in the proper network.

(ii) Real-time data access: With no delays, the real-time data access gives patients the information (Uma, S. 2023) they need about their drugs, which are updated in real-time by medical professionals. Since the computer- and paper-based systems fall short of this procedure, cloud computing client-server design offers this chance. Even yet, gaining safe access to data is a difficult undertaking.

(iii) Patients engagement: The medical records maintained by the health sector generally handled by the organization resources such as doctors, lab technicians or record maintenance section, or by the third party service providers. But, the patients or the close authorized relatives of the patients cannot handle the medical records as the participation of the patient is very less in the traditional management system. The advancements of cloud storage and IoT health monitoring systems helps in collecting the data from the patients, but direct accessing the information is still demanding task.

## 5. BLOCKCHAIN APPLICATIONS IN THE MEDICINE INDUSTRY

The arrival of BCT has sparked a huge interest in its potential applications, particularly in the realm of medicine. The extent to which it may mitigate worries about fraud in clinical trials is receiving a lot of attention. (Alsabah, M. et al. 2025) uses a review of 144 papers to find the possible benefits of using BCT to enhance hospital functionalities. By improving data efficiency and allaying concerns about data manipulation, this innovative technology has the capability to drastically change the hospitals. The data storage mechanism of blockchain ensures the highest security requirements, making it unique. BCT's flexibility, interconnectedness, accountability, and authentication for data access provide healthcare data with a trustworthy and decentralized protection. Researchers who have highlighted its potential to lower certain hazards include. A list of applications is shown in Figure 4.

### (i) Preserving Personal Health Data

Clinical research generates a huge quantity of patient data and healthcare data. This data is gathered by a variety of tests, assessments, estimates, and surveys, all of which involve evidence from documents and records. Medical professionals carefully examine this data, verifying its accuracy by comparing it to the primary data that was stored in the Blockchain framework. Modern encryption techniques used by blockchain provide secure and safe data exchanges. All pertinent patient data, including name, date of birth, detection, remedies, and medical history, are recorded and kept up to date using the Electronic Health Record (EHR) (Farahat, M.A., et al. 2023) format. After that, these documents are kept on cloud computing platforms or in traditional databases.

### (ii) Security and Openness

Healthcare providers may put patient care first by using BCT because of its unmatched safety and transparency features. It also speeds up the application procedure for funding for significant initiatives involving the study and treatment of uncommon illnesses. The efficiency of diagnosis, treatment, and overall cost-effectiveness in the medical framework can all be greatly enhanced by using a single distributed ledger to enable data exchange across various medical service providers.

### (iii) Management of Health Records

The management of medical records might be totally changed by BCT. It provides a number of benefits, including as simplifying administrative tasks, handling insurance, exchanging medical information, and storing electronic health records. Patients may now easily send their health data to a secure Blockchain network with the use of specialized software. The inclusion of digital Blockchain contracts enhances the effective cooperation of intelligent devices and sensors.

### (iv) Clinical Trials

The usage of BCT has shown its value in surmounting challenges that impede clinical studies. This cutting-edge technology efficiently addresses problems like erroneous data and disjointed information, guaranteeing consistency with study goals. Additionally, using Blockchain in clinical studies gives participants more faith in the outcomes. The healthcare sector is always changing, and by using business analysis tools, it can identify new possibilities and accurately analyze shifting market trends.

### (v) Career Observation

Medical professionals may confirm that patients have access to vital medical equipment and remotely monitor their health by using the trustworthy power of BCT. This sophisticated technology not only has the ability to track critical metrics like supply levels, bed utilization, and room temperature, but it also has the ability to entirely change the field of medical logistics. Blockchain and IoT (Hanumantharaju, R., et al. 2021) technology may be effortlessly integrated to create a strong healthcare network that promotes increased transparency and responsiveness that in turn ensures patient care and monitoring.

*Figure 5. Blockchain's Use in Healthcare Applications.*

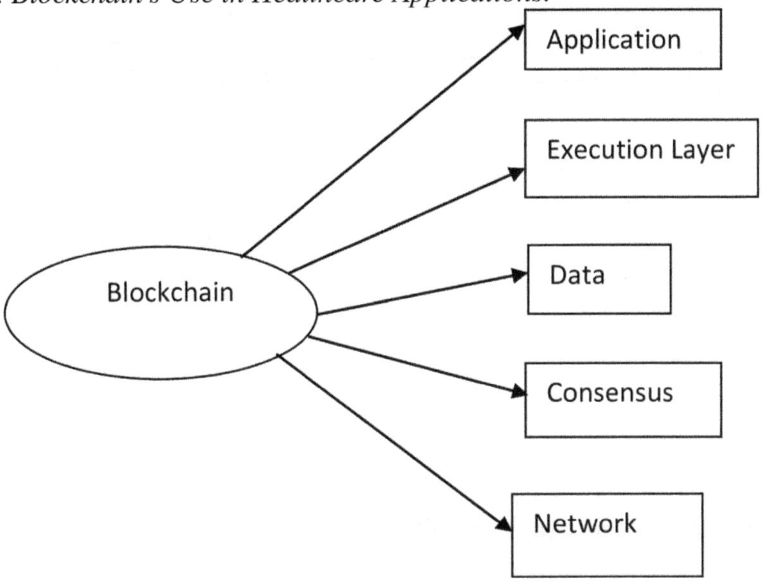


## (vi) Hospital Financial Records Management

Accurately preserving their financial accounts in their accounting processes is crucial for hospitals. Thankfully, clinical trials provide the perfect setting for effective operation and evaluation. Solutions to improve accounting and reporting in this area are now being developed, thanks to the rise of Blockchain enterprises. Potential blockchain-based fixes for the current healthcare system Blockchain is a distributed ledger which utilizes decentralized methods to store data so it is spread across several nodes or organizations and is very difficult to edit.

*Figure 6. Potential Applications of BCT in Medicine*

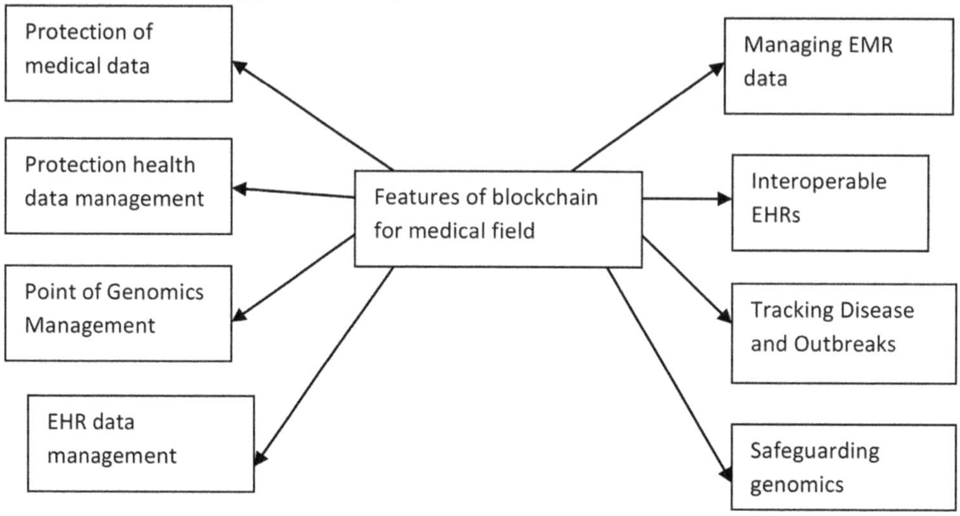


## (vii) Privacy and Security of Data

BCT may provide a safe, unhackable method of storing medical data. Encrypted and time-stamped patient data records are present at every point in the chain, guaranteeing data privacy and minimizing the likelihood of unauthorized access. Giving every patient a secure and unique identity may facilitate to minimize faults and assure that the right patient gets the treatment they need. Even if their records aren't available without the data in them, patients still have total control over them. Smart contracts on the blockchain may be used to handle patient consent.

## (viii) Cooperation

Blockchain facilitates the integration of patient records, which is especially useful when patients get treatment from many institutions and need to make sure that all relevant data is available to the whole healthcare system. BCT has the capability to encourage hospitals to follow standard operating procedures.

## (ix) Drug and logistical control monitoring

BCT ensures transparency and veracity of consumption by monitoring the whole medicine supply chain. It helps to prevent the sale of fake drugs. In 2023, (Kumari,

A., et al. 2024) documenting a drug's transfer on a blockchain, from production to patient, may increase transparency and accountability.

### (x) Clinical Trials and R&D

There has been an increase in R&D spending and the release of new medications within the last 20 years. By certifying the ethics of the data gathered, BCT safeguards the correctness of outcomes and prevents data tampering in clinical studies. Encouraging qualified patients to take part in clinical trials and protecting patient privacy are made easier by BCT. Blockchain acceptance in the medical domain will need overcoming technical challenges and regulatory constraints with the assistance of stakeholders. Although there can be benefits, it's crucial to thoroughly scrutinize the needs and specific circumstances of the healthcare system in question.

## 6. OBSTACLES RELATED TO IMMEDIATE CONSEQUENCES

- Scalability: Managing an immense flood of transactions in real-time is a critical problem for blockchain networks in the modern, fast-paced digital world. When the network's user base and transaction volume continue to grow rapidly, scalability and efficient data exchange become more important. It is a difficult task for blockchain networks to handle this demand while maintaining optimal performance and speed.
- Delay: Secure transaction verification and efficient data processing depend on minimizing delay in real-time circumstances. However, when it comes to blockchain networks, particularly public ones, consensus procedures and network congestion are the main reasons for delays in transaction confirmation. Low latency might be hard to accomplish without compromising network reliability and security.
- Interoperability: Many entities make up the contemporary healthcare system, such as government organizations, insurance companies, labs, hospitals, and clinics. Modern BCT may be difficult to incorporate into these established frameworks while maintaining smooth communication and compatibility with other systems and databases. Fast data transfer and seamless system compatibility are difficult to achieve.
- Regulatory Compliance: Ensuring data security while integrating BCT with government union legislation is a challenging task. The need for regulatory compliance complicates real-time data exchange and limits the usage of blockchain in the medical sector.

- Data Security: Using BCT has many integrated security elements, like hashing in cryptography and decentralized agreement. Even though these factors provide a strong foundation for data security, there are still topics which need to be answered for manifesting stability between secure and rapid data transmission. To fully secure sensible victim's data from illegitimate access, robust encryption methods and privacy-preserving techniques must be implemented
- Cost: The healthcare sector must make a sizable initial investment in BCT. This means allocating funds for building the necessary infrastructure, putting in place a robust network, and ensuring seamless system integration. To speed up data exchange, more expenses for hardware, software, and network resources will most likely also be needed for seamless, real-time utilization. Healthcare organizations need to carefully weigh the potential returns on investment against the initial installation costs when assessing this innovative equipment. For BCT to realize its full potential, a quantity of problems requires to be conveyed, consisting of interoperability, regulatory compliance, scalability, and standardization.

## Regulations' Effect on the Adoption of Blockchain

Applications that use BCT are now struggling with compliance and navigating the requirements of data security ordinance including the California Consumer Privacy Act, SEC, Health Insurance Portability and Accountability Act, and tax legislation, state legislation, anti-corruption legislation, and anti-money-laundering legislation. For innovation to proceed at a rapid rate, policymakers and corporate entities will need to work together on the laws and norms of engagement around blockchain. This raises the issue of whether new regulations for blockchain assets will be created or whether the current laws will be changed to accommodate blockchain. Since blockchain is based on immutability, transparency, and trust, several industries are implementing it into their operations. This distinct feature is also the cause of the regulators' opposition to it. Blockchain has the potential to be a new democratic instrument that gives consumers back control over their personal information and the ability to make money off of it. BCT adoption and innovation are being slowed down in a number of sectors and businesses due to a lack of governance, compliance, and appropriate rules. This is one of the main issues that new technologies like virtual reality (VR), 3D printing, the IoT, and AI are facing.

## Adoption Challenges for Blockchain in Medicine

Even though BCT is highly effective in fixing problems and gaps in healthcare management systems, integrating BC into HMS remains difficult. Various organizations and individuals are still hesitant to embrace BC technology.

The following point discusses a few of the crucial issues:

- Scalability and Data Storage

The growing volume of negotiations produces the blockchain to increase daily. Because of the higher demands on repository and processing power, the network can possess lesser nodes with the processing capability to control and verify data on the blockchain. Huge block dimensions, though, may cause blockchain branches and slow down propagation. Scalability and huge data repository are therefore challenging matters.

- Access to and dependability of data

There are advantages and disadvantages to BC's decentralized concept. Although a decentralized network removes the chance of a lone place of negligence, the blockchain moreover has difficulties with dependability and data access. This is because BC is susceptible to a cyber attack because to certain blockchain features. Data accessibility and dependability are therefore among the main issues with blockchain

- Security and privacy

Although encryption offers security and protection, healthcare stakeholders continue to view database accessibility—even when encrypted—as a serious issue. As a result, it is needed to properly govern access control in the blockchain environment. Numerous groups provide medical data that could direct to inadvertent, privacy and security breaches. Consequently, ahead of granting access control, the information must be examined and anticipated.

## 7. RESTRICTIONS AND PERFORMANCE EVALUATION OF BLOCKCHAIN USE IN MEDICINE

Adoption hurdles persist despite all the advantages BCT has to offer the medical aid.

- Secure and Confidential Information: The arrival of BCT has made it unnecessary for other organizations to step in and helps facilitate the security of patient data. In an emergency, patients may require to select several agents to access their healthcare history and data, potentially leading to a data security breach if there is no third party involved. The potential for destinations to have access to restricted data is a major restriction.
- In BCT, throughput—which is often measured in Transactions per Second (TPS)—measures a network's speed and ability to handle transactions. It shows the true percentage of completed, successful transactions over a certain period of time. For high-demand systems, higher throughput—typically attained via sophisticated consensus processes or scaling solutions like sharding—is essential for lowering transaction costs and network congestion.
- Difficulty in Expanding Capacity: One of the biggest drawbacks is the daily rise in transaction volume, which makes it very challenging to manage the massive amount of healthcare data, including patient records, which must be safely maintained and stored.
- Difficult to interface with present systems: Because healthcare technology is advancing more slowly than other industries, integrating with the present frameworks is more difficult. However, it is strenuous to promote medical expectations to go from research data to blockchain at the right time because of the low acceptability amount in the healthcare industry and the existing technology and rules.
- Cost and Resources: Using BCT might be difficult for small healthcare organizations since it requires a large financial outlay to integrate into the current system, which may leave them detached from their potential. It is very tough for fearful IT experts to apply BCT.
- Regulatory Barriers: The healthcare industry is subject to strict legal and regulatory obligations. While adhering to both national and international legal frameworks are very challenging, understanding these regulations and ensuring that the technology complies with them is essential for the integration of blockchain. Business plans to advance blockchain use in healthcare 4.0 as BCT is new to the healthcare sector, new business procedures will be needed to ensure a smooth transition.
- Clinical Trials: According to (Rejeb, A., et al. 2021), clinical trials are crucial in research domains for finding novel medications in a controlled setting. This method is more expensive, thus it must be done carefully to prevent fraud and improper use of the findings. Blockchain makes it easier to find the right people for clinical trials, streamlines the procedure, and encourages further research in the medical domains. A transparent process that makes it possible for everyone to assess the clinical reports is necessary to guarantee

that the trial results are not falsified. According to (Mastrantonas, A., et. al. 2024), blockchain is a mesh of nodes which ensures that no data may be altered without authorization. Transparency in documentation and a decentralized approach will support patient consent and record integrity.

- Cost-effectiveness: BCT produces the capability to reduce the need for duplicate data entry and effort across many healthcare institutions, which will save money on administrative and data management procedures. Blockchain may increase the traceability, authenticity, and consistency of commodities by introducing streamlined processes of smart contracts. This would definitely minimize personnel involvement and the paperwork and administrative expenditures. Recalls, issues with regulatory compliance, and counterfeit medicine may all be less expensive as a result. Increased billing process transparency may save costs linked to billing disputes, mistakes, and related administrative expenditures. It's crucial to have in mind that, even with these potential financial benefits, there are still upfront costs, technological difficulties, and regulatory thoughts related to implementing blockchain in the medical sector. The overall cost impact will depend on the particular condition, the implementation strategy, and the extent of industry acceptability. Forming partnerships may help reduce implementation-related challenges and promote the pooling of resources and expertise by offering financial incentives like financing possibilities or discounts for subsidiaries. All parties participating in the healthcare industry must be committed for a long time to the effective adoption of blockchain, and a multidisciplinary approach to improving the technology in the field is necessary.

## CONCLUSION

BCT use in the medical domain both has benefits and drawbacks. Blockchain's decentralization, increased security, and immutability have the facility to revolutionize the handling of healthcare data. It provides advantages including patient data protection, seamless data transfer, and assistance with a range of duties like managing medical records and processing insurance claims. To fully realize its advantages, however, obstacles including real-time implementation problems, interoperability constraints, and regulatory compliance need to be resolved. Upcoming developments in BCT, such as improvements in scalability and privacy-preserving methods, could spur further innovation and use in the medical domain. To fully use blockchain in medicine, strategic business approaches centered on collaboration, standardization, and regulatory alignment are essential. Healthcare organizations may find a secure, fruitful, and patient-focused medical ecosystem by using BCT.

## Future Research Directions

Every field is seeing widespread usage of the IoTs, and the medical domain is one that is extensively using the IoMT, a sub-domain of the IoT. This is crucial for healthcare institutions to provide high-quality treatment. We have suggested a framework and a blockchain integration to solve the troubles of the IoMT. Though, a number of aspects need to be thoroughly examined in further studies: In the healthcare industry, a thorough analysis of blockchain and IoMT integration performance concerns is necessary. Although some research has been done on blockchain execution in the IoT space, no specific job of this kind was done in IoMT architectures. In order to achieve very low latency and highly optimized energy efficiency, scheduling algorithm design and review should be researched. Even though this article has covered a theoretical analysis of the security issues with the blockchain-IoMT architecture and how a blockchain may address them, the effectiveness of these security solutions can be practically demonstrated by carrying out their implementation and demonstration.

## REFERENCES


Akhai, S., & Abbass, M. (2025). Smart Manufacturing for Better Healthcare: Integrating 3D Printing, Robotics, and IoT. In Singh, S. P., Jain, D. K., & Debayle, J. (Eds.), *Healthcare Recommender Systems*. Springer., DOI: 10.1007/978-3-031-80056-6_16

Alsabah, M., Naser, M. A., Albahri, A. S., Albahri, O. S., Alamoodi, A. H., Abdulhussain, S. H., & Alzubaidi, L. (2025). A comprehensive review on key technologies toward smart healthcare systems based IoT: Technical aspects, challenges and future directions. *Artificial Intelligence Review*, *58*(11), 343. DOI: 10.1007/s10462-025-11342-3

Amin, M. S., Ahmad, S., & Loh, W. K. (2025). Federated learning for Healthcare 5.0: A comprehensive survey, taxonomy, challenges, and solutions. *Soft Computing*, *29*(2), 673–700. DOI: 10.1007/s00500-025-10508-z

Ben Fekih, R., & Lahami, M. (2020). Application of BCT in Healthcare: A Comprehensive Study. In Jmaiel, M., Mokhtari, M., Abdulrazak, B., Aloulou, H., & Kallel, S. (Eds.), Lecture Notes in Computer Science: Vol. 12157. *The Impact of Digital Technologies on Public Health in Developed and Developing Countries. ICOST 2020*. Springer., DOI: 10.1007/978-3-030-51517-1_23

Cihan, S., Yılmaz, N., Ozsoy, A., & Beyan, O. D. (2025). A systematic review of the blockchain application in healthcare research domain: Toward a unified conceptual model. *Medical & Biological Engineering & Computing*, *63*(5), 1319–1342. DOI: 10.1007/s11517-024-03274-x PMID: 39789305

Dhingra, S., Raut, R. D., Yadav, V. S., Cheikhrouhou, N., & Naik, B. K. R. (2025). Blockchain adoption challenges in the healthcare sector: A waste management perspective. *Operations Management Research : Advancing Practice Through Research*, *18*(2), 518–536. DOI: 10.1007/s12063-023-00413-9 PMID: 40625400

Dlamini, Z., Miya, T. V., Hull, R., Molefi, T., Khanyile, R., & de Vasconcellos, J. F. (2023). Society 5.0: Realizing Next-Generation Healthcare. In Dlamini, Z. (Ed.), *Society 5.0 and Next Generation Healthcare*. Springer., DOI: 10.1007/978-3-031-36461-7_1

Esmaeilzadeh, P. (2022). Benefits and concerns associated with blockchain-based health information exchange (HIE): A qualitative study from physicians' perspectives. *BMC Medical Informatics and Decision Making*, *22*(1), 80. DOI: 10.1186/s12911-022-01815-8 PMID: 35346176

Farahat, M. A., Darwish, A., & Hassanien, A. E. (2023). The Implication of Metaverse in the Traditional Medical Environment and Healthcare Sector: Applications and Challenges. In Hassanien, A. E., Darwish, A., & Torky, M. (Eds.), *The Future of Metaverse in the Virtual Era and Physical World. Studies in Big Data* (Vol. 123). Springer., DOI: 10.1007/978-3-031-29132-6_7

Hammad, M., Panaousis, M., Ali, H., & Khan, W. A. (2026). Industry 4.0 in Pharmaceuticals: A New Era of Smart Manufacturing. In *Smart Manufacturing Blueprint: Navigating Industry 4.0 Across Diverse Sectors. Springer Series in Advanced Manufacturing*. Springer., DOI: 10.1007/978-3-032-00214-3_6

Hanumantharaju, R., Pradeep Kumar, D., Sowmya, B. J., Siddesh, G. M., Shreenath, K. N., & Srinivasa, K. G. (2021). Enabling Technologies for Fog Computing in Healthcare 4.0: Challenges and Future Implications. In Tanwar, S. (Ed.), *Fog Computing for Healthcare 4.0 Environments. Signals and Communication Technology*. Springer., DOI: 10.1007/978-3-030-46197-3_7

Ibrahim, A. M., Zoromba, M. A., Abousoliman, A. D., Zaghamir, D. E. F., Alenezi, I. N., Elsayed, E. A., & Mohamed, H. A. H. (2025). Ethical implications of artificial intelligence integration in nursing practice in arab countries: Literature review. *BMC Nursing*, *24*(1), 159. DOI: 10.1186/s12912-025-02798-3 PMID: 39934834

Kamel Boulos, M. N., Wilson, J. T., & Clauson, K. A. (2018). Geospatial blockchain: Promises, challenges, and scenarios in health and healthcare. *International Journal of Health Geographics*, *17*(1), 25. DOI: 10.1186/s12942-018-0144-x PMID: 29973196

Kashyap, V. R., Bhushan, B., Farhaoui, Y., & Alkhayyat, A. (2025). Digital Twin Robots for Securing IoT Based Healthcare 4.0 Application: Key Technologies, Integration Trends and Recent Advancement. In Sharma, R., & Jeon, G. (Eds.), *Data Analytics for Smart Robotics and Its Applications. Intelligent Systems Reference Library* (Vol. 272). Springer., DOI: 10.1007/978-3-031-87697-4_3

Khan, A. A., Laghari, A. A., Baqasah, A. M., Bacarra, R., Alroobaea, R., Alsafyani, M., & Alsayaydeh, J. A. J. (2025). BDLT-IoMT—a novel architecture: SVM machine learning for robust and secure data processing in Internet of Medical Things with blockchain cybersecurity. *The Journal of Supercomputing*, *81*(1), 271. DOI: 10.1007/s11227-024-06782-7

Khan, A. A., Shaikh, A. K., Alroobaea, R., Baqasah, A. M., Alsafyani, M., Alsufyani, H., & Laghari, A. A. (2025). Blockchain-enabled secure Internet of Medical Things (IoMT) architecture for multi-modal data fusion in precision cancer diagnosis and continuous monitoring. *Journal of Cloud Computing (Heidelberg, Germany)*, *14*(1), 58. DOI: 10.1186/s13677-025-00775-4

Kumari, A., Kumar, P., & Golyan, A. (2024). Introduction of Blockchain for Biomedical and Healthcare System. In Kumar, P., & Kumari, A. (Eds.), *Blockchain for Biomedical Research and Healthcare. Interdisciplinary Biotechnological Advances*. Springer., DOI: 10.1007/978-981-97-4268-4_1

Kumari, M., Gupta, M., & Ved, C. (2021). Blockchain in Pharmaceutical Sector. In Namasudra, S., & Deka, G. C. (Eds.), *Applications of Blockchain in Healthcare. Studies in Big Data* (Vol. 83). Springer., DOI: 10.1007/978-981-15-9547-9_8

Mackey, T. K., Kuo, T. T., & Gummadi, B.. (2019). 'Fit-for-purpose?' – challenges and opportunities for applications of BCT in the future of healthcare. *BMC Medicine*, *17*, 68. DOI: 10.1186/s12916-019-1296-7 PMID: 30914045

Mahajan, H. B. (2022). Emergence of Healthcare 4.0 and Blockchain into Secure Cloud-based Electronic Health Records Systems: Solutions, Challenges, and Future Roadmap. *Wireless Personal Communications*, *126*(3), 2425–2446. DOI: 10.1007/s11277-022-09535-y

Mastrantonas, A., Kokkas, P., Chatzopoulos, A., Papoutsidakis, M., Stergiou, C., Vairis, A., & Kanetaki, Z. (2024). Identifying the effects of Industry 4.0 in the pharmaceutical sector: Achieving the sustainable development goals. *Discover Sustainability*, *5*(1), 460. DOI: 10.1007/s43621-024-00716-2

Mukherjee, P., & Singh, D. (2020). The Opportunities of Blockchain in Health 4.0. In Rosa Righi, R., Alberti, A., & Singh, M. (Eds.), *BCT for Industry 4.0. Blockchain Technologies*. Springer., DOI: 10.1007/978-981-15-1137-0_8

Onur, D., & Özbakır, Ç. (2025). Pediatrics 4.0: The Transformative Impacts of the Latest Industrial Revolution on Pediatrics. *Health Care Analysis : HCA : Journal of Health Philosophy and Policy*. Advance online publication. DOI: 10.1007/s10728-025-00536-z PMID: 40690134

Orabi, M. M., Emam, O., & Fahmy, H. (2025). Adapting security and decentralized knowledge enhancement in federated learning using BCT: Literature review. *Journal of Big Data*, *12*, 55. DOI: 10.1186/s40537-025-01099-5

Raj, A., & Prakash, S. (2024). Privacy preservation of the internet of medical things using blockchain. *Health Services and Outcomes Research Methodology*, *24*(1), 112–139. DOI: 10.1007/s10742-023-00306-1

Rejeb, A., Treiblmaier, H., Rejeb, K., & Zailani, S. (2021). Blockchain research in healthcare: A bibliometric review and current research trends. *Journal of Data, Information and Management*, *3*(2), 109–124. DOI: 10.1007/s42488-021-00046-2

Uma, S. (2023). Blockchain and AI: Disruptive Digital Technologies in Designing the Potential Growth of Healthcare Industries. In Rai, B. K., Kumar, G., & Balyan, V. (Eds.), *AI and Blockchain in Healthcare. Advanced Technologies and Societal Change*. Springer., DOI: 10.1007/978-981-99-0377-1_9

Yuman, Y., Goyal, S. B., Rajawat, A. S., Kumar, M., Shankar, A., Alhayan, F., & Basheer, S. (2025). A blockchain-based solution for enhancing the efficiency and security of healthcare knowledge management systems in the era of industry 4.0. *Wireless Networks*, *31*(2), 983–1004. DOI: 10.1007/s11276-024-03770-w

# Chapter 8
# The Economics of Trust: Evaluating the Cost-Effectiveness of Cybersecure AI Systems in Healthcare Delivery

**Lawal Olamilekan Abdulwahab**
http://orcid.org/0000-0003-4955-244X
*School of Business and Economics, Universiti Brunei Darussalam, Brunei*

## ABSTRACT

*Artificial intelligence (AI) is increasingly embedded in healthcare, promising improvements in diagnosis, efficiency, and cost, but it faces rising cybersecurity risks, regulatory challenges, and trust issues following data breaches. Despite financial losses, cybersecurity remains a compliance cost rather than a strategic investment. This chapter introduces a new view by considering cybersecurity as key to trust and cost-effectiveness in AI healthcare. Using health, cybersecurity, and AI governance research, it presents an Economic Evaluation Framework for Cybersecure AI (EECAI) that applies cost-benefit, cost-effectiveness, and return-on-security-investment analyses to evaluate secure AI deployment. The chapter shows how cybersecurity investments deliver measurable economic, clinical, and organizational value, emphasizing cybersecurity as a trust-building asset rather than a cost. It offers key insights for healthcare managers, developers, and policymakers to sustain safe, viable AI healthcare.*

## 1. INTRODUCTION

Healthcare systems globally are rapidly transforming digitally, integrating AI into clinical, administrative, and operational areas. AI supports diagnostic imaging,

DOI: 10.4018/979-8-3373-9119-9.ch008

decision-making, predictive analytics, and remote monitoring, potentially reducing costs while enhancing care and efficiency. Economic studies indicate AI can save costs by optimizing resources, cutting hospital admissions, and boosting workforce productivity (Chakkaravarthy & Jaganathan, 2025; Ghosh et al., 2025). However, these anticipated gains increasingly depend on the security and integrity of the digital infrastructures that support AI-enabled healthcare delivery.

As AI adoption expands, cybersecurity threats against healthcare escalate. Healthcare is highly vulnerable due to the value of patient data, legacy systems, and interconnected devices. Cyberattacks like ransomware, breaches, and AI-specific threats are increasing in frequency and severity, imposing financial and operational burdens on healthcare institutions (Jourdain, 2026; Mbacop et al., 2025). These incidents disrupt clinical services, increase regulatory penalties, and undermine public confidence in digital health technologies.

The convergence of AI and cybersecurity creates new risks, expanding attack surfaces, and introducing vulnerabilities such as data poisoning, model inversion, and exploitation. Healthcare organizations' reliance on AI tools for threat detection adds complexity to the balance between innovation and risk management (Das et al., 2024; Rongali, 2025). This interdependence highlights the need to evaluate cybersecurity not only as a technical safeguard but as an economic enabler of AI-driven healthcare value creation.

## 1.1 Problem Statement

Despite cybersecurity's vital role in AI healthcare, investments remain reactive and compliance-focused. Spending is mainly driven by regulations, such as data privacy laws, rather than by economic analysis. Evidence shows poor investment links to more breaches, financial losses, and lost patient trust, but budget issues persist (Musa & Abdulfatai, 2024; Pratama et al., 2025). A key challenge is the lack of strong economic frameworks to assess cybersecurity investments in AI healthcare. While health economics offers tools for clinical interventions, these are seldom used for digital security. Cybersecurity economics mainly concentrates on general IT, providing a limited understanding of healthcare AI risks, regulations, and trust issues (Das et al., 2024). This disconnect leaves decision-makers without clear guidance on how to balance innovation, security, and cost-efficiency. The economic and cybersecurity dynamics shaping AI-enabled healthcare systems are multidimensional and interdependent. Table 1 summarizes the principal drivers influencing cost structures, risk exposure, and trust outcomes in digital healthcare environments.

*Table 1. Key Economic and Cyber Risk Drivers in AI-Enabled Healthcare Systems*

| Driver Category | Description | Economic Implication | Trust Implication |
|---|---|---|---|
| AI Efficiency Gains | AI-enabled diagnostics, predictive analytics, workflow automation, and remote monitoring | Reduced operational costs; improved productivity; optimized resource allocation | Increased clinician confidence and patient engagement when performance is reliable |
| Expanding Digital Infrastructure | Integration of EHRs, IoMT devices, cloud platforms, and AI decision-support systems | Higher capital and maintenance expenditure, and expanded digital dependency. | Increased reliance on system reliability and data integrity |
| Cyber Risk Exposure | Ransomware attacks, data breaches, adversarial AI manipulation, system compromise | Direct financial losses; remediation costs; downtime; regulatory penalties | Erosion of institutional credibility and patient trust following incidents |
| Regulatory & Compliance Pressure | Data protection laws, AI governance standards, and audit requirements | Compliance expenditure, potential liability, and legal costs | Enhanced trust when compliance is stable and transparent |
| Governance & Transparency Gaps | Limited explainability, weak accountability structures, and fragmented oversight | Hidden risk accumulation; inefficient allocation of security resources | Reduced adoption due to uncertainty and perceived opacity |
| Budget Constraints & Underinvestment | Reactive security spending; compliance-driven budgeting | Higher long-term expected losses; volatility in cost structure | Trust is unstable due to recurring disruptions |

**Source:** Developed by the authors based on the reviewed literature.

The table shows that AI healthcare systems operate in a complex environment where efficiency gains and cyber risks grow together. AI reduces costs and boosts productivity, but expanding digital infrastructure and cybersecurity threats create economic volatility. Regulatory pressures and governance gaps complicate resource decisions. Trust is a key outcome affected by security controls and institutional stability. These links highlight the need for an economic evaluation framework that accounts for all cost drivers, thereby justifying cybersecurity as essential for long-term sustainability.

## 1.2 Research Motivation and Rationale

Trust is a key economic asset in healthcare, influencing patient engagement with digital technology, clinician reliance on AI, and institutional legitimacy, all of which depend on system security and reliability (van Kessel et al., 2024). Studies increasingly emphasize that transparency, explainability, and governance of AI systems directly influence user trust and adoption, with measurable economic consequences (Mandava et al., 2025). Cybersecurity, therefore, plays a central role in sustaining trust, not merely by preventing losses but by enabling continued value realization from AI investments.

Cybersecurity investments serve as mechanisms for risk-adjusted value creation. Preventive measures lower expected losses, stabilize operations, and safeguard intangible assets like reputation and public confidence (Tick & Szabo-Harka, 2024). Evidence from multi-sectoral analyses shows that strategic cybersecurity investments can significantly improve cost-benefit outcomes and organizational resilience when compared to reactive incident response models (Moussa & Zine-Dine, 2025). In healthcare, where service disruptions and data breaches impact clinical outcomes, these economic benefits are especially significant. This chapter aims to bridge the fields of health and cybersecurity economics by developing an integrated AI-enabled healthcare framework. It repositions cybersecurity as a strategic investment that promotes trust, efficiency, and sustainability in digital healthcare.

## 1.3 Objectives of the Chapter

The chapter pursues the following objectives:

1. To conceptualize cybersecurity as an economic determinant of trust and performance in AI-enabled healthcare systems.
2. To integrate health economic evaluation techniques with cybersecurity investment analysis.
3. To develop a structured framework for assessing the cost-effectiveness of cybersecure AI deployment.
4. To demonstrate how cybersecurity investments enhance clinical, operational, and economic outcomes.
5. To provide evidence-based guidance for healthcare managers, software developers, and policymakers.

Following this, Section 2 reviews AI in healthcare, cybersecurity economics, and trust governance. Section 3 covers the foundations of trust economics. Section 4 details the methodology for the evaluation framework. Section 5 introduces the Economic Evaluation Framework for Cybersecure AI (EECAI). Section 6 applies the framework via scenario analysis. Sections 7 and 8 discuss stakeholder, policy, and governance implications. The chapter ends with future research and reflections on cybersecurity's role in AI healthcare.

## 2. LITERATURE REVIEW

This section synthesizes contemporary studies at the intersection of artificial intelligence, cybersecurity, health economics, and trust-based governance. It critically reviews recent contributions to identify conceptual advances, empirical findings, and persistent gaps that motivate the development of an integrated economic evaluation framework for cybersecure AI in healthcare.

### 2.1 Artificial Intelligence in Healthcare Delivery

Studies show that AI transforms healthcare through precise diagnostics, improved workflow efficiency, and data-driven decision-making. Economic evaluations indicate AI diagnostic systems save costs by reducing unnecessary procedures, improving early detection, and boosting clinician productivity (Kavitha et al., 2025). For example, cost-consequence analyses of AI diagnostic tools across cardiology, obstetrics, and gastroenterology indicate that AI can be cost-saving or cost-effective depending on clinical context and implementation design (Chatzikou et al., 2025). Beyond diagnostics, AI models boost healthcare efficiency via automation and analytics. Reviews highlight that AI's economic benefits depend on implementation, governance, and clinical workflows, not just performance (Leenen et al., 2025). These findings suggest that AI value realization is contingent on organizational readiness, data integrity, and sustained system reliability.

However, the literature also underscores that AI adoption introduces new dependencies on digital infrastructure and data availability. As healthcare systems scale AI usage, their exposure to systemic risks, particularly cyber risks, intensifies (Sindiramutty et al., 2025; Theilmann et al., 2025). This dependency creates a direct link between AI-enabled value creation and the robustness of cybersecurity controls, a relationship that is often underexplored in economic evaluations of AI in healthcare.

### 2.2 Cybersecurity Challenges in AI-Enabled Healthcare

Cybersecurity experts label healthcare as high-risk due to sensitive health data, outdated systems, and the rapid adoption of interconnected technologies such as IoMT. Rising ransomware, data breaches, and service disruptions threaten not just finances but also patient safety and care continuity (Nunez Migliorisi, 2025). AI integration complicates cybersecurity by introducing vulnerabilities such as adversarial manipulation, data poisoning, and exploits. Although collaborative intelligence and ensemble learning enhance threat detection, they also increase system complexity and governance requirements (Annie Silviya et al., 2025).

This dual AI role as both a security enhancer and a risk amplifier creates a paradox for traditional security management. AI cybersecurity solutions also raise concerns about transparency and explainability. Studies show that opaque, black-box AI systems can undermine trust among clinicians and IT professionals, hindering human–AI collaboration (Latif et al., 2026). These challenges highlight the need for cybersecurity strategies that not only improve technical resilience but also support trust, accountability, and informed decision-making within healthcare organizations.

## 2.3 Economics of Cybersecurity

The economic dimensions of cybersecurity have gained increasing attention across critical infrastructure sectors. Contemporary research demonstrates that preventive cybersecurity investments can significantly reduce expected losses by lowering breach probability and minimizing disruption severity (Boonen et al., 2025). Multi-sectoral economic analyses reveal that organizations adopting proactive security architectures, such as zero-trust models and AI-enhanced monitoring, achieve superior cost-benefit outcomes compared to those relying on reactive incident response (Butani, 2026; Vasilica et al., 2025). Cybersecurity economics literature emphasizes diminishing returns to security investment, underscoring the need for optimal allocation rather than maximal spending.

Studies show that targeted investments aligned with organizational risk profiles yield the highest economic efficiency, particularly in resource-constrained environments (Ngo & Wright, 2024). Most existing models are sector-agnostic and overlook healthcare-specific externalities, such as patient harm, service disruptions, and regulatory penalties. Cybersecurity failures cause indirect costs such as reputational damage, patient loss, and trust erosion, which are often omitted in traditional models, thereby underestimating cybersecurity's true value. Studies recommend sector-specific frameworks to include both tangible and intangible cybersecurity outcomes.

## 2.4 Balancing Cybersecurity Investment and Operational Efficiency

While literature supports increased cybersecurity investment to reduce risk, excessive spending may have diminishing or negative returns beyond an optimal point.

Too many controls can cause inefficiencies, administrative burdens, and workflow issues, potentially harming healthcare delivery (De Morais Rodrigues et al., 2025).

Within healthcare, strict authentication, frequent password updates, extensive access controls, and multilayered verification can boost security but may increase clinician workload and reduce time for patient care. Studies show poorly integrated protocols can cause alert fatigue, delays in EHR access, and lower user satisfaction (Al-Qahtani et al., 2025; Wosny, 2025). In such circumstances, the indirect costs associated with reduced productivity and workflow disruptions may partially offset the benefits from enhanced protection against cyber threats.

This view challenges the notion that greater cybersecurity spending always adds value. It proposes an optimal investment range where security gains outweigh operational costs. Beyond that, extra spending yields limited risk reduction and higher efficiency losses (Zhao et al., 2025). The economic problem, therefore, becomes one of optimization rather than maximization.

The emergence of AI-enabled healthcare systems further complicates this relationship. Advanced security mechanisms embedded in AI infrastructure may improve resilience against cyberattacks, but they may also increase computational overhead, implementation complexity, staff training requirements, and integration costs (Shukla, 2025). Evaluating cybersecurity only as risk reduction may miss key organizational value, revealing a gap in current research that often separately assesses cybersecurity effectiveness or healthcare outcomes. Few studies analyze trade-offs within a unified economic framework. This study introduces the EECAI framework, which considers both security benefits and organizational costs to evaluate the cost-effectiveness of cybersecure AI in healthcare.

## 2.5 Health Economics and Cost-Effectiveness Analysis

Health economics offers a solid foundation for evaluating healthcare interventions via cost-effectiveness and cost-utility analyses. Its application to digital health underscores the importance of context-specific assumptions, transparent modeling, and accounting for implementation costs (Nikolaev, 2025). These principles are directly applicable to the evaluation of cybersecurity interventions supporting AI-enabled healthcare.

Integrative reviews note that many AI-related economic evaluations remain theoretical, with limited consideration of system risks, governance costs, and long-term sustainability (Wu et al., 2025). This limitation highlights cybersecurity investment challenges, where benefits are uncertain and losses are avoided. Combining health economic methods with cybersecurity risk modeling allows a more comprehensive assessment. Discussions propose extending cost-effectiveness frameworks to include risk-adjusted outcomes, resilience metrics, and system reliability indicators (Shafrin et al., 2024). Such extensions are particularly relevant for AI-enabled healthcare systems, where failures can cascade across clinical, operational, and reputational domains.

## 2.6 Trust, Governance, and Economic Sustainability

Trust acts as a unifying theme in AI, cybersecurity, and healthcare governance. It affects clinicians' acceptance of AI, patient engagement with digital health, and organizations' willingness to invest in innovation (Ranwala & Andrade, 2025). Research on explainable and transparent AI systems demonstrates that trust-enhancing design features improve adoption and collaborative performance without sacrificing technical effectiveness (Bhushan & Dixit, 2024).

From a governance perspective, studies emphasize that ethical oversight, regulatory alignment, and cybersecurity compliance are not merely constraints but enablers of sustainable innovation (Abdulwahab & Azam, 2026). Legal and ethical analyses show that poor governance exposes healthcare organizations to liability, compliance costs, and reputational harm, with significant economic consequences (Ashrafi et al., 2025). The emerging scholars, therefore, position trust as an intangible yet economically consequential asset. Cybersecurity plays a central role in sustaining this asset by ensuring data integrity, system availability, and accountability (Onatuyeh et al., 2025). However, existing research rarely explicitly includes trust in economic models, missing how cybersecurity investments yield lasting economic and clinical value.

Studies show AI benefits healthcare economically, but only with a robust digital infrastructure. Cybersecurity research highlights the efficiency of preventive investments but lacks healthcare-specific value frameworks. Health economics provides tools rarely used for cybersecurity or trust outcomes. Governance studies stress transparency but do not quantify economic impacts, creating a research gap. An integrated framework is needed to evaluate cybersecurity as a cost-effective, trust-building investment in AI for healthcare. Bridging this gap requires combining insights from health economics, cybersecurity, and AI governance, motivating the development outlined next.

The reviewed literature spans multiple disciplinary domains, each contributing partial insights into the relationship between artificial intelligence, cybersecurity, and economic performance in healthcare. However, these streams remain fragmented in their treatment of trust and economic evaluation. Table 2 synthesizes the principal contributions, limitations, and research gaps identified across these domains.

*Table 2. Comparative Synthesis of Literature Streams Informing the Economics of Trust Framework*

| Literature Stream | Core Analytical Focus | Key Contributions | Conceptual or Methodological Limitations | Gap Addressed in This Chapter |
|---|---|---|---|---|
| Artificial Intelligence in Healthcare | Cost savings, diagnostic accuracy, and operational efficiency | Demonstrates potential for productivity gains and improved clinical outcomes | Often assumes stable digital infrastructure; limited integration of cybersecurity risk | Incorporates cybersecurity as a determinant of AI cost-effectiveness |
| Cybersecurity Economics | Risk modeling, breach probability, cost–benefit optimization | Shows that preventive security investment reduces expected losses | Typically sector-agnostic; undervalues healthcare-specific externalities | Develops a healthcare-specific cybersecurity valuation framework |
| Health Economics | Cost-effectiveness analysis (CEA), cost–benefit analysis (CBA), allocative efficiency | Provides structured economic evaluation methodologies | Rarely applied to digital security interventions or trust variables | Extends economic evaluation to cybersecurity-enabled AI systems |
| AI Governance & Trust Studies | Transparency, explainability, and accountability mechanisms | Demonstrates that trust enhances adoption and collaboration | Trust treated qualitatively; limited monetization or economic modeling | Operationalizes trust as a measurable economic mediator |
| Regulatory & Compliance Research | Legal exposure, data protection, audit stability | Highlights the financial and reputational consequences of weak governance | Compliance-focused rather than value-creation oriented | Reframes compliance as a strategic economic enabler |

**Source:** Developed by the authors from interdisciplinary literature synthesis.

The table shows that, despite significant scholarship in AI, cybersecurity economics, health economics, and governance, these fields remain disconnected. AI focuses on efficiency but neglects risk; cybersecurity models loss prevention but lacks healthcare-specific valuation; health economics offers evaluation tools but rarely applies them to digital security; governance studies recognize adoption but seldom quantify economic impacts. This fragmentation creates a gap, justifying an integrated framework that treats cybersecurity and trust as key to AI-enabled healthcare value.

## 3. THEORETICAL AND CONCEPTUAL FRAMEWORK

Building on prior literature, this chapter adopts an interdisciplinary approach combining health economics, cybersecurity economics, and AI governance to show how cybersecurity investments create value by fostering trust in AI healthcare systems. It establishes the conceptual foundation by viewing cybersecurity as a dynamic economic input rather than a static safeguard.

## 3.1 Health Economics Perspective on Digital Health Security

Health economics provides a rigorous framework for assessing the efficiency of healthcare interventions in resource-scarce settings. Key principles such as allocative efficiency, opportunity cost, and marginal benefit help determine whether an intervention provides sufficient value relative to its cost (Abdulwahab, 2026a). Methodological guidance emphasizes that economic evaluation is increasingly necessary for non-clinical digital health interventions, particularly those that indirectly influence patient outcomes through system-level performance (Zakiyah et al., 2024).

In AI-enabled healthcare, cybersecurity maintains AI effectiveness by ensuring data integrity, availability, and service continuity. Security failures can disrupt care, compromise diagnostics, and lead to costly recoveries (Abbou et al., 2024). Economic evaluations of AI diagnostic systems demonstrate that cost savings and efficiency gains are highly sensitive to system reliability and implementation risk (El Arab & Al Moosa, 2025). This sensitivity suggests that cybersecurity investments directly influence the incremental cost-effectiveness of AI technologies. From a health economics perspective, cybersecurity spending is a preventive investment that reduces downstream costs associated with adverse events. In cost-effectiveness analysis, secure AI systems should have lower expected costs per health outcome than insecure ones, despite higher initial costs. This supports including cybersecurity in health economic models.

## 3.2 Cybersecurity as an Economic Public Good

Cybersecurity economics views information security as a quasi-public good with positive externalities, information asymmetry, and underinvestment. Organizations bear the full cost of security, but benefits such as reduced systemic risk and increased trust are shared only partially among stakeholders (Posso & Altmann, 2025). This misalignment leads to continued underinvestment in cybersecurity. Economic analyses show that preventive strategies offer greater economic value than reactive ones, especially in highly interconnected and regulated sectors (Fotis, 2024). In healthcare, cybersecurity failures in interconnected systems can spread quickly, increasing losses beyond individual institutions.

Decision-theoretic studies highlight cost-effectiveness as a key criterion for cybersecurity investments, along with security effectiveness and compliance (Rattanapong et al., 2025). These findings suggest cybersecurity investments are economic choices balancing cost, risk, and performance. However, models often undervalue intangible benefits such as trust, reputation, and legitimacy, which are vital to the sustainability of the healthcare system (Tariq, 2024). The theoretical limitation of existing models thus lies in their inability to fully internalize trust-related outcomes, underscoring the need for an expanded economic framework.

## 3.3 AI Governance and the Economics of Trust

AI governance studies reveal how trust is built, maintained, and eroded in AI systems. Trust is vital for deploying AI in high-stakes domains such as healthcare, as it affects patient safety and accountability (Sirbu & Mercioni, 2024). Governance mechanisms, including transparency, explainability, and accountability, are shown to influence user confidence and system adoption significantly (Kim et al., 2026). Empirical studies demonstrate that explainable AI and human-in-the-loop governance models improve trust without compromising system performance, thereby enhancing both technical and organizational outcomes (Abdulwahab, 2026b; Oriaro & Mishra, 2025). From an economic perspective, trust reduces transaction costs by lowering resistance to adoption, minimizing oversight burdens, and enabling smoother human–AI collaboration (Daly et al., 2025). These reductions translate into measurable efficiency gains and improved return on investment.

Legal and regulatory studies highlight trust's economic importance by demonstrating the financial risks associated with governance failures. Poor oversight and cybersecurity weaken healthcare organizations, risking liability, penalties, and damage to reputation (Chavan & Shabadi, 2025). These external costs often significantly impact organizational performance and resource use. Trust is seen as intangible capital connecting cybersecurity investment to economic success. Cybersecurity not only mitigates risk but also builds trust, supporting the economic sustainability of AI healthcare systems.

## 3.4 Conceptual Model of the Economics of Trust Framework

The conceptual relationships underlying the Economics of Trust framework are illustrated in Figure 1. This conceptual framework illustrates how cybersecurity investment functions as a strategic economic input in AI-enabled healthcare systems. Through risk-reduction and trust-enhancement mechanisms, cybersecurity strengthens trust as a mediating variable, which, in turn, amplifies economic and clinical outcomes, including reduced expected losses, higher AI adoption, improved cost-effectiveness, and long-term institutional sustainability.

*Figure 1. The Economics of Trust Conceptual Model*

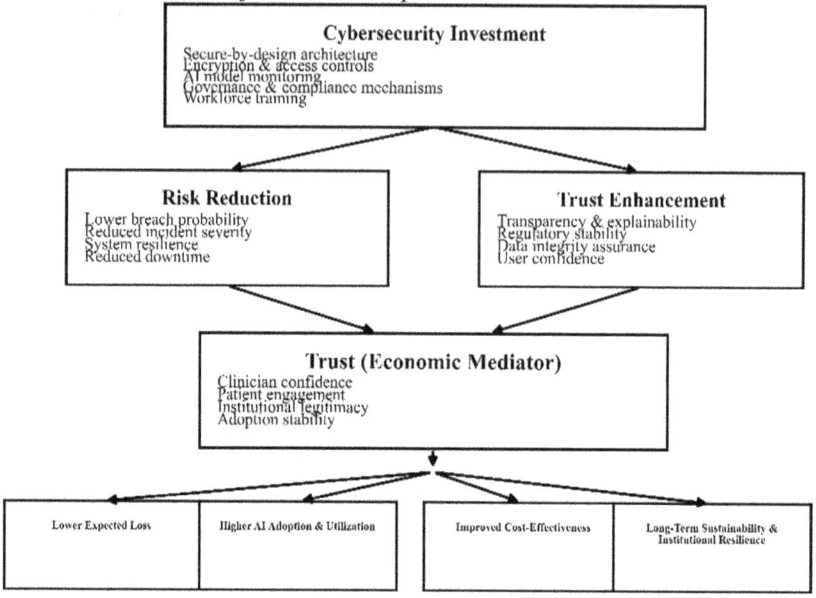


**Source:** *Developed by the authors.*

Synthesizing insights from health economics, cybersecurity economics, and AI governance, this chapter introduces the Economics of Trust Framework. It views cybersecurity as a value-generating investment within the AI healthcare lifecycle, grounded in three core ideas. First, cybersecurity reduces losses by lowering the risk of adverse cyber events. Second, it boosts trust among patients, clinicians, and regulators through transparency, reliability, and accountability. Third, increased trust improves AI adoption, use, and sustainability, boosting economic returns. Trust links cybersecurity efforts to economic and clinical outcomes, with secure AI systems outperforming insecure ones in value. This expands traditional ROI by emphasizing intangible, important outcomes. The framework guides cybersecurity investments by drawing on economic theory and trust dynamics, addressing research gaps and supporting strategic decisions in AI healthcare.

## 4. RESEARCH METHODOLOGY

Grounded in the interdisciplinary foundations from the previous section, this chapter uses a transparent approach to assess the economic value of cybersecurity in AI-enabled healthcare. As in earlier chapters, the methodology emphasizes analytical rigor, replicability, and policy relevance rather than primary data collection.

## 4.1 Research Design

This chapter employs a conceptual–analytical design with scenario analysis, ideal for economic evaluations of emerging AI cybersecurity with limited data. Healthcare AI research emphasizes the value of conceptual synthesis and scenario models when evidence is fragmented or context-dependent (Alghamdi et al., 2025; Choudhury & Goel, 2025). The research comprises three parts: a synthesis of recent studies on AI, cybersecurity, and economic evaluation; the development of the Economic Evaluation Framework for Cybersecure AI (EECAI); and case-based simulations demonstrating healthcare use. This approach links theory and practice while maintaining clarity.

## 4.2 Data Sources and Literature Synthesis

The chapter relies on peer-reviewed studies from Scopus- and ABDC-indexed journals (2022-2026) on healthcare AI economics, cybersecurity, digital governance, and regulation, prioritizing open-access for transparency. It stresses that economic evaluations of digital health tech should integrate insights from regulatory reports, cybersecurity incidents, and risk assessments to reflect real-world use accurately (Santos, Sampaio, et al., 2025; Santos, von Hafe, et al., 2025). This chapter blends academic and industry research on cyber risk, compliance costs, and resilience. Using a narrative synthesis, it integrates insights across disciplines to identify key cost drivers, benefits, and trust outcomes in AI-enabled healthcare systems.

## 4.3 Economic Evaluation Techniques

To operationalize the Economics of Trust Framework, the chapter adapts economic evaluation techniques for cybersecurity. Cost-Benefit Analysis (CBA) compares cybersecurity investment costs with expected reductions in incident losses, penalties, and disruptions. Studies show preventive investments have favorable cost-benefit ratios when risk exposure is high (Abdulwahab, 2026c; Chong et al., 2025). Cost-Effectiveness Analysis (CEA) is employed to assess the efficiency of secure versus non-secure AI systems relative to defined outcomes, such as system availability, data integrity, and continuity of care.

By framing cybersecurity as an enabling intervention, CEA enables comparison of incremental costs per unit of improved system performance. ROSI metrics, capturing organizational financial performance, are used as decision-support tools for managers managing limited resources under uncertainty (Barik et al., 2023; He et al., 2025). These techniques offer a multidimensional assessment of cybersecurity value, capturing tangible and risk-adjusted economic outcomes. Table 3 outlines the core evaluation methods, their purposes, and their applications in AI-enabled healthcare, clarifying the methodological structure of the EECAI framework.

*Table 3. Economic Evaluation Techniques Applied in the EECAI Framework*

| Evaluation Technique | Analytical Purpose | Application Within EECAI | Managerial Decision Insight |
|---|---|---|---|
| Cost–Benefit Analysis (CBA) | Compares the total monetary costs and benefits of cybersecurity investment | Quantifies expected reduction in breach-related losses, regulatory penalties, and downtime relative to security expenditure | Determines whether cybersecurity investment generates positive net economic value |
| Cost-Effectiveness Analysis (CEA) | Assesses incremental cost per unit of defined outcome | Compares secure versus non-secure AI deployment in terms of system availability, reliability, and trust-adjusted utilization | Identifies the economically efficient level of security investment |
| Return on Security Investment (ROSI) | Calculates financial return relative to cybersecurity expenditure | Estimates the percentage return generated through avoided incident costs and stabilized operational performance | Supports budget justification and strategic allocation decisions |
| Risk-Adjusted Expected Loss Modeling | Incorporates probability and impact of cyber incidents into cost estimation | Evaluates lifecycle cost divergence between secure and insecure AI systems | Enables long-term financial planning under uncertainty |
| Trust-Adjusted Performance Metrics | Measures the indirect economic value of trust variables | Operationalizes adoption rates, patient engagement, and compliance stability as economic proxies | Internalizes intangible benefits into a formal economic evaluation |

**Source:** Developed by the authors, drawing on health economics and cybersecurity investment literature.

The Table shows that the EECAI framework combines traditional health economics with cybersecurity valuation to assess multidimensional AI performance. Cost–benefit and cost-effectiveness analyses assess investment efficiency, while ROSI and risk-adjusted modeling account for probabilistic losses. Trust-adjusted metrics extend evaluations by including intangible yet valuable outcomes. These methods enable a comprehensive view of cybersecurity as both risk mitigation and a strategic investment in AI healthcare systems.

## 4.4 Scenario-Based Case Simulation

Given ethical and practical constraints in live healthcare system experiments, the chapter uses hypothetical, realistic scenario simulations. This method, common in cybersecurity and healthcare AI research, explores system behavior under different risk and investment conditions without harming institutions (Brohi & Mastoi, 2025; Sajid et al., 2025). The simulation compares two AI deployment scenarios: Scenario

A, with minimal cybersecurity controls, and Scenario B, with integrated, trust-focused cybersecurity measures. It analyzes costs, breach likelihood, downtime, regulatory risk, adoption, and retention, based on current cybersecurity and healthcare studies.

### 4.5 Assumptions and Analytical Scope

The analysis relies on clear assumptions: healthcare organizations aim to minimize long-term costs, cybersecurity investments have diminishing returns, and proxies like system use, service continuity, and compliance measure trust. The scope focuses on organizational decision-making in healthcare, emphasizing management and policy outcomes affecting AI sustainability and system resilience.

## 5. ECONOMIC EVALUATION FRAMEWORK FOR CYBERSECURE AI (EECAI)

This section introduces the Economic Evaluation Framework for Cybersecure AI (EECAI), an integrative decision-support model designed to assess the cost-effectiveness of cybersecurity investments in AI-enabled healthcare systems. The framework operationalizes the Economics of Trust perspective by translating cybersecurity, trust, and AI governance into measurable economic variables that support strategic decision-making.

### 5.1 Framework Overview

The EECAI framework views cybersecurity as a fundamental part of the AI healthcare lifecycle, not just compliance costs. It emphasizes that AI performance depends on the security, integrity, and trustworthiness of the digital environment, and that these factors affect economic outcomes through three pathways: Risk Reduction, Trust Enhancement, and Value Amplification. This integration allows comparison of secure versus non-secure AI strategies in healthcare.

### 5.2 Cost Components of Cybersecure AI Systems

The structural components and evaluation logic of the EECAI framework are presented in Figure 2. This framework operationalizes the Economics of Trust perspective by integrating cybersecurity controls across the AI healthcare lifecycle and linking them to formal economic evaluation techniques, including cost-benefit analysis (CBA), cost-effectiveness analysis (CEA), and return on security investment (ROSI). The framework demonstrates how embedded cybersecurity investments translate into measurable economic and organizational outcomes, ultimately supporting long-term sustainability and institutional resilience.

*Figure 2. Economic Evaluation Framework for Cybersecure AI (EECAI).*

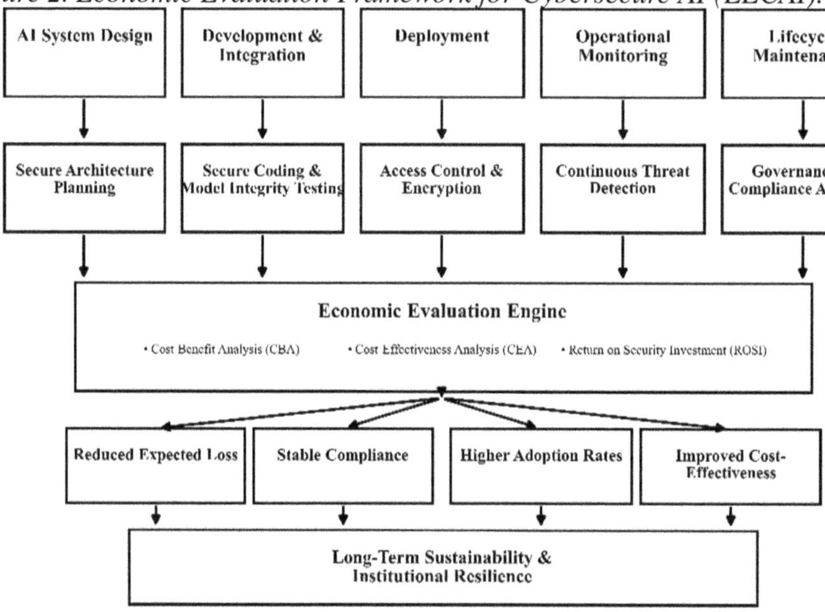


**Source:** *Developed by the authors.*

The framework classifies cybersecurity costs in AI healthcare into direct, indirect, and opportunity costs. Direct costs include security infrastructure, software, encryption, controls, AI monitoring, audits, and training, and are usually reflected in IT budgets. Indirect costs include operational changes such as system delays, workflow redesign, and productivity dips during security setup. Opportunity costs are the forgone opportunities, such as delayed AI deployment or reduced investment in other innovations due to limited resources. EECAI views these costs as upfront investments, justifiable when balanced against long-term system performance and prevented losses, not just short-term budgets.

## 5.3 Benefit Components and Value Creation Mechanisms

EECAI highlights cybersecurity benefits beyond preventing losses, including financial savings, regulatory compliance, and operational stability. It also boosts trust, system reliability, and adoption of AI tools, reinforcing organizational value. Cybersecurity thus acts as a strategic enabler, supporting sustainable value in AI-powered healthcare systems. To operationalize the Economic Evaluation Framework for Cybersecure AI (EECAI), it is necessary to systematically distinguish between the categories of costs and benefits associated with cybersecurity investments. Table 4 outlines the principal cost components and value-creation mechanisms embedded in the framework.

*Table 4. Cost and Benefit Components in the EECAI Framework*

| Category | Sub-Component | Description | Economic Relevance |
|---|---|---|---|
| **Direct Costs** | Security Infrastructure | Encryption systems, intrusion detection tools, and secure cloud architecture | Upfront capital expenditure required to reduce breach probability |
| | Secure Development Practices | Model validation, adversarial testing, and secure coding protocols | Reduces AI system vulnerability and long-term remediation costs |
| | Workforce Training | Cybersecurity awareness, AI governance training | Enhances human-layer resilience and reduces operational risk |
| **Indirect Costs** | Workflow Adjustment | Temporary productivity decline during system integration | Short-term operational impact during implementation |
| | Governance & Compliance Management | Audit preparation, documentation, and reporting systems | Stabilizes regulatory exposure and prevents penalty costs |
| **Opportunity Costs** | Capital Allocation Trade-Off | Resources diverted from alternative innovation projects | Reflects strategic investment prioritization decisions |
| **Tangible Benefits** | Breach Loss Avoidance | Reduced incident remediation costs and downtime losses | Direct financial savings through risk mitigation |
| | Regulatory Stability | Lower fines, legal exposure, and liability claims | Predictable compliance environment reduces financial volatility |
| | Operational Continuity | Reduced service disruption and workflow interruption | Protects productivity and revenue streams |
| **Intangible Benefits** | Clinician Trust & Adoption | Increased reliance on AI-supported decisions | Improves AI utilization and return on investment |
| | Patient Engagement & Retention | Greater confidence in data protection and system reliability | Sustains long-term institutional reputation and digital participation |
| | Institutional Credibility | Enhanced regulatory and stakeholder confidence | Strengthens strategic positioning and competitive advantage |

**Source:** Developed by the authors within the EECAI conceptual framework.

The table shows that cybersecurity investment in AI-enabled healthcare involves multiple cost layers, beyond visible infrastructure costs. While direct and indirect costs are measurable, opportunity costs involve strategic trade-offs. Benefits include not only loss avoidance but also trust and reputation, which impact long-term economic success. The EECAI framework categorizes these elements, capturing both tangible and intangible value, reinforcing the economic case for proactive cybersecurity investment.

## 5.4 Operational Measurement Specification for EECAI Implementation

To make the EECAI framework practically implementable, Table 5 is extended through an operational measurement specification that identifies the minimum data required to evaluate cybersecure AI investments in healthcare. This specification translates the cost and benefit categories into measurable inputs, institutional responsibilities, and review timelines.

*Table 5. Operational Data Dictionary for EECAI Implementation*

| EECAI Variable | Required Input Data | Data Source | Responsible Stakeholder | Measurement Frequency | Minimum Viable Dataset |
|---|---|---|---|---|---|
| Direct cybersecurity costs | Security software, encryption tools, monitoring systems, and cloud security costs | Procurement and finance records | Finance unit, CIO, CISO | Quarterly | Annual cybersecurity expenditure |
| Indirect implementation costs | Staff training time, workflow disruption, and temporary productivity losses | HR and operational reports | HR, clinical operations | Quarterly | Training hours and deployment disruption records |
| Opportunity costs | Projects delayed or investments forgone due to cybersecurity spending | Strategic planning and budget documents | Executive management | Annually | Capital allocation records |
| Breach loss avoidance | Estimated reduction in breach costs, downtime, remediation, and legal exposure | Incident reports and risk assessments | CISO, risk management team | Quarterly | Baseline and post-investment incident estimates |
| Operational continuity | System uptime, service disruption, recovery time | IT monitoring logs | IT department | Monthly | Uptime and downtime records |
| Regulatory stability | Audit findings, penalties avoided, compliance status | Compliance reports | Compliance officer | Annually | Audit and compliance records |

continued on following page

*Table 5. Continued*

| EECAI Variable | Required Input Data | Data Source | Responsible Stakeholder | Measurement Frequency | Minimum Viable Dataset |
|---|---|---|---|---|---|
| Clinician trust and adoption | AI usage rates, clinician confidence, and acceptance surveys | System usage logs and staff surveys | Clinical leadership, quality assurance | Semi-annually | AI utilization data and clinician survey results |
| Patient trust and engagement | Patient satisfaction, digital service use, and privacy confidence | Patient surveys and service records | Patient experience office | Semi-annually | Patient satisfaction and digital engagement data |

**Source:** Developed by the authors from interdisciplinary literature synthesis.

The EECAI framework should include an explicit investment-stopping rule: cybersecurity investment continues only until the marginal benefits, including Expected Loss Reduction, Trust Benefit, and AI Performance Benefit, equal the marginal cost. When costs surpass combined benefits, spending should be reconsidered or redirected. This prevents overinvestment, which can cause friction, administrative burden, and inefficiency.

## 5.5 Measuring Trust as an Economic Variable

The EECAI framework uniquely views trust as a measurable economic mediator, operationalized through proxies like AI adoption, system uptime, regulatory stability, and patient engagement. It embeds trust into economic evaluation, capturing overlooked value streams in cost–benefit analyses. This helps decision-makers see how cybersecurity and governance investments improve efficiency, credibility, and long-term returns.

To strengthen operational measurement, the EECAI framework proposes the use of trust proxies that can be monitored alongside traditional economic indicators. These proxies include patient retention rates, digital health service utilization, clinician adoption rates of AI-supported recommendations, patient satisfaction scores, complaint frequencies, and survey-based trust indices. Changes in these indicators can be linked to economic outcomes such as revenue stability, service utilization, implementation success, and operational efficiency.

A healthcare organization experienced a decline in trust after a cybersecurity breach, with patient retention dropping from 90% to 85% among 20,000 patients, each worth $500 annually, resulting in over $500,000 in revenue loss. Improved trust from secure AI systems can boost patient engagement, adoption of digital services, and AI-enabled care. While trust is partly intangible, its impact is measurable through organizational performance indicators. The EECAI framework views trust as an economic variable rather than a purely qualitative concept.

## 5.6 Risk-Adjusted Economic Evaluation Logic

EECAI adopts a risk-adjusted valuation approach that recognizes the inherently probabilistic nature of cyber threats and AI system failures. Rather than treating cyber incidents as isolated or exceptional events, the framework integrates expected loss calculations that account for both the likelihood of a breach and the severity of its potential impact. Within this logic, secure AI systems, although potentially requiring higher upfront investment, demonstrate a lower expected total cost over time due to reduced exposure to financial, operational, and reputational risks. In contrast, insecure systems may appear cost-efficient in the short term but ultimately generate significantly higher long-run costs as risk accumulates. This approach reframes cybersecurity expenditure as a strategic investment aligned with long-term financial sustainability and resilience, rather than as a short-term cost to be minimized.

## 5.7 Managerial and Decision-Support Utility

The EECAI framework helps healthcare leaders and policymakers make practical AI decisions. It compares deployment strategies, finds optimal cybersecurity investments, and justifies security budgets with economic reasoning. The framework aligns cybersecurity with organizational goals, framing it as a strategic investment in trust and value. It moves organizations from reactive compliance to proactive, economically governed AI healthcare systems. The next section shows its real-world use through scenario analysis, comparing secure and insecure AI strategies in healthcare.

## 5.8 Procedural Algorithm for EECAI Implementation

To strengthen the operational applicability of EECAI, the framework can be implemented through a stepwise procedural algorithm that converts conceptual evaluation into an executable decision model. The process begins by defining the AI use case, clinical scope, evaluation period, and deployment alternatives. Decision-makers then identify the relevant cost inputs, including direct cybersecurity costs, indirect implementation costs, operational friction costs, and opportunity costs. These inputs are obtained from finance records, IT budgets, procurement documents, workforce training estimates, and clinical workflow assessments.

The second step estimates risk exposure for each deployment scenario by assigning values to breach probability, financial loss, downtime costs, penalties, recovery expenses, and reputation damage. Expected loss is calculated as: Expected Loss = Probability of Cyber Incident × Impact. The third step assesses the economic benefits of secure AI deployment, including avoided cyber losses, reduced downtime, improved service, higher clinician adoption, and stronger patient engagement. When trust is hard to price, EECAI uses proxies like patient retention, service use, AI adoption, satisfaction scores, and care continuity. The fourth step computes net economic value: Net Economic Value = Total Expected Benefits − Total Expected Costs.

The fifth step applies sensitivity analysis by varying key assumptions, including breach probability, incident severity, cybersecurity cost, patient retention effects, downtime duration, and adoption rates. This allows decision-makers to test whether the preferred option remains economically justified under conservative, moderate, and high-risk assumptions. The final step applies a decision threshold. A cybersecure AI investment should be approved when its expected loss reduction, trust-related gains, and AI performance benefits exceed its total incremental cost. Additional investment should continue only until: Marginal Expected Loss Reduction + Marginal Trust Benefit + Marginal AI Performance Benefit = Marginal Investment Cost.

This procedural algorithm makes the EECAI framework traceable and usable for hospital finance committees. It clarifies what data are required, how calculations proceed, which assumptions must be tested, and where the investment stopping point occurs.

## 5.9 Executive Decision Walkthrough: Evaluating a Cybersecure AI Deployment

To illustrate how EECAI supports managerial decision-making, consider a hypothetical executive committee meeting at a mid-sized hospital evaluating whether to deploy an AI-assisted diagnostic platform supported by enhanced cybersecurity controls. The executive team consists of the Chief Executive Officer (CEO), Chief Information Officer (CIO), Chief Information Security Officer (CISO), Chief Financial Officer (CFO), and Clinical Director. The proposed project requires an initial investment in AI infrastructure, cybersecurity enhancements, staff training, and ongoing monitoring capabilities.

The CFO focuses on costs, including software, cybersecurity, integration, and training, and questions whether the benefits justify the investment, requesting an economic analysis. The CISO reports rising cyber threats, such as ransomware and data breaches, and uses EECAI to estimate annual losses and the reduction achievable with cybersecure AI. The Clinical Director evaluates operational implications. Benefits include improved diagnostic accuracy, faster decision support, reduced clinician workload, and better patient outcomes. Concerns involve implementation complexity, staff adaptation, and workflow disruptions during deployment. The CEO emphasizes organizational reputation and patient trust. A major cyber incident could harm reputation, lower patient engagement, and damage trust in AI-supported care. EECAI includes these trust-related effects in the overall value assessment.

The executive committee applies a framework organizing information into EECAI categories, including costs, benefits, performance, trust, and compliance. These inputs are evaluated collectively to assess the total economic impact. The framework provides three decision indicators: net economic value (comparing costs and benefits), risk-adjusted returns (including reductions in cyber losses), and trust-related value (patient confidence, reputation, stakeholder acceptance). The committee concludes that the projected reduction in cyber losses, along with improved diagnostics and trust, outweighs the cost. The investment is approved, subject to the EECAI stopping rule for ongoing reassessment. EECAI turns broad tech, cybersecurity, and trust factors into a structured decision process, helping healthcare leaders evaluate these areas within a unified economic model.

## 6. APPLICATION AND CASE-BASED ANALYSIS

This section demonstrates the practical applicability of the Economic Evaluation Framework for Cybersecure AI (EECAI) through a structured, scenario-based analysis. The objective is to illustrate how healthcare decision-makers can apply the framework to compare the economic performance of secure and non-secure AI deployment strategies under realistic operating conditions.

### 6.1 Scenario Description

This analysis examines a mid-sized healthcare institution implementing an AI-enabled decision-support system to improve diagnostics and patient management. The system uses large patient data, integrates with electronic health records (EHRs), and supports clinicians across departments. Two deployment strategies are evaluated. Scenario A (Minimal-Security AI Deployment) involves basic cybersecurity controls mainly for compliance, with limited AI-specific safeguards. In contrast, Scenario B (Cybersecure AI Deployment) adopts a secure-by-design framework, integrating advanced cybersecurity controls, continuous monitoring mechanisms, explainable AI governance structures, and workforce training initiatives aligned with trust, transparency, and accountability objectives. Both scenarios assume identical AI functionality, clinical scope, and operational goals, ensuring that differences in outcomes can be attributed primarily to variations in cybersecurity investment and governance strategy.

## 6.2 Cost Structure Comparison

Under Scenario A, initial implementation costs are lower due to reduced expenditure on cybersecurity infrastructure, governance mechanisms, and training. However, this cost advantage is offset by higher expected downstream costs associated with increased vulnerability to cyber incidents, system downtime, and regulatory instability. In contrast, Scenario B incurs higher upfront costs driven by investments in secure software practices, AI model monitoring, resilience planning, and trust-oriented governance. These costs are treated within EECAI as preventive investments rather than overhead expenses. When evaluated over a multi-year horizon, Scenario B exhibits a more stable cost trajectory, while Scenario A shows greater cost volatility due to risk exposure and reactive incident management.

To facilitate structured comparison between the two AI deployment strategies, Table 6 summarizes their differential economic, operational, and trust-related implications across key evaluation dimensions.

*Table 6. Comparative Economic Evaluation of Minimal-Security and Cybersecure AI Deployment*

| Evaluation Dimension | Scenario A: Minimal-Security Deployment | Scenario B: Cybersecure Deployment | Short-Term Effect | Long-Term Effect | Strategic Economic Implication |
|---|---|---|---|---|---|
| Initial Implementation Cost | Lower upfront investment due to limited security integration | Higher upfront investment due to secure-by-design architecture | Budget efficiency advantage (A) | Lifecycle stability advantage (B) | Short-term savings vs long-term sustainability |
| Breach Probability | Elevated exposure to cyber incidents | Significantly reduced probability through layered controls | Risk underestimation (A) | Risk containment (B) | Divergence in expected cumulative losses |
| Incident Severity & Recovery Cost | High remediation expenses and extended downtime | Contained impact due to resilience mechanisms | Cost volatility (A) | Cost predictability (B) | Reduced financial shock exposure |
| System Downtime | Frequent disruption affecting clinical workflows | High availability and continuity | Operational instability (A) | Sustained productivity (B) | Protection of service revenue and workforce efficiency |
| Regulatory & Compliance Stability | Greater likelihood of audit findings and penalties | Stable compliance environment with proactive governance | Monitoring burden (A) | Lower liability exposure (B) | Reduced legal and reputational risk |

continued on following page

*Table 6. Continued*

| Evaluation Dimension | Scenario A: Minimal-Security Deployment | Scenario B: Cybersecure Deployment | Short-Term Effect | Long-Term Effect | Strategic Economic Implication |
|---|---|---|---|---|---|
| Clinician & Patient Trust | Reduced confidence due to system vulnerabilities | Higher confidence driven by transparency and reliability | Adoption hesitation (A) | Sustained AI utilization (B) | Amplified return on AI investment |
| Overall Cost-Effectiveness | Appears efficient in the initial phase | Demonstrates superior lifecycle cost-effectiveness | Perceived affordability (A) | Economic dominance over time (B) | Trust-adjusted efficiency gain |

**Source:** Developed by the authors (scenario-based analytical modeling).

The table shows the lifecycle differences between minimal-security and cybersecure AI strategies. Scenario A offers short-term savings but risks accumulation, cost volatility, and trust issues. Scenario B requires higher initial costs but proves more cost-effective in the long term by mitigating risks, ensuring stability, and promoting adoption. This comparison supports the Economics of Trust, emphasizing that cybersecurity investments improve AI performance by protecting long-term value rather than just cutting initial costs.

## 6.3 Risk and Loss Exposure Analysis

Using a risk-adjusted valuation approach, the framework estimates the expected financial losses arising from cyber incidents under each scenario. Scenario A is characterized by a higher probability of data breaches, service disruptions, and AI model compromise, resulting in substantial direct recovery costs as well as indirect losses associated with clinical interruptions, regulatory penalties, and reputational damage. In contrast, Scenario B significantly reduces both the likelihood and potential impact of such events through the implementation of layered security controls and proactive monitoring mechanisms. The EECAI framework illustrates that even modest reductions in breach probability can yield considerable economic benefits within healthcare environments, where regulatory obligations and clinical consequences significantly amplify the overall cost of incidents.

## 6.4 Trust and Adoption Outcomes

Trust-related outcomes distinguish the two scenarios. In Scenario A, security concerns reduce clinician confidence and limit AI integration, with patient engagement hindered by privacy issues and system unreliability. In Scenario B, better transparency and reliability boost clinician adoption and patient engagement, leading to improved AI utilization, higher ROI, and stable operations. EECAI measures these effects through adoption rates, continuity, and governance, reinforcing trust as an economic factor. To illustrate the economic importance of trust, consider a hospital with 20,000 patients annually. Under minimal security, security incidents lower trust, causing a 5% drop in retention and a 10% drop in digital service use. With an average patient value of $500, this results in about $500,000 in lost revenue each year. The cybersecure scenario maintains trust and engagement, ensuring continued use of AI services. Although trust itself is not directly monetized, its effects impact the cost-effectiveness of AI deployment.

## 6.5 Cost-Effectiveness Comparison

The lifecycle divergence in cumulative risk-adjusted costs between secure and non-secure AI deployment strategies is illustrated in Figure 3. This figure illustrates the lifecycle economic divergence between AI systems implemented with minimal cybersecurity controls and those deployed using integrated, trust-oriented security measures. While minimal-security deployment appears less costly initially, cumulative risk exposure and incident-related losses result in significantly higher long-term costs. In contrast, cybersecure deployment demonstrates greater lifecycle cost stability and superior long-term economic performance.

*Figure 3. Risk-Adjusted Cost Trajectory of Minimal-Security versus Cybersecure AI Deployment.*

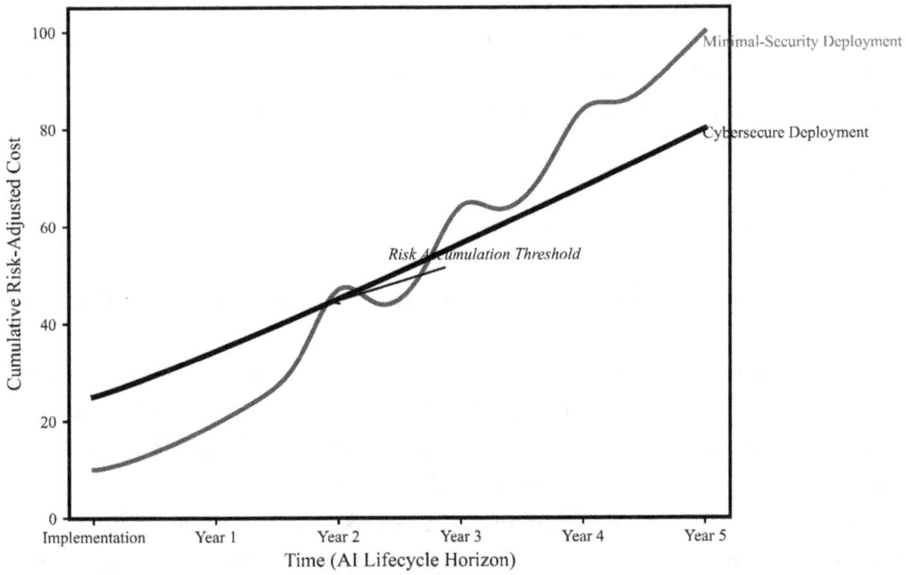


**Source:** *Developed by the authors (conceptual lifecycle modeling).*

Joint evaluation of costs and outcomes shows a clear long-term divergence between the two scenarios. While Scenario A may seem cost-efficient short-term, rising risk exposure makes it less economical over time due to escalating losses. Conversely, Scenario B proves more cost-effective with lower total costs per system performance and trust-adjusted outcome. This underscores a key insight of the Economics of Trust: cybersecurity investments enhance AI cost-effectiveness by protecting and amplifying long-term value, not just reducing operational costs.

From a managerial view, the findings offer key strategic insights. Cybersecurity investments in AI healthcare systems should be viewed across the entire technology lifecycle, not as one-time costs. This approach considers long-term maintenance, upgrades, risk mitigation, and breach costs. Trust-building security measures like strong data protection, transparent governance, and compliance enhance user confidence, boost adoption, and improve system stability, collectively benefiting organizational performance and sustainability. Focusing only on short-term cost cuts may cut expenses initially but increases long-term financial, reputational, and operational risks. The EECAI framework helps healthcare organizations see the economic impacts of insecure AI, guiding cybersecurity investments for long-term value and resilience. Case analysis shows cybersecurity is vital for AI healthcare system sustainability. The next section explores how cybersecure AI benefits stakeholders like managers, developers, policymakers, and patients.

## 7. IMPLICATIONS FOR STAKEHOLDERS

The application of the Economic Evaluation Framework for Cybersecure AI (EECAI) reveals that cybersecurity investment decisions have differentiated but interconnected implications across the healthcare ecosystem. This section translates the analytical findings into actionable insights for key stakeholder groups whose decisions collectively shape the sustainability, trustworthiness, and economic performance of AI-enabled healthcare systems.

### 7.1 Implications for Healthcare Managers and Administrators

For healthcare leaders, the findings highlight the urgent need to view cybersecurity as a strategic investment rather than just IT spending. Short-term cost cuts increase long-term risks, disrupt operations, and harm trust. The EECAI framework provides a structured, economic basis for decision-making by justifying cybersecurity budgets through cost-effectiveness and risk metrics rather than solely on compliance. It aligns cybersecurity with organizational goals like service continuity, patient retention, system reliability, and AI use. The framework also integrates cybersecurity into digital transformation and capital planning. It supports moving from reactive to proactive risk management, with strong economic evidence to advocate for investments at all levels.

## 7.2 Implications for Software Developers and AI Practitioners

For AI developers and practitioners, the analysis highlights the economic value of secure-by-design and trust-aware practices. Cybersecurity features such as explainability, monitoring, and resilience should be core, not optional, components of AI systems. EECAI advises incorporating security from data collection through deployment and maintenance, emphasizing transparency and auditability to build trust, meet regulatory requirements, and stabilize institutions. Collaboration with healthcare organizations is vital to align security with economic and operational needs. Understanding economic principles helps developers demonstrate the value of secure AI and strengthen their market position.

## 7.3 Implications for Policymakers and Regulators

The findings impact policymakers and regulators in AI and cybersecurity in healthcare. Cybersecurity mandates create economic value by reducing risk, boosting resilience, and building trust. The EECAI framework helps assess the proportionality and justification of cybersecurity regulations. These incentives encourage proactive security investments and align AI governance, data protection, and cybersecurity policies with shared economic and trust goals. Viewing cybersecurity as a strategic enabler, regulators can foster innovation while maintaining safety and efficiency, shifting away from punitive models towards balanced policy architectures.

## 7.4 Implications for Clinicians and Healthcare Professionals

For healthcare professionals, cybersecurity impacts workflow, decision-making, and accountability. Insecure AI systems can erode trust, slow adoption, and increase burdens. Vulnerable systems cause data errors and disruptions, reducing confidence and efficiency. Secure AI boosts trust, reduces outages, and supports safer patient care. Viewing cybersecurity as essential to usability helps healthcare organizations improve clinician engagement and integration and maximize digital health benefits.

## 7.5 Implications for Patients and Society

Cybersecurity investments in AI healthcare strengthen trust, protect data, and ensure equitable access. Secure, transparent systems boost patient engagement. Trust erosion from cyber incidents causes long-term costs, but proactive investments boost confidence, safeguard health info, and maintain service continuity. Cybersecure AI enhances resilience, societal welfare, digital inclusion, and modernization of the health system. Stakeholder implications demonstrate practical relevance, but broader regulatory context shapes implementation. The next section explores the impacts of policy and governance, emphasizing how economic evaluation can guide sustainable strategies. The implications of cybersecure AI investment vary across stakeholder groups but remain interconnected within the broader healthcare ecosystem. Table 7 synthesizes the differentiated economic and trust-related impacts for key actors involved in AI-enabled healthcare delivery.

*Table 7. Stakeholder-Specific Economic and Trust Implications of Cybersecure AI Investment*

| Stakeholder Group | Economic Impact of Minimal-Security AI | Economic Impact of Cybersecure AI | Trust Implication | Strategic Action Recommended |
|---|---|---|---|---|
| Healthcare Managers & Administrators | Increased financial volatility due to breach exposure and reactive spending | Stabilized lifecycle costs and improved risk-adjusted financial planning | Strengthened institutional legitimacy and governance credibility | Integrate cybersecurity into long-term capital planning and performance metrics |
| AI Developers & Technical Practitioners | Higher liability exposure and reputational risk | Competitive differentiation through secure-by-design architecture | Enhanced user confidence and adoption | Embed security and explainability throughout the AI lifecycle |
| Policymakers & Regulators | Increased enforcement burden and systemic instability | Reduced systemic risk and predictable compliance environment | Greater public confidence in digital health governance | Align regulatory incentives with proactive cybersecurity investment |
| Clinicians & Healthcare Professionals | Workflow disruption, reduced confidence in AI outputs | Reliable system performance and improved decision-support integration | Increased professional trust in AI-assisted care | Participate in governance and trust-building initiatives |
| Patients & Society | Risk of data misuse and service interruption | Enhanced data protection and continuity of care | Greater engagement with digital health services | Promote transparency and digital literacy initiatives |

**Source:** Developed by the authors based on a framework application.

The Table demonstrates that cybersecurity investment generates distributed economic and trust benefits across the healthcare ecosystem. While minimal-security deployment increases financial volatility, operational instability, and systemic risk, cybersecure AI implementation produces stabilizing effects that extend beyond individual organizations. By enhancing institutional credibility, regulatory predictability, professional confidence, and patient engagement, cybersecurity functions as a cross-cutting enabler of sustainable digital health innovation. These stakeholder-specific dynamics reinforce the chapter's central argument that cybersecurity constitutes a strategic economic asset rather than a peripheral technical safeguard.

## 8. POLICY AND GOVERNANCE IMPLICATIONS

The economic evaluation of cybersecure AI systems has important implications for how healthcare institutions and regulators design governance structures, allocate resources, and balance innovation with risk management. This section examines how the Economics of Trust framework can inform policy and governance strategies that promote sustainable, secure, and economically efficient AI adoption in healthcare.

### 8.1 Aligning Cybersecurity Policy With Economic Incentives

A central implication of the EECAI framework is that cybersecurity policies should be aligned with economic incentives rather than minimum compliance thresholds. Traditional regulatory approaches often emphasize prescriptive controls or punitive enforcement, which can encourage organizations to adopt a checklist mentality focused on cost minimization rather than value creation. By contrast, economic evaluation reveals that proactive cybersecurity investment generates positive returns by reducing long-term risk exposure and stabilizing AI-enabled healthcare delivery. Policymakers can leverage this insight by designing incentive-based mechanisms such as funding support, reimbursement adjustments, or certification advantages that reward organizations for adopting economically efficient, trust-enhancing security practices. Aligning policy instruments with economic outcomes encourages healthcare institutions to internalize the long-term value of cybersecurity rather than treating it as an externally imposed burden.

### 8.2 Regulatory Compliance as Value Creation

The framework also reframes regulatory compliance as a source of economic value rather than a constraint on innovation. Compliance with data protection, AI governance, and cybersecurity standards reduces uncertainty, limits liability, and enhances institutional credibility with patients, clinicians, and technology partners. From an economic perspective, stable compliance environments lower transaction costs by reducing audit friction, legal disputes, and reactive remediation expenses. When cybersecurity governance is embedded early in AI system design, compliance costs are more predictable and less disruptive, contributing to smoother operational performance. This reframing has important implications for regulators: policies that emphasize integration of cybersecurity and AI governance throughout the system lifecycle are more likely to support innovation while maintaining safety and trust.

## 8.3 Integrating Economic Evaluation Into AI Governance Frameworks

A critical governance implication is the explicit integration of economic evaluation into AI and cybersecurity governance frameworks. Existing governance models often emphasize ethical principles and technical safeguards, yet they frequently overlook systematic assessment of economic trade-offs. The EECAI framework addresses this gap by embedding cost-effectiveness analysis, risk-adjusted valuation, and trust-based performance metrics directly into governance decision-making processes. Through this integration, organizations and regulators can compare alternative governance strategies based on economic efficiency, determine optimal levels of cybersecurity investment, and justify policy interventions using transparent, evidence-based criteria. By aligning ethical and technical objectives with measurable economic outcomes, incorporating economic evaluation enhances accountability, strengthens institutional legitimacy, and promotes more rational and sustainable governance of AI systems.

## 8.4 Institutional Governance and Cross-Functional Coordination

Effective governance of cybersecure AI systems requires cross-functional coordination across clinical leadership, IT security, compliance, and executive management. The framework highlights that fragmented governance structures undermine both security effectiveness and economic performance by creating misaligned incentives and accountability gaps. Institutions that adopt integrated governance models that jointly address cybersecurity, AI strategy, and economic planning are better positioned to manage systemic risk and sustain trust. Governance structures should therefore support shared responsibility for AI security outcomes and enable continuous learning and adaptation as technologies and threats evolve.

## 8.5 Toward Sustainable and Trust-Centered AI Regulation

The Economics of Trust advocates a shift toward trust-centered AI regulation, viewing trust as an economically significant outcome that can be cultivated through governance and cybersecurity investments. Secure, reliable AI enhances public confidence in digital healthcare, increasing adoption, utilization, and long-term value. Sustainable AI healthcare depends on maintaining this trust, enabling policymakers to balance innovation, safety, accountability, and fiscal responsibility by integrating trust dynamics and economic evaluation. Cybersecurity plays a crucial role in economic sustainability and trust, and the chapter concludes by summarizing key points and outlining future research directions.

## 9. FUTURE RESEARCH DIRECTIONS

While this chapter offers a structured economic framework for assessing cybersecure AI in healthcare, future research is necessary to refine it and support decision-making. Empirical validation of the EECAI framework using real-world healthcare data, including longitudinal studies on cybersecurity investments, AI adoption, and economic outcomes, is needed to estimate cost-effectiveness and to test trust proxies more effectively. Cross-jurisdictional research is vital, as healthcare systems differ in their regulations, cultures, and economies, which in turn affect cyber risk and trust. International comparisons could show how policies influence the economic performance of cybersecure AI. Additionally, integrating behavioral economics and decision theory would improve model predictions by understanding healthcare leaders' perceptions of risk and trust. Lastly, expanding focus to societal and equity issues is crucial, as cybersecurity failures can harm vulnerable populations by disrupting services and enabling data misuse. Future studies should explore how cybersecurity investments that preserve trust can foster not only financial efficiency but also equitable access, social welfare, and public confidence in AI healthcare.

## 10. CONCLUSION

This chapter argues that cybersecurity protects the economic value of healthcare AI by stabilizing trust, reducing risks, and supporting sustainable innovation. The rapid integration of AI has transformed healthcare delivery, with benefits dependent on secure, reliable digital infrastructure. Cybersecurity should be viewed as a strategic economic investment, not just a technical or regulatory requirement. Using insights from economics and AI governance, it introduces the Economics of Trust and the EECAI framework. The analysis shows cybersecurity adds value by reducing losses, building trust, and stabilizing adoption, leading to better long-term AI returns. Scenario analysis confirms secure AI outperforms insecure systems on a risk-adjusted, lifecycle basis.

The implications extend beyond individual organizations. For healthcare managers, the framework provides an economic rationale for proactive cybersecurity investment. For developers, it reinforces the value of secure-by-design and trust-aware AI systems. For policymakers, it offers a basis for aligning regulation with economic sustainability rather than minimum compliance. Ultimately, for patients and society, cybersecure AI systems represent a foundation for safe, reliable, and trustworthy digital healthcare. In an era where trust has become a critical currency of innovation, cybersecurity emerges as its principal guarantor. By reframing cybersecurity as a driver of economic and ethical resilience, this chapter contributes to a more holistic understanding of how AI can be deployed responsibly, efficiently, and sustainably in healthcare delivery.

## Conflict of Interest Declaration

The authors declare that they have no conflicts of interest regarding the publication of this chapter.

## AI Use Declaration

The authors acknowledge that artificial intelligence tools were used solely to improve language clarity and readability. The authors reviewed and approved all content and are fully responsible for the final version of this chapter.

## REFERENCES


Abbou, B., Kessel, B., Ben Natan, M., Gabbay-Benziv, R., Dahan Shriki, D., Ophir, A., Goldschmid, N., Klein, A., Roguin, A., & Dudkiewicz, M. (2024). When all computers shut down: The clinical impact of a major cyber-attack on a general hospital. *Frontiers in Digital Health*, *6*, 1321485. Advance online publication. DOI: 10.3389/fdgth.2024.1321485 PMID: 38433989

Abdulwahab, L. O. (2026a). Designing Inclusive and Economically Sustainable Health Reforms in the Digital Era: A Phygital Approach to Equity, Efficiency, and Engagement. In Phygital Insights on National Health Reform: Economics, Marketing, and Leadership (pp. 191–232). IGI Global Scientific Publishing. https://www.igi-global.com/chapter/designing-inclusive-and-economically-sustainable-health-reforms-in-the-digital-era/409192

Abdulwahab, L. O. (2026b). Governing Health Equity: The Political Economy of Public Health Investment and Access in the Global South. In The Political Economy of Global Healthcare Industries: States, Markets, and Power (pp. 117–158). IGI Global Scientific Publishing. https://www.igi-global.com/chapter/governing-health-equity/404997

Abdulwahab, L. O. (2026c). Health System Sustainability and Labor Market Participation in an Aging Workforce: Economic Implications and Policy Options. In The Economics of an Aging Workforce: Challenges, Opportunities, and Policy Perspectives (pp. 245–288). IGI Global Scientific Publishing. https://www.igi-global.com/chapter/health-system-sustainability-and-labor-market-participation-in-an-aging-workforce/409708

Abdulwahab, L. O., & Azam, H. (2026). Platform Work in Europe's Green and Care Economies: Regulatory Pathways for Sustainability, Social Protection, and Fair Work. In Regulating the Gig Economy in the European Union: Challenges, Innovations, and Global Impacts (pp. 99–124). IGI Global Scientific Publishing. https://www.igi-global.com/chapter/platform-work-in-europes-green-and-care-economies/395612

Al-Qahtani, L. A. S., Alsomali, M. M., Al-Hadad, A. M., Alfaraj, Z. A., Almutairi, S. T., Al-Anazi, T. A., Alshehri, S. A., Al-Fifi, N. J., & Alharbi, S. F. (2025). FACTORS AFFECTING THE INTEGRATION OF ELECTRONIC HEALTH RECORD WORKFLOWS AMONG NURSES, MIDWIVES, MEDICAL SECRETARIES, AND HEALTH INFORMATICS SPECIALISTS IN RIYADH HOSPITALS. Scientific Culture, 11(3.1), 565–574. DOI: 10.5281/zenodo.11032569

Alghamdi, S., Mehmood, R., Alqurashi, F. A., & Alzahrani, A. (2025). Paving the Roadmap for XAI and IML in Healthcare: Data-Driven Discoveries and the FIXAIH Framework. *IEEE Access : Practical Innovations, Open Solutions, 13*, 174393–174427. DOI: 10.1109/ACCESS.2025.3616353

Annie Silviya, S. H., Hilda Jerlin, C. M., Anirudh, G., Indresh Kumar, E., Renuka Devi, S., & Dilli Babu, M. (2025). Enhancing Host-Based Intrusion Detection: A NEAT-Optimized Ensemble Learning Approach. Int. Conf. Next Gener. Comput. Syst.: Intell. Syst. Sustain. Dev., ICNGCS - Conf. Proc. 2025 International Conference on Next Generation Computing Systems: Intelligent System for Sustainable Development, ICNGCS 2025 - Conference Proceedings. DOI: 10.1109/ICNGCS64900.2025.11183188

Ashrafi, E., Mosadeghrad, A. M., & Arab, M. (2025). Analysis of administrative health policies in healthcare organizations. *Journal of Health Administration, 28*(1), 56–75. DOI: 10.61882/jha.28.1.56

Barik, K., Misra, S., Fernandez-Sanz, L., & Koyuncu, M. (2023). RONSI: A framework for calculating return on network security investment. *Telecommunication Systems, 84*(4), 533–548. DOI: 10.1007/s11235-023-01039-9

Bhushan, S., & Dixit, S. (2024). Explainable AI for Shaping Adoption of Artificial Intelligence. Asian Conf. Intell. Technol., ACOIT. 2024 Asian Conference on Intelligent Technologies, ACOIT 2024. DOI: 10.1109/ACOIT62457.2024.10939416

Boonen, T. J., Feng, Y., & Tong, Z. (2025). Cybersecurity investments and cyber insurance purchases in a non-cooperative game. *ASTIN Bulletin, 55*(2), 426–448. DOI: 10.1017/asb.2024.40

Brohi, S., & Mastoi, Q.-U.-A. (2025). AI Under Attack: Metric-Driven Analysis of Cybersecurity Threats in Deep Learning Models for Healthcare Applications. *Algorithms, 18*(3), 157. Advance online publication. DOI: 10.3390/a18030157

Butani, J. B. (2026). AI-Based Zero Trust Security Models for Cloud Computing. Commun. Comput. Info. Sci., 2669 CCIS, 509–518. DOI: 10.1007/978-3-032-07373-0_37

Chakkaravarthy, A. P., & Jaganathan, D. (2025). Intersecting AI and Medicine for Improved Care and Administrative Efficiency. In Ali, O., Amini, A., & Al-Ahmad, A. (Eds.), *Intersecting AI and Medicine for Improved Care and Administrative Efficiency* (pp. 39–58). IGI Global., DOI: 10.4018/979-8-3373-1772-4.ch002

Chatzikou, M., Latsou, D., Apostolidis, G., Billis, A., Charisis, V., Rigas, E. S., Bamidis, P. D., & Hadjileontiadis, L. (2025). Economic Evaluation of Artificially Intelligent (AI) Diagnostic Systems: Cost Consequence Analysis of Clinician-Friendly Interpretable Computer-Aided Diagnosis (ICADX) Tested in Cardiology, Obstetrics, and Gastroenterology, from the HosmartAI Horizon 2020 Project. *Healthcare (Basel), 13*(14), 1661. Advance online publication. DOI: 10.3390/healthcare13141661 PMID: 40724686

Chavan, R., & Shabadi, S. (2025). Cyber Security in Healthcare. In Mahalle, P. N., Shinde, G. R., Wasatkar, N. N., & Anerao, P. R. (Eds.), *Industry 5.0 for Society 5.0: Advancing Medical IoT and Smart Healthcare* (pp. 165–175). Bentham Science Publishers., DOI: 10.2174/97988988104501250100011

Chong, W. F., Feng, R., Hu, H., & Zhang, L. (2025). Cyber risk assessment for capital management. *The Journal of Risk and Insurance, 92*(2), 424–471. DOI: 10.1111/jori.12504

Choudhury, P., & Goel, P. (2025). Interface of Artificial Intelligence with Conventional Biostatistics in Healthcare Research. In *Methods in Molecular Biology* (Vol. 2952, pp. 411–428). Humana Press Inc., DOI: 10.1007/978-1-0716-4690-8_22

Daly, S. J., Hearn, G., & Papageorgiou, K. (2025). Sensemaking with AI: How trust influences Human-AI collaboration in health and creative industries. *Social Sciences & Humanities Open, 11*, 101346. Advance online publication. DOI: 10.1016/j.ssaho.2025.101346

Das, P., Gupta, I., & Mishra, S. (2024). Artificial intelligence driven cybersecurity in digital healthcare frameworks. In Gupta, D., & Hassanien, A. E. (Eds.), *Securing Next-Generation Connected Healthcare Systems: Artificial Intelligence Technologies* (pp. 213–228). Elsevier., DOI: 10.1016/B978-0-443-13951-2.00002-7

De Morais Rodrigues, L. E., Santos, G. N., Bonamigo, A., Garza-Reyes, J. A., Calado, R. D., & Santos, A. B. (2025). Empirical Evaluation of the Emergency Care Ecosystem Using Artificial Intelligence for Decision-Makers' Support. IEEE Int. Conf. Ind. Appl., INDUSCON - Proc., 1012–1018. DOI: 10.1109/INDUSCON66435.2025.11241784

El Arab, R. A., & Al Moosa, O. A. (2025). Systematic review of cost effectiveness and budget impact of artificial intelligence in healthcare. *NPJ Digital Medicine, 8*(1), 548. Advance online publication. DOI: 10.1038/s41746-025-01722-y PMID: 40858882

Fotis, F. (2024). Economic Impact of Cyber Attacks and Effective Cyber Risk Management Strategies: A light literature review and case study analysis. *Procedia Computer Science*, *251*, 471–478. DOI: 10.1016/j.procs.2024.11.135

Ghosh, O., Kumar, B., & Roy, P. K. (2025). Role of AI in revolutionizing clinical care. In Tariq, M. U. (Ed.), *Emerging Multisector Applications of AI and IoT* (pp. 69–102). IGI Global., DOI: 10.4018/979-8-3373-4332-7.ch003

He, Y., Xin, T., & Luo, C. (2025). Enhancing Cybersecurity Investment with FAIR-ROSI: A Responsible Cybersecurity Approach to Digital Society. *Information Systems Frontiers*. Advance online publication. DOI: 10.1007/s10796-025-10625-y PMID: 42206284

Jourdain, D. (2026). Cybersecurity for Interventional Radiologists: A Clinical Imperative for Protecting Patient Data and Imaging Systems. *Journal of Vascular and Interventional Radiology*, *37*(3), 107920. Advance online publication. DOI: 10.1016/j.jvir.2025.107920 PMID: 41270935

Kavitha, N., Nivethitha, T., Deebanchakkarawarthi, G., & Shakthipriya, P. (2025). Transforming Healthcare: Unleashing the Power of Artificial Intelligence of Things (AIoT). In Rajasekaran, A. S., Al-Turjman, F., & Suganyadevi, S. (Eds.), *AIoT: Artificial Intelligence of Things* (pp. 99–129). CRC Press., DOI: 10.1201/9781003482338-5

Kim, Y. J., Park, Y. S., & Park, S.-P. (2026). Enhancing data governance through transparency: An empirical study of the data trust model. *Technological Forecasting and Social Change*, *225*, 124551. Advance online publication. DOI: 10.1016/j.techfore.2026.124551

Latif, R. M. A., Mamarasulov, S., Farhan, M., Ullah, F., & Ahmad, J. (2026). Explainability of AI in Multimedia Security: Bridging the Gap between Complexity and Trust. In Srivastava, V. K., Khare, P., Awasthi, D., & Garg, L. (Eds.), *Multimedia And Multimodal Intelligence For Sustainable Development* (pp. 1–22). CRC Press., DOI: 10.1201/9781003634522-1

Leenen, J. P. L., Hiemstra, P., Ten Hoeve, M. M., Jansen, A. C. J., van Dijk, J. D., Vendel, B., Versteeg, G., Hakvoort, G. A., & Hettinga, M. (2025). Exploring the complex nature of implementation of Artificial intelligence in clinical practice: An interview study with healthcare professionals, researchers and Policy and Governance Experts. PLOS Digital Health, 4(5 May). DOI: 10.1371/journal.pdig.0000847

Mandava, R., Vellela, S. S., Gorintla, S., Dalavai, L., Malathi, N., & Haritha, K. (2025). Evaluating the Impact of Explainable AI on User Trust in Financial Decision-Support Systems. Int. Conf. Comput. Robot., Test. Eng. Eval., ICCRTEE. International Conference on Computational Robotics, Testing and Engineering Evaluation, ICCRTEE 2025. DOI: 10.1109/ICCRTEE64519.2025.11052919

Mbacop, T. L., De La Cruz, E., Nadella, G. S., Le, H., De La Cruz, A. M., & Oni, O. (2025). Exploring Cybersecurity Challenges, Strategies, and Implications in Healthcare: A Qualitative Study. IEEE Integr. STEM Educ. Conf., ISEC. 2025 15th IEEE Integrated STEM Education Conference, ISEC 2025. DOI: 10.1109/ISEC64801.2025.11147260

Moussa, F. Z., & Zine-Dine, K. (2025). The impact of cyber-attacks on cybersecurity investment game model. *Chaos, Solitons, and Fractals*, *200*, 117040. Advance online publication. DOI: 10.1016/j.chaos.2025.117040

Musa, A., & Abdulfatai, A. O. (2024). Artificial intelligence for secured cybersecurity in emerging healthcare systems. In A. L. Imoize, C. Meshram, J. B. Awotunde, Y. Farhaoui, & D.-T. Do (Eds.), Cybersecurity in Emerging Healthcare Systems (pp. 203–240). Institution of Engineering and Technology. DOI: 10.1049/PBHE064E_ch7

Ngo, C., & Wright, C. B. (2024). EFFECTIVE INTEGRATION OF COMMERCIAL AND OPERATIONAL RISKS. Proc. Bienn. Int. Pipeline Conf. IPC, 5. DOI: 10.1115/IPC2024-134036

Nikolaev, A. A. (2025). An integrative model for health technology assessment: Perspectives for the Russian healthcare system. *Health Care of the Russian Federation*, *69*(5), 416–422. DOI: 10.47470/0044-197X-2025-69-5-416-422

Nunez Migliorisi, T. N. (2025). Healthcare Data Breaches: Diving in the Dark. Lect. Notes Networks Syst., 1424 LNNS, 587–602. DOI: 10.1007/978-3-031-92605-1_36

Onatuyeh, E. A., Oghorodi, D., Okpako, E. A., Ojei, E., Osakwe, G., Chinedu, N. B., Okoh, S. K., Odu, V. C., Chinedu, P. U., & Nwankwo, W. (2025). CYBERSECURITY AND BUSINESS SURVIVAL IN NIGERIA: BUILDING CUSTOMER'S TRUST. *African Journal of Applied Research*, *11*(1), 786–813. DOI: 10.26437/ajar.v11i1.882

Oriaro, S., & Mishra, S. (2025). Improving cybersecurity through explainable artificial intelligence: A systematic literature review. *Issues in Information Systems*, *26*(3), 387–400. DOI: 10.48009/3_iis_2025_2025_131

Posso, R., & Altmann, J. (2025). Trust and Trust-Building Policies to Support Cybersecurity Information Sharing: A Systematic Literature Review. Lect. Notes Comput. Sci., 15358 LNCS, 212–228. DOI: 10.1007/978-3-031-81226-2_19

Pratama, I. P. A. E., Widyantara, I. M. O., Linawati, L., & Gunantara, N. (2025). Bibliometric Analysis of AI-Based Prototype Proposal for User Security Awareness in Healthcare. *JOIV: International Journal on Informatics Visualization, 9*(3), 982–994. DOI: 10.62527/joiv.9.3.3319

Ranwala, R. A. D. L. M. K., & Andrade, A. Q. (2025). Enhancing AI Clinical Decision Support Trust: Design Workshop Insights from General Practitioners. *Studies in Health Technology and Informatics, 329*, 593–597. DOI: 10.3233/SHTI250909 PMID: 40775927

Rattanapong, P., Sukma, N., & Darakorn Na Ayuthaya, S. (2025). Determinants of cybersecurity investment in ASEAN organizations: An integrated structural equation modeling approach. *Frontiers in Communications and Networks, 6*, 1594554. Advance online publication. DOI: 10.3389/frcmn.2025.1594554

Rongali, S. K. (2025). AI-Powered Threat Detection in Healthcare Data. Int. Conf. Artif. Intell. Mach. Vis., AIMV. 2025 International Conference on Artificial Intelligence and Machine Vision, AIMV 2025. DOI: 10.1109/AIMV66517.2025.11203733

Sajid, S. Nazir, Mohd., & Aijaz, M. (2025). Beyond Severity: Tactical Risk Scoring for Healthcare Vulnerabilities. Int. Conf. Multidiscip. Res. Innov. Eng., MRIE, 427–432. DOI: 10.1109/MRIE66930.2025.11156632

Santos, A. R., Sampaio, F., Londral, A. R., & Perelman, J. (2025). Mapping methodologies for economic assessment of digital health technologies: A scoping review protocol. *BMJ Open, 15*(7), e099933. Advance online publication. DOI: 10.1136/bmjopen-2025-099933 PMID: 40750290

Santos, A. R., von Hafe, F., Sampaio, F., Londral, A. R., & Perelman, J. (2025). Mapping Methodologies for Economic Evaluation of Digital Health Technologies: A Scoping Review. *Value in Health : The Journal of the International Society for Pharmacoeconomics and Outcomes Research*. Advance online publication. DOI: 10.1016/j.jval.2025.09.012 PMID: 41015334

Shafrin, J., Kim, J., Cohen, J. T., Garrison, L. P., Goldman, D. A., Doshi, J. A., Krieger, J., Lakdawalla, D. N., Neumann, P. J., Phelps, C. E., Whittington, M. D., & Willke, R. (2024). Valuing the Societal Impact of Medicines and Other Health Technologies: A User Guide to Current Best Practices. *Forum for Health Economics & Policy, 27*(1), 29–116. DOI: 10.1515/fhep-2024-0014 PMID: 39512185

Shukla, A. (2025). AI for Healthcare Security: The Intersection of Innovation and Resilience. Commun. Comput. Info. Sci., 2404 CCIS, 109–127. DOI: 10.1007/978-3-031-85558-0_6

Sindiramutty, S. R., Jhanjhi, N. Z., & Khan, N. A. (2025). AI in healthcare safeguarding patient privacy and confidentiality. In Hussain, K. (Ed.), *Vulnerabilities Assessment and Risk Management in Cyber Security* (pp. 369–404). IGI Global., DOI: 10.4018/979-8-3693-6135-1.ch015

Sirbu, C. L., & Mercioni, M. A. (2024). Fostering Trust in AI-Driven Healthcare: A Brief Review of Ethical and Practical Considerations. Int. Symp. Electron. Telecommun., ISETC - Conf. Proc. 2024 16th International Symposium on Electronics and Telecommunications, ISETC 2024 - Conference Proceedings. DOI: 10.1109/ISETC63109.2024.10797264

Tariq, M. U. (2024). Enhancing cybersecurity protocols in modern healthcare systems: Strategies and best practices. In Garcia, M. B., & de Almeida, R. P. P. (Eds.), *Transformative Approaches to Patient Literacy and Healthcare Innovation* (pp. 223–241). IGI Global., DOI: 10.4018/979-8-3693-3661-8.ch011

Theilmann, K., Dahlem, N., Steffny, L., Podevin, D., Hartnik, J., & Greff, T. (2025). Towards Effective AI in Healthcare: Identifying Success Factors and the Potential of Human-in-the-Loop. IFIP Advances in Information and Communication Technology, 755 IFIPAICT, 173–188. DOI: 10.1007/978-3-031-96239-4_13

Tick, A., & Szabo-Harka, N. (2024). Analysis of Information Security in a Corporate Environment-a Human Perspective. IEEE World Symp. Appl. Mach. Intell. Informatics, SAMI - Proc., 469–474. DOI: 10.1109/SAMI60510.2024.10432889

van Kessel, R., Ranganathan, S., Anderson, M., McMillan, B., & Mossialos, E. (2024). Exploring potential drivers of patient engagement with their health data through digital platforms: A scoping review. *International Journal of Medical Informatics*, *189*, 105513. Advance online publication. DOI: 10.1016/j.ijmedinf.2024.105513 PMID: 38851132

Vasilica, B.-V., Anton, F. D., Mocanu, S., & Chiriac, B. N. (2025). Implementation and Evaluation of a Zero-Trust Security Model in Distributed Industrial Networks. Proc. - Int. Conf. Control Syst. Comput. Sci., CSCS, 243–250. DOI: 10.1109/CSCS66924.2025.00044

Wosny, M. (2025). Understanding the Root Causes of Healthcare Professionals' Frustration with Digital Tools. *Studies in Health Technology and Informatics*, *323*, 344–348. DOI: 10.3233/SHTI250109 PMID: 40200506

Wu, W.-T., Chao, Y.-W., Lin, T.-K., Huang, C.-K., & Hsieh, P.-H. (2025). Economic evaluation of AI-assisted technologies in healthcare: A systematic review. *Journal of Food and Drug Analysis*, *33*(4), 487–500. DOI: 10.38212/2224-6614.3570 PMID: 41525195

Zakiyah, N., Marulin, D., Alfaqeeh, M., Puspitasari, I. M., Lestari, K., Lim, K. K., & Fox-Rushby, J. (2024). Economic Evaluations of Digital Health Interventions for Patients With Heart Failure: Systematic Review. *Journal of Medical Internet Research*, *26*, e53500. Advance online publication. DOI: 10.2196/53500 PMID: 38687991

Zhao, L., Wu, X., Li, J., & Tong, H. (2025). Economics of Cybersecurity Investment and Information Sharing: Firm Decision Making Under Policy Constraints. *Systems*, *13*(2), 83. Advance online publication. DOI: 10.3390/systems13020083

# Chapter 9
# Designing for Compassion Through Emotional and Artificial Intelligence to Enhance Workforce Wellbeing in Healthcare

**Krishnaveni Subramani**
http://orcid.org/0009-0000-9785-4595
*SR University, India*

**Geetha Manoharan**
http://orcid.org/0000-0002-8644-8871
*SR University, India*

## ABSTRACT

*The health care systems are increasing both emotional and operational pressures that affect the clinical workforce's well-being and patient care quality. Compassion, which has always been seen as the symbol of the healthcare practice, tends to worsen when the workload pressure was high, time runs out, and the complexity of the administration was overwhelming. Simultaneously, artificial intelligence was being deployed more often in clinical decision support, workflow organization, and communication. This change provides possibilities and threats to the continuity of human contact in care settings. The principles of emotional intelligence used to inform the application of AI towards the practices that would safeguard the role of clinicians, relational sensitivity, and psychological resilience. The chapter draws on*

DOI: 10.4018/979-8-3373-9119-9.ch009

*the idea of Compassion-Centered Hybrid Intelligence (CCHI), which was a model that integrates both emotional intelligence and artificial intelligence to enhance compassionate practice and support the well-being of the workforce.*

## INTRODUCTION

Healthcare settings exist under a constant load of pressure due to the increase in the number of patients, complicated medical conditions, and constant reorganization of the organizations (Morrow et al., 2023). The clinical roles require long-term attention, quick clinical decision-making, and emotional contact with people who have lost, are in pain, or are feeling uncertain (Dey, 2024). Such a mixture generates an environment in which emotional work stable and severe (Graves and Compson, 2024). The traditional understanding of compassion has been considered the fundamental aspect of professional identity and therapeutic practice that implies awareness of suffering, emotional needs, and supportive response (Cinar & Bilodeau, 2024). Studies are still showing that humane communication can help to increase patient satisfaction, trust in providers, and anxiety in the treatment process (Hernandez, 2024; Cho et al., 2024). Nevertheless, organizational facilities tend to be more focused on quantifiable efficiency, speed in the execution of tasks, and uniformity of procedural processes at the cost of time that can be used in relational communication. Compassionate expression forced due to documentation requirements, staffing constraints, and pressures of shifts, not because it was unintended but because the system does not support it (Dailah et al., 2024; Kleinrichert, 2024). Such degradation of relational presence was a factor that leads to emotional burnout and lowers empathy ability in the long term (Arora et al., 2024).

The concept of digital transformation in healthcare exposes healthcare to new technologies in the workflow of diagnoses, treatment planning, communication systems, and administrative activities (George et al., 2024). Artificial Intelligence (AI) also adds predictive analytics, schemes, image recognition, and robotic documentation capabilities that have the potential to lessen mental load and redundancy (Papadopoulos and Lazzarino, 2024). These systems have the promise of reprioritizing clinician efforts on direct-patient care. Nevertheless, AI implementation produces another effect on communication relationships and emotional bond perceptions (Mitsea et al., 2024). Automated interfaces can be associated with depersonalization of care in case the emotional context was not deliberately included (Gyrard et al., 2023). Subtle affective cues, tone modulations, and empathic attunements are some of the elements of clinical interactions that do not necessarily receive high priority during computational processes (DeTore et al., 2024). Thus, the development of emotional sensitivity should be a central part of AI because it was the only way to preserve the quality of relations and ethical delivery of care (He et al., 2023).

Emotional Intelligence (EI) involves the ability to identify one's own feelings, understand the feelings of other people, manage the internal feelings, and approach interpersonal communication considerately (Jonas et al., 2024). In healthcare, EI aids teamwork, patient relationships, conflict management, and survivability in the most stressful situations (Creed et al., 2022). Enhancing EI at organizational levels was associated with leadership modeling, reflective practice, training, and policies that ensure that emotional labor was recognized as a professional skill (Peng et al., 2022). Once emotional intelligence was implemented in the organizational culture, clinicians are more attentive and empathic with equal measure and less moral distress (Levin et al., 2024). This promotes psychological safety and sustainable practices of compassionate care (Higgins et al., 2024).

Compassion-Centered Hybrid Intelligence was a model that suggests that AI and EI be used together to support the provision of compassionate care (Levin et al., 2024). Hybrid intelligence acknowledges that AI could be efficient, identify patterns, and make predictions, whereas humans can judge, be emotional, and have an ethical sense (Sharma et al., 2023). Al, it can help to be compassionate by reducing administrative workload, detecting emotional distress indicators, or encouraging supportive communication patterns. Clinicians still be in charge of relational connection and empathic interpretation. By making technological innovation in line with the ability of the human emotion, compassion can be kept at the center of healthcare identity and practice.

To maintain the standards of compassionate care, organizational support of well-being, reflective learning, and relational practice, therefore, was needed (Vial and Almon, 2023). A combination of Compassion-Centered Hybrid Intelligence into the workflow design, professional development, and assessment systems facilitate the coexistence of clinical excellence and human understanding. This framework creates the environment where compassion was not an extra undertaking but a reinforced and renewable part of everyday practice.

## CONCEPTUAL FOUNDATIONS OF COMPASSION-CENTERED HYBRID INTELLIGENCE (CCHI)

### Defining Compassion in Clinical Practice

Compassion in clinical practice was a dynamic and deliberate reaction to the misery of patients based on understanding, feeling, and a promise to act in their support. It includes identification of vulnerability, distress recognition, and meaningful interaction that upholds dignity. Compassion goes beyond sympathetic comprehension and was a relational one that was developed through listening attentiveness, presence, and responsiveness. In healthcare, compassion was a fundamental professional value that shapes therapeutic alliances, trust and healing experiences with patients. It was a human-to-human relationship, which facilitates psychological comfort and clinical results, as shown in figure 1.

Clinical practices often imply complicated emotional environments in which illness, uncertainty, and fear come together with individual backgrounds and cultural significance. Compassion-oriented practice was a combination of cognitive knowledge about the needs of the patients and the affective, ethical care. It calls on clinicians to be present and open even in stressful circumstances, which can be both verbal and non-verbal displays of concern. This meaning of compassion was neither an emotional over-identification nor a form of empathy but rather a felt harmony between empathy and a sound professional judgment. This balance was a healthy source of a caring environment that complies with patient autonomy but fosters comfort and reassurance.

*Figure 1. Defining Compassion in Clinical Practice*

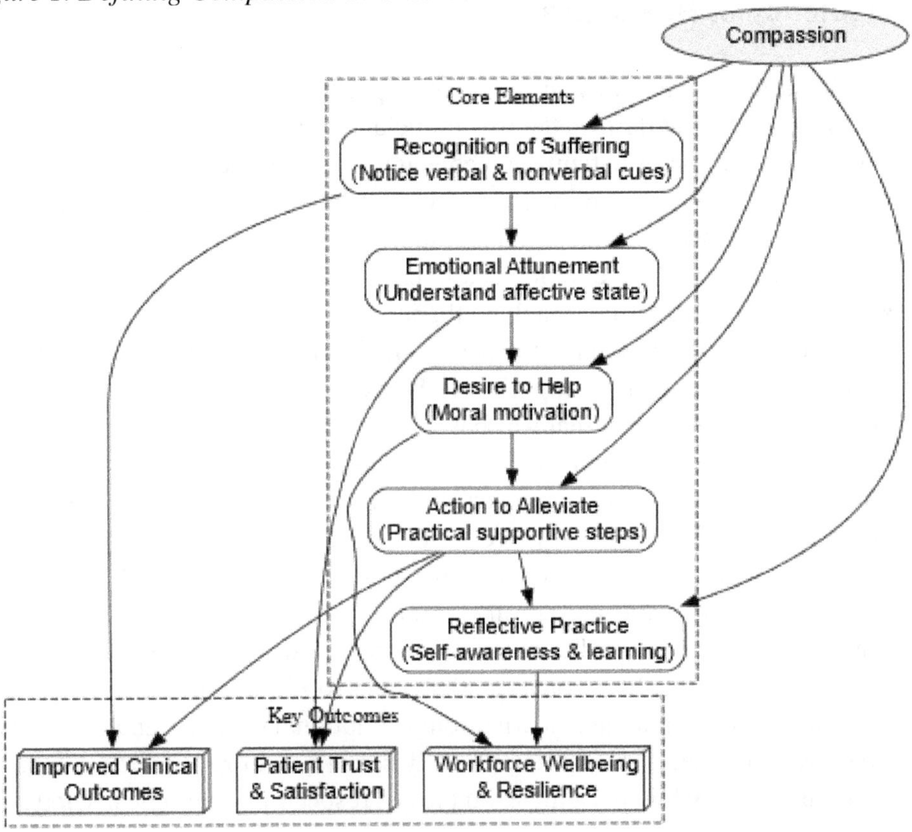


Maintaining the compassion was contingent on the environmental factors, organizational culture, and the working loads. Compassion was not merely an individual character but occurs in systems that either support or inhibit emotional availability. Busy timetables, heavy workloads, and inadequate time to engage in reflective practice undermine caring presence, which causes emotional exhaustion and impersonality. In order to maintain compassionate care as a collective clinical norm, supportive infrastructures, reflective spaces, and relational communication practices are used. With the help of training, leadership modeling, and workflow design, compassion as an inseparable part of healthcare delivery reinforced, leading to strengthened patient experience and workforce well-being.

## Emotional Intelligence as a Professional Competency in Healthcare

Emotional intelligence was an important aspect of professional competence in health care settings that defines the way clinicians perceive, interpret, and react to the emotional situation of patients and colleagues. The clinical work was the constant interpersonal interaction in cases of vulnerability, uncertainties, and human suffering. The ability to detect emotional responses, control the inner responses, and stay calm in the face of the complicated interactions facilitates building trust and therapeutic relationships. Emotional intelligence thus leads to the provision of care that recognizes the personhood of the patient, maintaining the dignity and safety of the relationship in the clinical experience. This competency was a relational skill set and an ethical orientation that was based on attentiveness and presence.

Healthcare teams operate in challenging and uncertain conditions where moral tension, stress, and time-constrained decision-making are often present. Emotional intelligence helps in building resilience, as it helps the professionals to take the distressing events without losing empathic engagement. Clinicians who have strongly developed emotional awareness are likely to be more effective in conveying their messages, responding to conflict more patiently, and working more efficiently in multidisciplinary teams. Emotional intelligence also plays a role in the reflective practice, as it helps a clinician to learn through emotional response and not be overwhelmed by it. Leaders who are emotionally sensitive in organizational contexts shape culture at work by providing examples of respect, psychological safety, and compassionate accountability.

Emotional Intelligence Training as a planned professional skill was in line with combating burnout, compassion fatigue, and labor instability. The conditions provided by structured reflection programs, peer support models, mentorship, and relational communication training make clinicians more emotionally resilient. The presence of emotional intelligence in the curricula, within performance systems, and among leadership approaches was an indication of acknowledging emotional labor as a valid and critical part of healthcare work. Emotional intelligence training maintains a healthier workforce, as it assists in ensuring the quality of human care as well as professional engagement sustainability. This ability therefore plays a central role in the creation of healthcare systems that emphasize compassion and well-being as well as technical and procedural excellence.

## ARTIFICIAL INTELLIGENCE IN CONTEMPORARY HEALTHCARE SYSTEMS

AI has been integrated into numerous healthcare processes to complement diagnostic processes and predictive analytics, office operations, and patient-facing applications. Machine learning algorithms to interpret the images, risk stratification, drug discovery, and real-time tracking of physiological indicators are now incorporated in clinical settings. Digital systems assist clinicians to analyze data quickly and identify patterns that allow them to act immediately and also minimize delays that come with manual review. Figure 2 illustrate the rise of AI-based tools depicts the transition to data-enhanced care systems where computational intelligence was used in conjunction with human judgment.

The use of AI in the infrastructure of healthcare organizations has become a common trend in the pursuit of operational efficiency and lessening cognitive load among clinical staff. Algorithms used to automate routine documentation and improve schedule optimization and supply chain coordination, which allow spending time on direct contact with patients. Decision-support platforms combine significant amounts of medical histories, clinical guidelines, and population-wide data to help in the creation of evidence-based treatment plans. This integration allows the creation of more structured care environment where information flows across departments and across care teams.

*Figure 2. Artificial Intelligence in Contemporary Healthcare Systems*

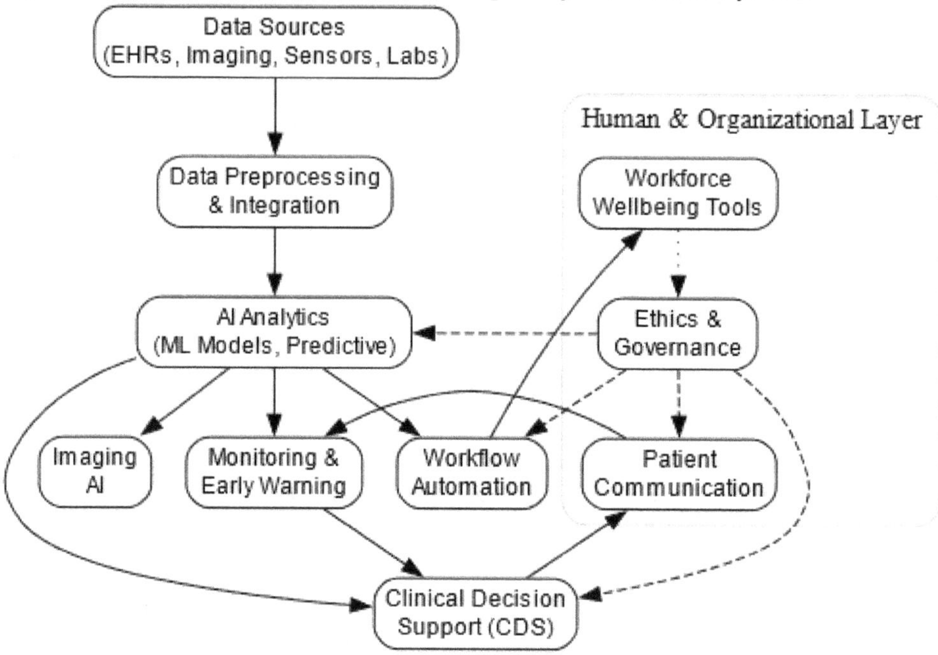


The growth of AI applications in the healthcare setting was also associated with concerns about the maintenance of humanistic principles in clinical practice. The automated decision layers have the ability to modify the relational relationship between clinicians and patients, especially where there was a shift to screen-based communication. Devoid of a reflexive design based on caring and ethical accountability, the digital systems are likely to promote efficiency-driven working processes that decrease chances of emotional interaction. The solution to the issue was a balance between technical possibilities and the humanistic principle of patient care so that AI should be viewed as an empowering ally that enhances, but does not weaken, the quality of face-to-face care.

## RISKS OF DEPERSONALIZATION AND OVER-RELIANCE ON AUTOMATION

The patterns of interaction between healthcare workers and patients are frequently redesigned by the artificial intelligence introduced into clinical workflows. In situations where digital systems are involved in communication, triage, or documentation, the personal connection changed to a norm-based interaction based on automated requests. Task-oriented interactions can be transferred to the past practices where clinical encounters were built on active listening, presence, and mutual emotional grasp. Depersonalization occurs when interfaces begin to filter human experience in such a way that efficiency was prioritized over relations. An environment where automation was the main influence decrease the room to express emotion, develop narrative, and respond to the nuances that culminate in compassion.

Increased automation distorts professional judgment because it promotes automatic acceptance of the results provided by algorithms without thoughtful consideration. The emergence of decision support platforms that seem more accurate and definitive compel clinicians to follow the outputs of the system even in complicated scenarios that require subtlety. With machine direction in the assessment and care plan, professional identity and autonomy are limited. There was also emotional work, which was relocated as technology eliminates some types of interpersonal interaction, leaving unexpressed psycho-emotional burdens out of high-stakes circumstances. The concept of sustainable compassionate practice demands the spaces where digital tools are not used as a defining factor of interaction but as supportive resources. The alignment of AI applications with relational care values ensures the protection of the human aspect of the clinical encounter and the emotional presence of the clinical encounter that ensures meaningful caregiving.

## HYBRID INTELLIGENCE: COLLABORATIVE HUMAN–MACHINE DECISION-MAKING

Hybrid intelligence was a model where the human cognitive, ethical, and emotional abilities collaborate with the computational processing, pattern recognition, and automated support facilities. In the healthcare settings, such a hybrid role introduces clinical prudence, experience, and humane expertise into the discussion with evidence-based analysis, forecasting, and constant observation opportunities. This kind of integration provides the opportunity to conduct decision-making processes based on the strengths of human professionals and artificial systems, which creates conditions of balanced, context-sensitive, and relationally sensitive care delivery.

Human-machine decision-making was a process of collaboration that occurs in a set of systematic interaction points by means of which clinicians make judgments based on the recommendations provided by AI and evaluate the nuances of the situation and employ moral arguments that are based on patient-focused values and priorities of care. AI elements bring on board large-scale data inference and quick identification of a sophisticated pattern that not be noticed by the human clinician. Narrative knowledge, emotional sensitivity, and social, cultural, and relational understanding are all provided by human professionals. This reciprocal complementarity contributes to clinical practices that are scientifically knowledgeable and compassionate. Successful teamwork means having system feedback available, easy-to-follow explanation channels, and training that instills a sense of confidence to interpret algorithmic results.

Compassion integration into hybrid intelligence settings requires purposeful system design by putting an emphasis on emotional awareness, supportive communication, and relational sensitivity. The elements of AI can be utilized to decrease cognitive load, give reflective cues in the case of an emotionally taxing interaction, and give stress warning signs to a team of healthcare providers. The clinicians still have the responsibility of acting in a manner that demonstrates professional empathy, ethical sensitivity, and patient-centered care values. Distributing both cognitive and emotional loads among human and machine actors, hybrid intelligence spaces open the possibility of the workforce maintaining compassionate interactions even under the influence of challenging clinical loads. This practice makes compassion not a solitary individual action but an assisted, group, and technologically facilitated practice in the healthcare delivery process.

## THE ETHICAL IMPERATIVE FOR COMPASSION-ORIENTED DIGITAL INNOVATION

Digital innovation in healthcare should be compassion-centered and therefore needs a value base of recognizing the emotional, relational, and moral aspects of clinical practice. Technology was often introduced to the care setting with a focus on efficiency, productivity, and standardization of procedures. These priorities define working habits, the expectations of professionalism, and the way of interacting with the patient. Figure 3 showing the emotional meaning of caregiving experiences has been underestimated when technological systems are used to focus on measurable outputs only. Competent compassion-based digital innovation aims to balance the technological growth with the ethical culture of healthcare by protecting human dignity, emotional presence, and trustful relationships. This congruence suggests that compassion was not a subjective emotion but rather a fundamental value that can be used to design the system and make decisions in the organization.

Artificial intelligence tools are still used in the field of diagnosis, workflow coordination, monitoring systems, and communication procedures. Such instruments determine the relationship of healthcare professionals to their patients and peers, the development of emotional labor, and the formation of clinical judgments in stressful situations. When digital systems fail to consider the compassionate aspect, clinical interactions tend to assume transactional patterns that restrict empathy, reflective awareness, and understanding. An empathetic design strategy motivates software developers, medical organizations, and policymakers to incorporate emotional intelligence skills into digital systems. This tactic reinforces enabling conditions in which clinicians do not lose the ability to respond sensitively, patiently, and with moral satisfaction.

*Figure 3. The Ethical Imperative for Compassion-Oriented Digital Innovation*

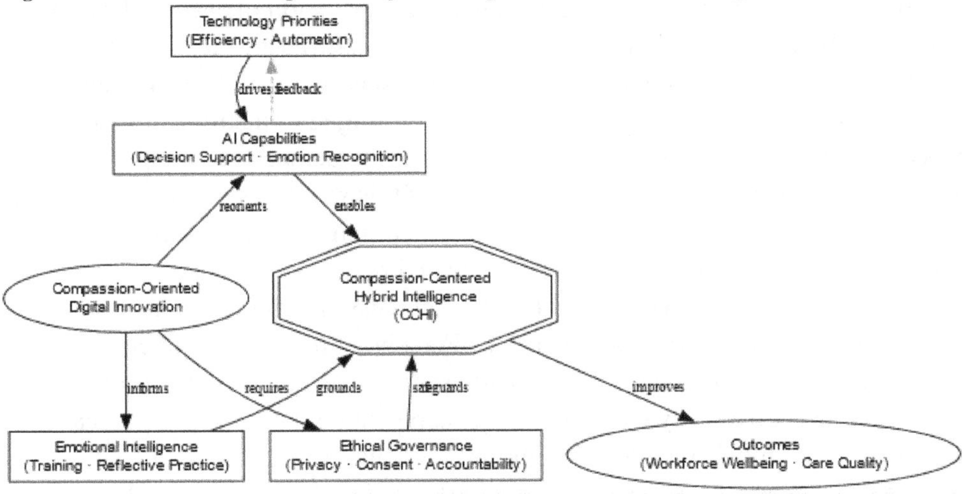


Digital healthcare ethics entails ethical duty that considers the vulnerability that exists within the process of patient experience and the emotions that healthcare providers bear with it. Compassion-oriented innovation fosters organizational cultures in which emotional expression was validated, reflective practice was institutionalized, and technology can help and not hurt relational care. The moral duty goes beyond the avoidance of harm; it demands the positive development of circumstances that foster health, decency, and human relationships. A compassionate culture helps to sustain a healthy workforce morale, build therapeutic relationships, and remember the primary goal of healthcare, to relieve suffering in both clinical and emotional aspects.

# EMOTIONAL INTELLIGENCE IN HEALTHCARE WORKFORCE WELLBEING

## Emotional Labor and Relational Demands in Clinical Work

Clinical practice was long-term emotional contact, constant interpersonal sensitivity, and paying attention to patients, families, and colleagues. Healthcare professionals often find themselves in care setups suffering, uncertain, fearful, and grieving and have to control their emotions consistently and present empathic messages. Even when the inside emotions are of fatigue or distress, emotional expressions are usually required to be altered to suit the demands of professionalism, reassurance, and compassion. The expression of this work was often interpreted as emotional labor, which goes well beyond the accomplishment of clinical work and directly adds to the perceived quality of care and patient experience.

Clinical relationships require a continuous process of striking a balance between decision-making and emotional sensitivity. Perceiving the nuances of communication, the ability to react to emotional manifestations, and the skill to communicate the comprehension are key elements in the therapeutic relationships. Clinical staff have to work with different cultural groups, personal backgrounds, and emotional reactions, and must have adaptive empathy and situational sensitivity. Such relational responsibilities are experienced in the context of busy schedules that are conditioned by time, workload, and institutional demands on employees, and which impose constant pressure on emotional resources. The commodity of compassion has a tendency of being used over and over again without some systematic replenishment.

The emotional work that lacks proper organizational support also be a contributor to compassion fatigue, depersonalization, and low levels of psychological well-being. The thing was that, as the emotional demands accumulate without the possibility of recovery, reflection, and relational reinforcement, the clinicians experience a decreasing ability to be present and connected. The given dynamic has an impact not only on personal well-being but also on team communication, patient trust, and quality of care outcomes. Understanding emotional labor as inherent to clinical practice, and not an incidental by-product of technical skill, motivates healthcare systems to create conditions, technologies, and policies that ensure and enhance the emotional resilience of the workforce.

## Components of Emotional Intelligence Relevant to Patient Care

Emotional intelligence in the healthcare practice involves the abilities that help comprehend, interpret, and react to emotional dynamics in the clinical interactions. Self-awareness was an underlying element, as it allows clinicians to be aware of emotional reactions to severe, doubtful, or stressful clinical scenarios. Given personal responsiveness, one can consciously modify the tone, language, and presence to respond to a patient. The next capacity was self-regulation, which was the complementary capacity, which directs the clinician to deal with internal stress and avoid emotional overload that disrupt judgment, communication, and clear vision of the therapeutic process. These abilities are some of the reasons why these settings are characterized by suffering, critical decision-making, and time-constrained interventions needed to be stable and emotionally steady as showed in figure 4.

*Figure 4. Components of Emotional Intelligence Relevant to Patient Care*

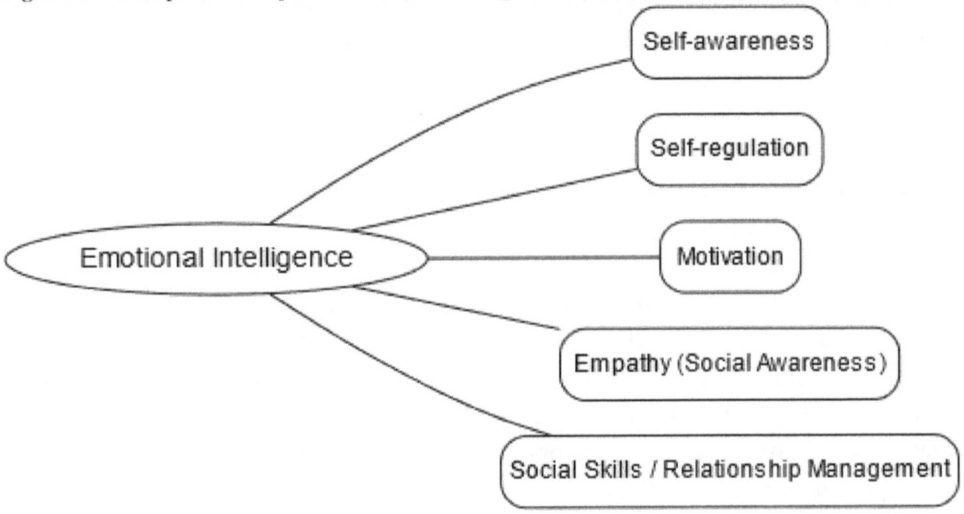


Empathy was one of the key concepts that takes the center of patient care, as it was the ability to perceive and comprehend the emotional conditions of patients, families, and colleagues. A compassionate approach promotes clinicians to receive the experiences, fears, and hopes of lived experiences that are articulated during clinical dialogues. Empathy builds trust and creates a good environment where patients feel appreciated and heard. Social awareness goes beyond the individual level of caring by helping to make the clinician sensitive to the cultural context, interpersonal clues, and emotional climate of clinical settings. This kind of awareness enables providing care responses that are responsive to patient needs, sensitivities, and expectations.

The relationship management puts the emotional intelligence framework in patient care into completion. This element entails communication style, which promotes clarity, relational trust, and respectful communication. Good relationship management facilitates teamwork in the course of care plan, understanding each other in education or counseling, and providing emotional support in painful situations. In teams, relationship management promotes positive working conditions for professionals who interact freely and seamlessly. All of these aspects of emotional intelligence maintain a humane philosophy of clinical practice, reinforcing patient confidence, professional satisfaction, and personal emotional health of the medical community.

## Role of EI in Managing Stress, Burnout, and Compassion Fatigue

Medical workers are faced with prolonged experiences of misery, ambiguity, and the heavy workload expectations, which create a mental burden. Emotional intelligence helps to be conscious of inner emotional signals and, as a result, to recognize a first sign of tension, irritability, or emotional exhaustion by the clinician. The awareness of these cues can lead to strategic uses of emotional regulation, including reflective pause, reframing, grounding methods, or facilitative conversation with coworkers. The emotional consciousness acts as a safeguard mechanism for staying calm, rational, and present in a stressful clinical encounter. Once emotional regulation was learned, stress responses become more organized and predictable instead of growing out of control into intense emotional conditions.

Burnout tends to occur in situations where emotional demands surpass the resources available to cope with them over a long duration. Emotional intelligence helps to maintain individual resilience by consciously setting boundaries, achieving emotional clarity, and adjusting to coping. Clinicians who have high emotional awareness usually use relational support networks, peer reflection, and mindful recovery practices to restore psychological energy. Strong empathy with suffering was commonly associated with compassion fatigue that limits the ability to empathically stay and develop emotional distancing. Emotional intelligence grants a moderated response to empathy by attunement without over-identification to pay compassionate action without breaking emotional stability and professional persistence.

Emotional reflection practices, formalized peer support, and work-related leadership behaviors that legitimize emotional experience are common in healthcare settings that recognize emotional intelligence as a key workforce competency. This creates a sense of collective resilience and collective responsibility for the well-being of such environments. Emotional intelligence training motivates clinicians to practice self-observation, consultation, and seeking help early in scenarios where emotional strain arises. By creating the conditions to combat the accumulation of stress, slow down the development of burnout, and safeguard the compassionate care through the long-term focus on the emotional skills, the healthcare systems create the conditions that oppose the development of burnout.

Longitudinal research further highlights the importance of emotionally intelligent system design. Studies tracking healthcare professionals over extended periods show that sustained exposure to high documentation demands and screen-mediated communication is associated with gradual declines in empathic engagement and increases in emotional exhaustion. In contrast, healthcare environments that implement supportive digital tools, reflective debriefing systems, and emotionally intelligent leadership practices demonstrate more stable empathy levels and lower burnout trajectories over time. These findings suggest that the long-term impact of AI on compassion depends less on the technology itself and more on the design philosophy, organizational culture, and integration of emotional intelligence competencies within digital systems.

## Enhancing Team Communication and Psychological Safety through EI

Healthcare environments are the fields where team communication has a heavy implication on clinical performance, coordination, and shared decision-making. EI facilitates better understanding of the interpersonal experience through a better sense of the tone, patient context, and the emotional conditions among individuals. Empathic-based communication enhances teamwork and minimizes conflict when it was time to put in the extra effort or in an emergency. The moment the members of the team are sensitive to the emotional signals of each other, the discussion becomes free and honest, and people can express their issues or seek help without any apprehension. These patterns of communication contribute to shared accountability and the relationship bonds that support the presence of effective clinical practice, showed in figure 5.

Psychological safety was a term that was used to describe a team climate where people can feel free to show their doubts, ask questions, and admit mistakes without the fear of being accused or criticized. Emotional intelligence plays a role in psychological safety, as attitudes of respect, curiosity, and patience would be developed in the common work settings. Leaders who are highly emotionally aware foster conversation thinking, recognize the emotional burden, and facilitate non-punitive reactions to problems. This was a workplace that promotes truthfulness about workloads, ethical issues, or clinical demands that influence well-being among healthcare professionals. Psychological safety helps to decrease emotional burden and maintain the long-term ability to be compassionate.

*Figure 5. Enhancing Team Communication and Psychological Safety through EI*

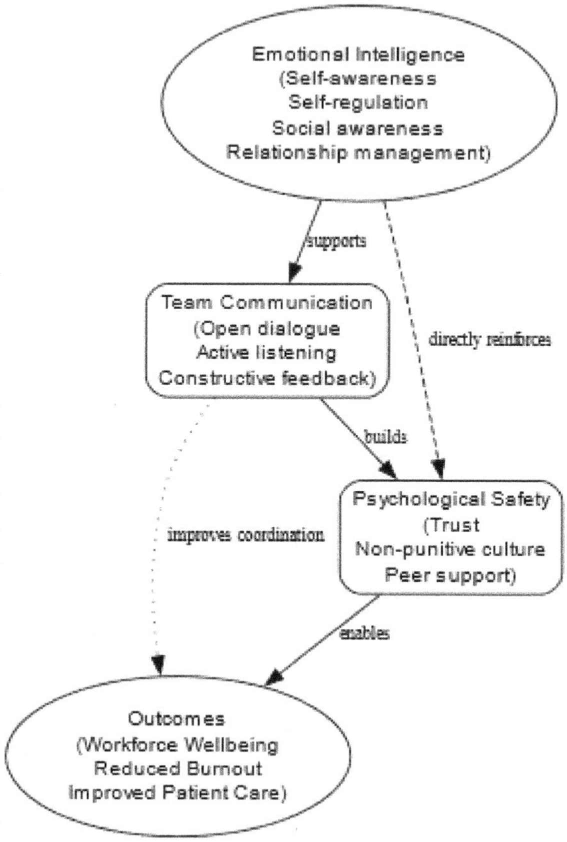


Professional teams that develop emotional intelligence can provide the conditions under which compassion and clinical expertise are mutually reinforcing. Empathic communication patterns result in better patient interactions, less confusion, and better continuity of care. The presence of emotions in the team context facilitates resilience in a group environment, which allows clinicians to cope with stressful circumstances without feeling emotionally depleted and disengaged. Positive psychological safety fosters good cultures whereby responsibility was shared by the individuals to ensure maintenance of caring care. These circumstances foster a balanced working environment where well-being, confidence, and ethical adherence are some of the values that lead to quality patient outcomes.

## ORGANIZATIONAL STRATEGIES FOR CULTIVATING EMOTIONALLY INTELLIGENT WORK ENVIRONMENTS

Development of emotionally intelligent working conditions within the healthcare institutions requires a commitment of the organization to the structures that promote reflective practices, awareness of interpersonal relationships, and supportive communication. The leader was at the forefront of providing an example of empathy, having open and honest discussions, and recognizing the emotional aspects of clinical practice. Emotional awareness, conflict management, relationship communication, and stress identification training programs would lead to a more stable and firmer workforce. The employment of workflows that allow moments to rest and check-ins among the team and collective decision-making encourage the creation of the environment in which emotional expression can be considered as legitimate instead of held back. Once organizational goals correspond to relational values, healthcare workers still have the ability to establish meaningful relationships with patients and fellow workers.

Environmental sustainability requires culturally acceptable norms that respect the sense of compassion as a group attribute rather than a personal one. Psychological safety was cultivated in institutions with peer support networks, reflective debriefing customs, and cultures of non-punitive feedback. Systems of recognition that appreciate empathy and collaborative care can strengthen the importance of emotional contributions and technical competence. Time management policies are designed to offset the cumulative stress generated by clinical environments of high intensity by means of rest, emotional processing, and mentorship. By implementing these measures, emotional intelligence was rendered a part of workplace identity, motivating the healthcare professionals to persist with relational presence when addressing the complex care needs.

## ARTIFICIAL INTELLIGENCE AS A SUPPORT MECHANISM FOR COMPASSIONATE PRACTICE

### AI for Reducing Documentation and Administrative Burden

The paperwork and administration often take a considerable amount of clinical time, putting pressure to the point of overlooking therapeutic presence and compassionate interaction. The tools of artificial intelligence that automatize the processes of routine data entry, organize clinical notes, and facilitate the digital records management bring about a decrease in cognitive load and task fragmentation. Intelligent form completion, speech-to-text systems, and predictive charting capabilities enable clinicians to focus on the screen instead of the patient. The workflow become more fluid when the administrative processes need less manual repetition, and space in care encounters created to provide emotional awareness and measured communication, as showed in figure 6.

*Figure 6. AI for Reducing Documentation and Administrative Burden*

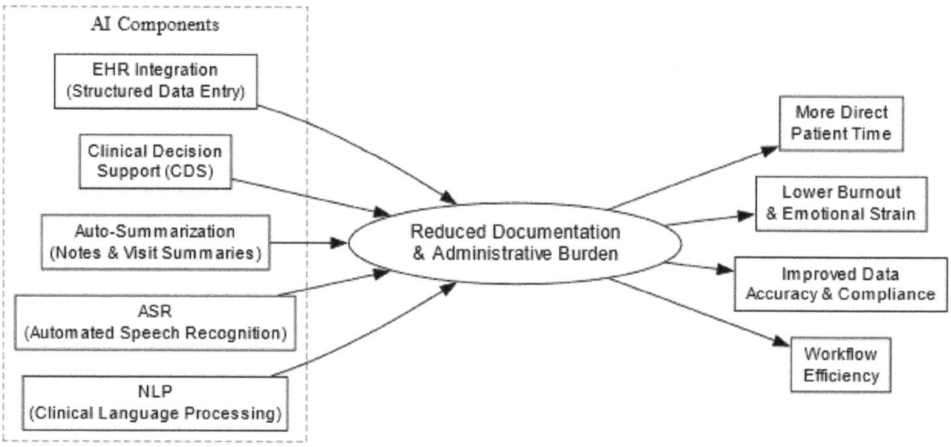


As the system design was consistent with clinical rhythms and professional judgment, a supportive role of AI in documentation appears. Intelligent triage documentation support, automatic recording systems, and intelligent data retrieval interfaces are used to help clinicians without disrupting interpersonal relationships. The lightened burden of bureaucracy allows medical workers to maintain an emotional ability to provide caring care. The fact that AI-based documentation relief was supported by organizations implies the feeling that there was emotional work involved in healthcare. These conditions promote empathetic sustainability, reflective presence, and relational attentiveness, strengthening the compassionate practice as one of the core aspects of quality care.

## Clinical Decision Support Systems and Cognitive Load Reduction

Clinical decision support systems also make contributions to the care settings by providing structured information that can help clinicians make decisions with complex information during the time pressures. Clinical data, diagnostic variables, treatment guidelines, and patient histories in large volumes tend to merge in the situations of making decisions, causing cognitive strain. Decision support tools provide systematized ways in which clinicians can narrow down the right information, identify clinical patterns, and evaluate risk in a better way. Assistive digital interfaces support prioritization and alleviate mental strain in clinicians as well as enable them to be more attentive when interacting with patients. Emotional presence was allowed to take space when cognitive burden was reduced so that compassion was released in communication and care behaviors.

Decision support systems also support reflective awareness in the sense that the presentation of information was done in forms that encourage understanding and not congestion. Robotic alerts, systematic record keeping, and task-related instructions help to streamline workflow more efficiently, reducing the chances of making mistakes because of distraction or fatigue. Smoother decision-making channels provide the environment where clinicians can devote more attention to relational communication as opposed to administrative clarification. Clinical decision support tools, through this role, can be informational resources as well as a tool that protects the emotional and cognitive capacity of healthcare professionals, both to help to maintain a compassionate practice that was active and sustainable.

## Emotion Recognition Technologies in Patient Interaction

Emotion recognition technology was a mechanism that can be used to recognize emotional states by analyzing vocal density, facial expression, gesture patterns, and language in order to detect the moods of patients when dealing with them. The systems are based on the affective computing models, machine learning techniques that group emotional cues in a more and more narrow way. Such technologies can be used in clinical settings where assist practitioners to gain an understanding of emotional distress, anxiety, confusion, or discomfort that not be communicated verbally. Emotion-aware interfaces, when incorporated into communication processes, provide the chance of prompt reassurance, empathic clarification, and relational presence. The utility of such technologies comes in the ability of the technologies to emphasize emotional strata in clinical interactions that silent because of time constraints, cultural influences, or finickiness on the part of patients.

The implementation process requires adherence to the principles of compassionate care as opposed to surveillance or judgment of behavior. Emotion recognition devices help to create conditions in which emotional conditions are recognized and given a portion of importance to match the physiological signals. Such systems, complemented with clinician skill, reflective listening, and contextual awareness, improve comprehension instead of substituting human sensitivity. Ethical rules and training make certain that the emotional insights that are formed by means of technology are used to support the respectful interaction, rather than to impact decision-making in reductive or prescriptive ways. The final objective was based on enhancing relational awareness, promoting patient dignity, and equipping clinicians with a more profound interpretive framework for addressing emotional needs in care interactions.

## Cultural Sensitivity and Algorithmic Bias in Emotion Recognition

Emotion recognition systems rely on training data that reflect facial expressions, vocal tones, and behavioral cues. However, emotional expression varies significantly across cultures, age groups, and social contexts. Gestures, eye contact, speech tempo, and facial affect that signal distress in one cultural setting may represent politeness, respect, or neutrality in another. When AI systems are trained on limited or culturally homogeneous datasets, they risk misinterpreting emotional cues, leading to inaccurate or inappropriate empathic responses.

Algorithmic bias in emotion-recognition systems may disproportionately affect patients from underrepresented ethnic, linguistic, or cultural backgrounds. Such bias can result in misclassification of emotional states, reduced trust in digital interfaces, and inequitable care experiences. To address this challenge, designers must ensure diverse and representative training datasets, culturally adaptive emotion models, and continuous validation across global populations.

Compassion-centered design requires that emotion-recognition technologies be sensitive to cultural variation and context. Co-design approaches involving patients, clinicians, and culturally diverse user groups can help ensure that emotional analytics reflect real-world experiences. By embedding cultural awareness into AI development, healthcare systems can promote equitable empathic support and avoid reinforcing systemic biases in digital care environments.

## AI-Assisted Communication Tools for Empathic Engagement

AI-assisted communication tools aid in empathic interaction by helping clinicians and patients have more direct and effective interactions by making them more attentive to each other. Cognitive digital platforms with natural language processing, sentiment analysis, and context-driven response generation are meant to help build environments in which emotional indicators are given equal consideration to clinical data. These are the tools that accompany and help the clinicians in the dialogue as direct them on how to express themselves in a way that brings in an understanding, comfort, and respect. Conversation support systems are able to identify when a patient shows signs of confusion, fear, or emotional distress, and the clinician can respond with language that was empathetic. It was through this type of augmented communication that clinical interaction experiences a level of relational richness and does not demand cognitive load on a healthcare professional. It is showed in figure 7.

*Figure 7. AI-Assisted Communication Tools for Empathic Engagement*

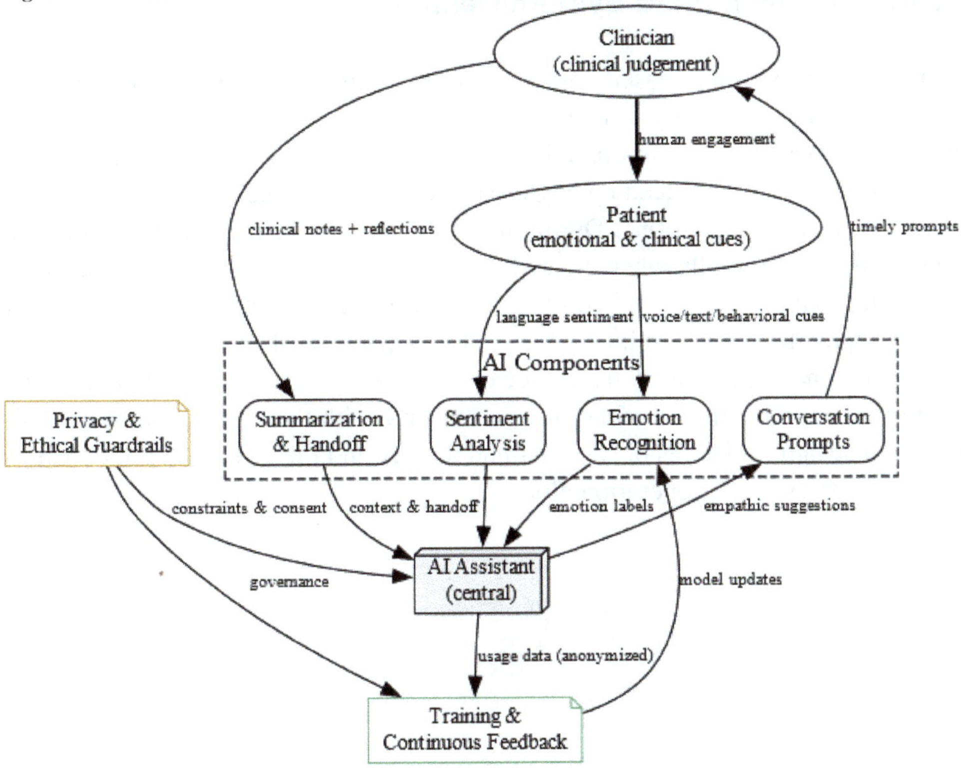


There are also AI-assisted communication strategies that are used in training and professional development. Computer-based dialogue settings allow their clinicians to practice responding to emotionally complex situations and get real-time guidance based on the emotional intelligence framework. This encourage cognitive awareness and build the habit of patient-centered communication. Empathic communication support tools that are integrated into the electronic health records prompt clinicians to be mindful of emotional aspects of care despite high-efficiency workflow pressures. In conjunction with organizational cultures that embrace empathy and psychological safety, these tools are a part of a healthcare system where empathic interaction was both sustainable and resilient.

# DESIGNING THE COMPASSION-CENTERED HYBRID INTELLIGENCE (CCHI) FRAMEWORK

## Principles of Human-Centered and Compassion-Oriented System Design

The design of human-based compassionate systems needs the vision of healthcare as a relational activity founded on trust, presence, and emotional sensitivity. Processes of designing are improved when it was understood that clinicians operate in settings that are influenced by cognitive needs, professional conduct, and ongoing interpersonal interactions. Digital technologies that help deliver care of high quality operate optimally when created with a close consideration of lived clinical experience, subtle patterns of communication, and the emotional importance of patient interactions. System interfaces, pathways, and displays of information add to the emotional tone in the delivery of care, steering the interactions towards being supportive or procedural. Technology was in tune with the original ethos of healing when design initiatives observe human dignity and the quality of relationships instead of efficiency of operation alone.

*Figure 8. Principles of Human-Centered and Compassion-Oriented System Design*

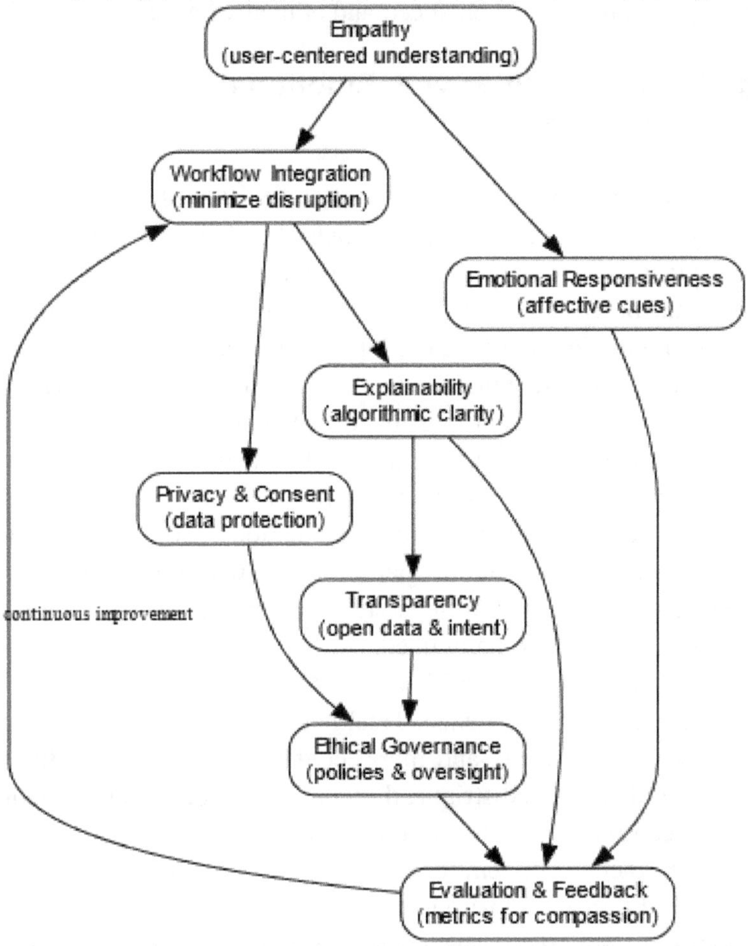


Figure 8 illustrate the compassion-based design focuses on community-driven development by including clinicians, patients, designers, and organizational leaders. Co-design methodologies promote discussion of emotional load, the moral friction, and the insidious aspects of care that emerge beyond quantifiable activities. This partnership serves in the development of digital apps that augment enabling dialogue, contemplative cognizance, and professional autonomy. The predetermined workflows designed in such a way that can pause, share interpretation, and provide relational recognition help clinicians to stay emotionally engaged even in the demanding conditions. Measures of evaluation, including well-being, the quality of interaction, and continuity of the relations, support continuous improvement. The system environment as a result of it was conducive to caring presence and incorporates technological support in a balanced and ethically based way.

## Aligning AI Functionalities with Emotional and Relational Needs

Correlating AI capabilities and emotional and relational requirements necessitates a strategy to consider compassion as one of the main design considerations and not a secondary factor. Digital systems usually work on the tasks, which are connected with the processing of data, with the organization of workflows, and with the clinical documentation, but the emotional interaction develops in the sphere of less obvious, context-sensitive indicators. A caring design philosophy asks system designers, clinical executives, and organizational decision-makers to think of ways in which digital technologies can encourage active listening, empathetic presence, and narrative comprehension in care interactions. Relational-oriented interfaces, prompts, and decision-support output foster reflection, recognition of patient emotion, and respectful communication when designed with relational priorities. The use of technology does not serve to separate people but rather as a medium through which human interaction was maintained.

The sensitivity to clinician well-being was also attached to AI functions that are based on emotional intelligence. Healthcare workplaces involve unceasing emotional stress, mental strain, and moral conflict. The use of digital tools that emphasize stress indicators, redistribute the workload, or encourage supportive team communication can be part of the culture of perceiving emotional labor as a part of the caregiving practice. Systems created in this orientation maintain a feeling of collective responsibility and sensitivity to emotional limits, as well as sensitivity to human susceptibility. A marked fit between technology and relational needs promotes the conditions in which compassion stay alive, be supported, and express itself to mean that health professionals able to maintain presence and emotional clarity in the context of the multifaceted requirements of clinical care.

## Integration of EI-Based Competencies into AI Algorithms and Interfaces

To incorporate emotional intelligence abilities into AI, a human experience, relational significance, and context sensitivity should be maintained as a technological design. AI systems crafted based on data with emotional manifestations, tone variations, behavioral indicators, and interactional patterns have the potential to aid in identifying stress, disorientation, or emotional distress in users. Elements of the interface that promote thoughtful pauses, empathetic language, and conversational flow that focuses on the patient contribute to maintaining the intensity of relationships during digital interactions. Open results, natural dialogue in language generators, and suggestions to seek clarification or soft investigation lead to human interaction and not robot delivery of responses. AI usage in the context of communication and empathy Design thinking Design attention focused on emotional subtleties enables AI implementations to operate in accordance with communicative and empathetic expectations of a healthcare environment, as shows in figure 9.

*Figure 9. Integration of EI-Based Competencies into AI Algorithms and Interfaces*

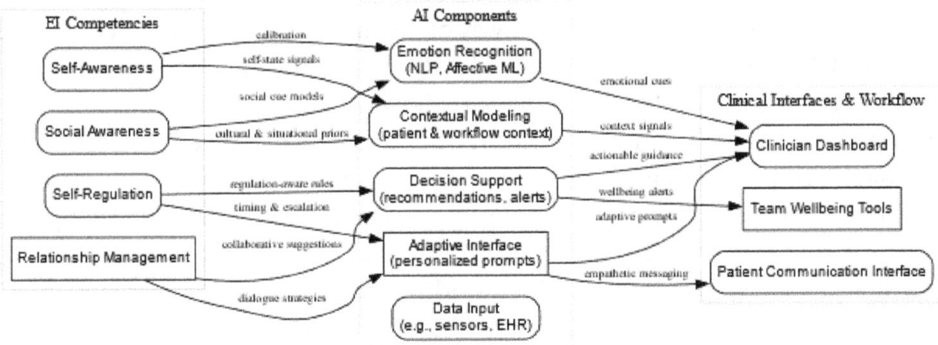


Such competencies are implemented not only in algorithmic training but also in interface structure, location of workflow, and management of interaction. The embedded systems in clinical routines have the advantage of an adaptive feedback loop, which responds to environmental stimuli and practitioner workload conditions. The AI that was informed with emotional intelligence helps to minimize emotional overload by assisting clinicians in critical decision-making and transitions of care. Human agency interfaces that capture the reflective choice-making and foreground the agency assert a collaborative relationship as opposed to a directive one. Environments of care where such AI integrations are implemented make the state of compassion the focus, clinical judgment still in-depth, and workforce wellbeing structurally strengthened by technological collaboration.

Explainable AI plays a critical role in ensuring trust and ethical accountability within compassion-centered hybrid intelligence systems. When AI tools identify emotional distress or recommend communication strategies, clinicians must understand the reasoning behind these outputs. Explanation interfaces that describe which behavioral cues, language patterns, or contextual signals triggered an alert allow clinicians to interpret the system's suggestions critically rather than follow them automatically. Transparent feedback channels reinforce professional autonomy and reduce the risk of blind reliance on algorithmic outputs. By making emotional insights interpretable and contextually grounded, explainable AI strengthens collaboration between human judgment and machine intelligence while preserving the ethical core of compassionate care.

## Workflow-Level Implementation Strategies for Hybrid Intelligence

The Compassion-Centered Hybrid Intelligence can be implemented on a workflow level, which requires that digital systems can be synchronized with the rhythm of clinical practice, the emotional needs of the patient, and the dynamics of cooperation between care teams. The most effective way of integration was the support of natural decision-making points by AI tools instead of disrupting clinical flow. The process of documentation, finding information, and predictive monitoring can be transferred to automation as the clinician's focus was left on interpersonal interaction. Contextual, emotional, and patient-centered interface designs can coerce clinicians to remain present and personally aware during discussions of care. The hybrid intelligence becomes stronger when there was a sense of balance between the efficiency of the workflow and the responsiveness of the workflow that was compassionate.

Maintaining a hybrid practice means that it should be adapted continuously, which guided by the response of frontline healthcare workers. Structured reflective discussions, repeated assessment of technology, and cross-disciplinary discourse promote the refinement on a basis of lived clinical experience. The training programs, which can show the way emotional intelligence competencies can interconnect with AI-driven processes, help to reach an understanding and build collective confidence. Clear communication between technical staff and healthcare personnel create trust and motivate ethical behavior in the design and implementation. When workflows mirror operational effectiveness and human relationships, hybrid intelligence facilitates clinician well-being, develops relational continuity, and reinforces the caring nature of healthcare practice.

## Evaluation Metrics for Compassion, Wellbeing, and Care Quality

To evaluate compassion-based hybrid intelligence, it was necessary to consider such measures reflecting emotional presence, the quality of relationships, and workforce well-being support. Clinical settings are known to utilize efficiency metrics and throughput statistics to assess performance, but these metrics fail to reflect the level of human relationship and the emotional nature of care relationships. Compassion assessment entails monitoring of communication voice, responsiveness when interacting with patients, sensitivity to emotions, and responsiveness to distress. Patient stories, staff reflective narratives, and qualitative feedback can provide a glimpse of the dynamics of relationships that cannot be captured by numerical measures only. Such practices allow the identification of the emotional aspect of providing care as a vital part of the healthcare quality instead of the abstract ideal. These evaluation metrics showed up in the figure 10.

Wellbeing assessment was aimed at psychological safety, stress load, and level of support in the normal and high-stress clinical work of the staff. The organizational climate was capable of supporting the emotional resilience of staff as demonstrated by regular debriefing structures, availability of peer support, and workload balance. The wellbeing climate can be comprehended through surveys of the workforce, sentiment analysis based on the patterns of clinical communications, and behavioral health screening instruments. Wellbeing evaluation in this context recognizes the reasoning that compassionate care thrives when staff members sense a sense of backing, identification, and significance in work-related capacities.

*Figure 10. Evaluation Metrics for Compassion, Wellbeing, and Care Quality*

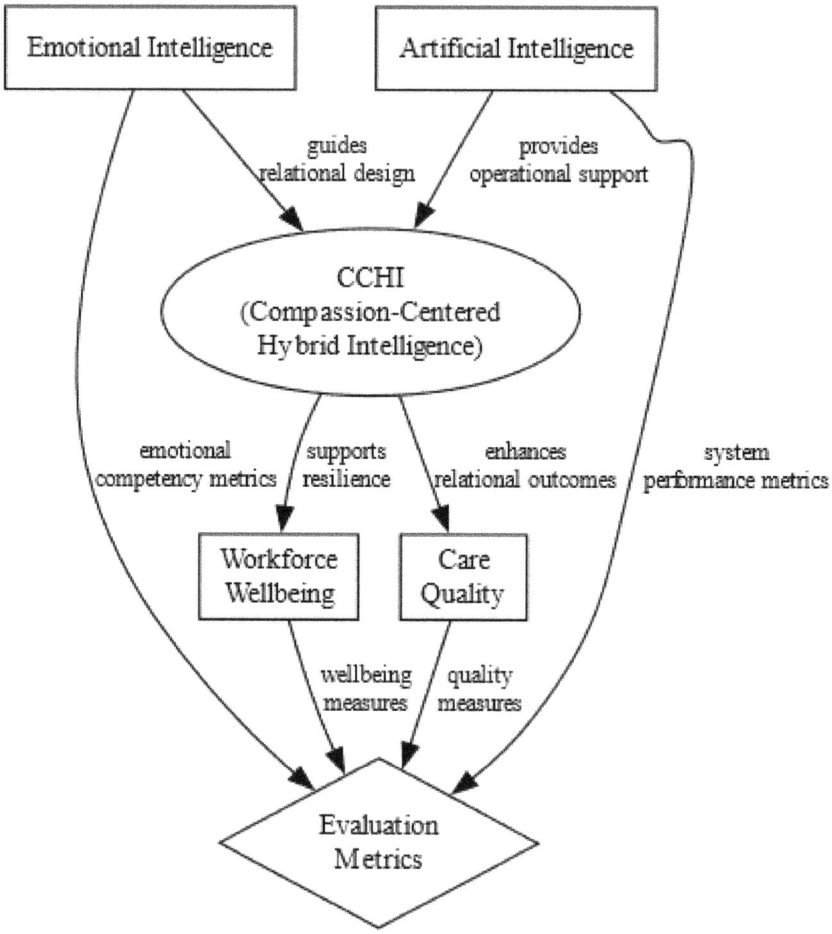


The quality of care in a Compassion-Centered Hybrid Intelligence model needs to have measures that combine clinical results with relational results. The recovery process in patients, treatment adherence, and minimization of preventable complications are valuable in addition to trust, comfort, and emotional reassurance indicators, which patients and families report on. These are achieved by the presence of hybrid intelligence systems that ease the workload, support cognitive processes, and increase situational awareness, but the human clinician was the source of compassionate presence. Assessment, which includes compassion, well-being, and quality of care, was built in to provide a global view of healthcare excellence, helping systems to move towards the environment in which emotional bonding and clinical efficacy form harmoniously rather than antagonistically.

# APPLICATION SCENARIOS AND CASE-BASED ILLUSTRATIONS

## AI-Enabled Clinical Debriefing and Emotional Support Systems

Clinical debriefing environments powered by AI provide a structured environment where healthcare professionals are able to process emotionally colored experiences that occur during the process of attending to the patient. Constant exposure to high-stress situations can create within an individual a strain that cannot be addressed when clinical practices proceed quickly from one task to the other. AI-assisted support systems have the potential to facilitate reflective communication by providing prompts to facilitate the expression of emotions, discovery of emotional triggers, and identification of individual coping strategies. These systems are based on language models, sentiment interpretation, and contextual response patterns to help convey the feeling in such a way that promote understanding of emotion instead of suppressing it. These environments encourage the normalization of emotional expression in the clinical culture, which minimizes isolation and strengthens the collective humanity among the healthcare staff.

Collaborative meaning-making in the clinical team can be promoted by the use of emotional support systems that include AI-guided reflection. Digital facilitation Group debriefing sessions help participants to voice their opinions, share ethical dilemmas, and maneuver an emotional residue of complicated cases. Pattern awareness using AI can reflect common stress signals in the team communication to draw organizational interest in the workload strain or strained relationship. The use of emotional support practices based on compassion-based principles enhances resilience, promotes professional identity, and maintains empathetic ability in the long term. These systems can work to build a clinical culture where mental well-being, mutual support, and compassionate presence are central to everyday practice by developing organizing channels of integration of emotions.

## Compassion-Aware Digital Conversational Agents for Patient Interaction

Digital conversational agents with compassion awareness are the communication interfaces that react to patients based on the emotional tone, life stories, and relationship needs. These agents can be used based on natural language processing models that are trained to identify statements of anxiety, uncertainty, or distress and provide a chance to engage in a supportive conversation. There are most of the time the emotional undertones involved in patient interactions that are not confined to imparting medical information. Compassionately designed conversational agents consider pacing, word choice, and thoughtful recognition, which allow patients to feel that their voices are heard during the time when clinical staff was under time pressure. This style of designing applies communication as a therapeutic process and not a mere exchange of facts.

*Figure 11. Compassion-Aware Digital Conversational Agents for Patient Interaction*

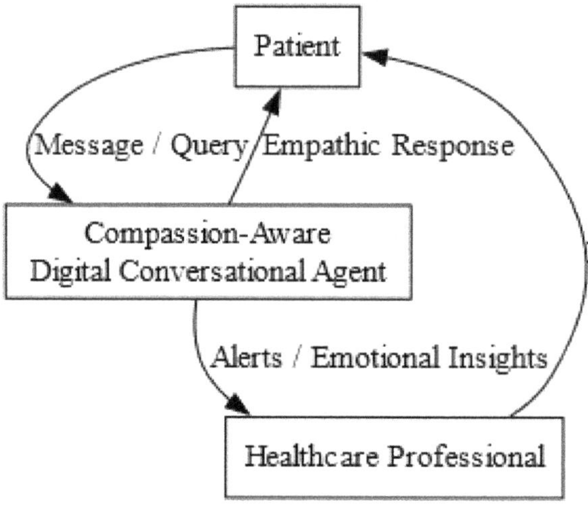


Figure 11 illustrate the introduction of compassion-conscious agents into medical settings promotes emotional support continuity. Patients usually endure excessive waiting time, uncertainty in treatment, or lack of continuity in communication between care teams. An agent that can chat with patients during these transitions can help them feel assured, get their instructions right, and encourage them to think about their problems or questions to be talked over with clinicians. This continuity enhances the involvement of the patient and helps to make the emotional experience in the process of care more stable. The agent was not meant to replace human dialogue but rather to act as an auxiliary to continuing relations in cases of clinical staff being required to do urgent errands.

## Staff Wellbeing Dashboards Using Affective and Behavioral Analytics

Affective and behavioral analytics-based staff wellbeing dashboards serve as reflective instruments that indicate emotional patterns, workload stresses, and interaction patterns in clinical settings. These dashboards are based on communication tone, patterns of shift lengths, frequency of task switching, and signs of stress-related behavior to create the overall view of the workforce emotional climate.

Rising cognitive strain was commonly indicated in real-time signals, e.g., more documentation anomalies or reduced interactions with patients. Visualization of these types of indicators promotes awareness of the emotional burden and promotes an appropriate conversation between the members of the clinical team in a timely manner. The dashboard space promotes the acknowledgment of emotional forces as serious aspects of career life but not an inner conflict that was being hidden.

Affective analytics, which are integrated into the routine of an organization, assist in timely intervention and joint problem-solving. When emotional patterns are discussed by the team, the psychological safety was reinforced, and the shame about fatigue or emotional pain was reduced. Leadership was better informed of what was required of the staff and can make staffing changes, schedule restorative breaks, or create specific peer support programs. Employees also acquire a common language to talk about emotional experience and help to create the atmosphere in which compassion flows between members of the team, not only clinicians to patients. The dashboard model can contribute to relational and emotional sustainability by strengthening the notion that caring workplaces need to take care of the emotional health of caregivers.

## Hybrid Intelligence Support in Intensive and Palliative Care Settings

The intensive and palliative care settings are highly emotional, decision-making was complicated, and often face the aspects of vulnerability, pain, and end-of-life realities. The clinical teams working in such settings deal with physiological instability and emotional aspects of patients and families in need of reassurance, clarity, and presence. The implementation of hybrid intelligence support brings about the use of digital systems to help in terms of constant monitoring, pattern identification, and coordinating workloads so that clinicians can focus more on engaging in compassionate communication and understanding. The machine-based assessment provides warning signs and anticipatory results as clinicians derive meaning, context, and human meaning. This mutual role construct provides room to enable relational care even in the instances of urgent response needs showed in figure 12.

*Figure 12. Hybrid Intelligence Support in Intensive and Palliative Care Settings*

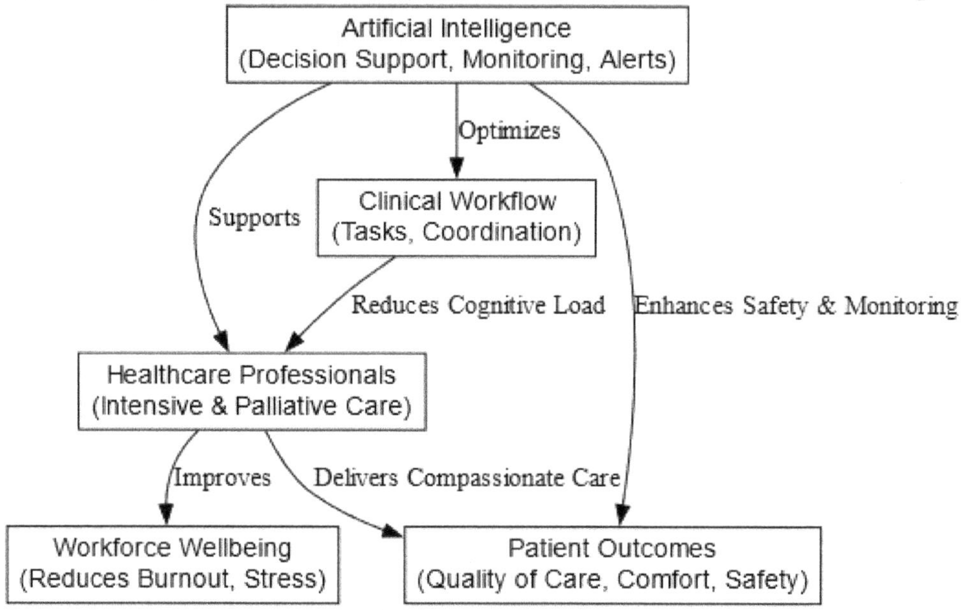


The mode of palliative care focuses on the comfort, dignity, and emotional attachment in the late life stages. Hybrid intelligence platforms also have a contribution through monitoring symptom trends, detecting distress signals, and planning interdisciplinary care. Such functions lessen administrative pressure and cognitive exhaustion and allow clinicians the time to be present, listen well, and respond aptly to emotional gestures by patients and families. The qualities of compassion in palliative situations are reflected in the presence of relationships, the sensitivity to individual stories, and the awareness of existential issues. Online assistance in such situations does not displace human compassion but only maintains the ability to provide it.

The intensive care environment requires accurate timing, rapid response, and team effort. Hybrid intelligence helps by integrating real-time information feeds, which have the capacity to saturate individual cognition. A better ground on which clinical teams rely on making calm, grounded decisions was provided when continuous data interpretation was handled by digital systems. The emotional stability of the critical care builds a better way of communicating with families who are in fear and uncertainty. The support of the hybrid intelligence allows creating the conditions under which compassion was not only possible, but also quite common even when urgency was the key feature of the environment. Emotional awareness, both in the design of the system and the medical practice, enhances the capability of delivering care that was both respectful of human experience and of medical necessity.

## Training and Simulation Programs Using Compassion-Centered AI Models

The compassion-based AI models in training and simulation programs play an auxiliary role in shaping relational awareness, emotional attunement, and reflective decision-making in healthcare professionals. These programs provide organized settings in which clinical teams are exposed to patient situations with an emotional complexity, ethical tension, and different communication requirements. Simulation platforms containing AI elements process verbal cues and patterns of interaction and response timing to provide information on the occurrence of compassion in care encounters. The participants are involved in practice that enhances listening presence, emotional recognition, and therapeutic communication and getting feedback based on behavioral and affective aspects. Compassionate response was a competency that was learned through repetition and instruction and was no longer a presumed personal inclination.

Professional development pathways that incorporate such simulation programs help to ensure sustainable compassionate care through the enhancement of relational skills in addition to clinical expertise. The AI-supported reflexive approach also allow the participants to analyze not only the outcomes of the procedure but also the affective space created in the clinical interaction. Compassion-focused simulation training as an organizational culture helps to create an environment in which emotional intelligence was still appreciated and developed. Such initiatives can help professionals to identify emotional burden early, give supportive communication, and coordinate care activities with the original purpose of relieving suffering. Through the development of compassionate presence based on systematic and technologically enabled practice, medical environments create robust teams that can provide humane and attentive care in the stressful clinical environments.

# CONCLUSION

The healthcare systems are undergoing changes as strive to meet the rising demands of service, varying needs of patients, and the rapid change in technology. The sustainability and integrity of healthcare delivery are still priorities within this dynamic environment where compassion and workforce well-being must be preserved. Compassion was also known to not only enhance the therapeutic relationships but also patient trust, adherence, emotional comfort, and patient satisfaction with the care. Meanwhile, clinicians operate in conditions that often increase emotional stress, cognitive burden, and moral distress. Such pressures may reduce the ability to stay present, be attentive, and be relationally involved. To overcome these issues, it was necessary to find ways that would support the emotional and physical health of medical workers and the organizational culture on the basis of which care was provided.

Emotional intelligence combined with artificial intelligence can provide the way to these objectives. Emotional intelligence helps to become aware, to be empathetic, to communicate reflectively, and to manage emotions effectively while working in a clinical situation. Artificial intelligence provides support to decisions, predictive workflow optimization, and administrative relief. In a harmonious development based on the Compassion-Centered Hybrid Intelligence (CCHI) framework, these two areas complement each other in such a way that it maintains a compassionate interaction and enhances operational efficiency. CCHI places technology as a facilitator of human connection but not a replacement of it. Through the crafting of AI systems that are responsive to the context of relationships, emotional variables, and lived experiences of patients and clinicians, digital innovation strengthen but not undermine the humane pillars of healthcare.

The execution of this framework requires institutional dedication, ethical governance, and continuous assessment. Organizational practices that promote reflective conversation, systematic emotional assistance, and appreciation of compassionate practice can be used to achieve psychological safety and workforce stability. Simulation, directed debriefing, and AI-assisted reflective feedback training programs assist clinicians to enhance emotional competence alongside technical expertise. Compassion, well-being, and quality of care measures are evaluated and combined to be sure that improvements are based on the fundamental healthcare principles.

The future of humane healthcare lies in the solution that merge technological progress with human knowledge. The Compassion-Centered Hybrid Intelligence model confirms that compassion was still an ethical and practical requirement. Through the promotion of system designs that maintain emotional presence, healthcare environments able to maintain continued care that was dignified, trustful, and of help to those who are the caregivers and those who are the care receivers.

## REFERENCES


Arora, S., Rai, M., & Gupta, M. (2024). Importance of industry 5.0 in understanding emotional intelligence. In *Human-Machine Collaboration and Emotional Intelligence in Industry 5.0* (pp. 205–219). IGI Global Scientific Publishing., DOI: 10.4018/979-8-3693-6806-0.ch011

Cho, A., Cha, C., & Baek, G. (2024). Development of an artificial Intelligence–Based tailored mobile intervention for nurse burnout: Single-Arm trial. *Journal of Medical Internet Research, 26*, e54029. DOI: 10.2196/54029 PMID: 38905631

Cinar, A. B., & Bilodeau, S. (2024). Incorporating AI into the inner circle of emotional intelligence for sustainability. *Sustainability (Basel), 16*(15), 6648. DOI: 10.3390/su16156648

Creed, T. A., Salama, L., Slevin, R., Tanana, M., Imel, Z., Narayanan, S., & Atkins, D. C. (2022). Enhancing the quality of cognitive behavioral therapy in community mental health through artificial intelligence generated fidelity feedback (Project AFFECT): A study protocol. *BMC Health Services Research, 22*(1), 1177. DOI: 10.1186/s12913-022-08519-9 PMID: 36127689

Dailah, H. G., Koriri, M., Sabei, A., Kriry, T., & Zakri, M. (2024, December). Artificial intelligence in nursing: technological benefits to nurse's mental health and patient care quality. In *Healthcare* (Vol. 12, No. 24, p. 2555). MDPI. https://doi.org/DOI: 10.3390/healthcare12242555

. DeTore, N. R., Balogun-Mwangi, O., Eberlin, E. S., Dokholyan, K. N., Rizzo, A., & Holt, D. J. (2024). An artificial intelligence-based virtual human avatar application to assess the mental health of health care professionals: A validation study. *Journal of Medical Extended Reality, 1*(1), jmxr-2024. https://doi.org/DOI: 10.1089/jmxr.2024.0016

Dey, D. N. C. (2024). Harmonizing the threads of well-being: AI (artificial intelligence), spirituality, healthcare, and management. *Spirituality, Healthcare, And Management* (April 24, 2024). DOI: 10.2139/ssrn.5002655

George, A. S., George, A. H., & Baskar, T. (2024). Artificial intelligence and the future of healthcare: Emerging jobs and skills in 2035. *Partners Universal Multidisciplinary Research Journal, 1*(1), 1–21. DOI: 10.5281/zenodo.11176554

Graves, M., & Compson, J. (2024, October). Compassionate AI for moral decision-making, health, and well-being. In *Proceedings of the AAAI/ACM Conference on AI, Ethics, and Society* (Vol. 7, No. 1, pp. 520-533). https://doi.org/DOI: 10.1609/aies.v7i1.31655

Gyrard, A., Tabeau, K., Fiorini, L., Kung, A., Senges, E., De Mul, M., Giuliani, F., Lefebvre, D., Hoshino, H., Fabbricotti, I., Sancarlo, D., D'Onofrio, G., Cavallo, F., Guiot, D., Arzoz-Fernandez, E., Okabe, Y., & Tsukamoto, M. (2023). Knowledge engineering framework for IoT robotics applied to smart healthcare and emotional well-being. *International Journal of Social Robotics*, *15*(3), 445–472. DOI: 10.1007/s12369-021-00821-6 PMID: 34804257

He, X., Zheng, X., & Ding, H. (2023). Existing barriers faced by and future design recommendations for direct-to-consumer health care artificial intelligence apps: Scoping review. *Journal of Medical Internet Research*, *25*, e50342. DOI: 10.2196/50342 PMID: 38109173

Hernandez, J. P. T. (2024). Compassionate care with autonomous AI humanoid robots in future healthcare delivery: A multisensory simulation of next-generation models. *Biomimetics*, *9*(11), 687. DOI: 10.3390/biomimetics9110687 PMID: 39590259

Higgins, O., Chalup, S. K., & Wilson, R. L. (2024). Artificial Intelligence in nursing: Trustworthy or reliable? *Journal of Research in Nursing : JRN*, *29*(2), 143–153. DOI: 10.1177/17449871231215696 PMID: 39070561

Jonas, D., Maria, E., Widiasari, I. R., Rahardja, U., & Wellem, T. (2024). Design of a tam framework with emotional variables in the acceptance of health-based iot in indonesia. *ADI Journal on Recent Innovation*, *5*(2), 146–154. DOI: 10.34306/ajri.v5i2.1005

Kleinrichert, D. (2024). Empathy: An ethical consideration of AI & others in the workplace. *AI & Society*, *39*(6), 2743–2757. DOI: 10.1007/s00146-023-01831-w

Levin, C., Naimi, E., & Saban, M. (2024). Evaluating GenAI systems to combat mental health issues in healthcare workers: An integrative literature review. *International Journal of Medical Informatics*, *191*, 105566. DOI: 10.1016/j.ijmedinf.2024.105566 PMID: 39079316

Mitsea, E., Drigas, A., & Skianis, C. (2024). Artificial intelligence, immersive technologies, and neurotechnologies in breathing interventions for mental and emotional health: A systematic review. *Electronics (Basel)*, *13*(12), 2253. DOI: 10.3390/electronics13122253

Morrow, E., Zidaru, T., Ross, F., Mason, C., Patel, K. D., Ream, M., & Stockley, R. (2023). Artificial intelligence technologies and compassion in healthcare: A systematic scoping review. *Frontiers in Psychology*, *13*, 971044. DOI: 10.3389/fpsyg.2022.971044 PMID: 36733854

Papadopoulos, I., & Lazzarino, R. (2024). Developing, delivering, and evaluating an online course on socially assistive robots in culturally competent and compassionate healthcare: A sequential multiphase, mixed-method study. *Digital Health, 10*, 20552076241271792. DOI: 10.1177/20552076241271792 PMID: 39493631

Peng, M. L., Wickersham, J. A., Altice, F. L., Shrestha, R., Azwa, I., Zhou, X., Halim, M. A. A., Ikhtiaruddin, W. M., Tee, V., Kamarulzaman, A., & Ni, Z. (2022). Formative evaluation of the acceptance of HIV prevention artificial intelligence chatbots by men who have sex with men in Malaysia: Focus group study. *JMIR Formative Research, 6*(10), e42055. DOI: 10.2196/42055 PMID: 36201390

Sharma, A., Lin, I. W., Miner, A. S., Atkins, D. C., & Althoff, T. (2023). Human–AI collaboration enables more empathic conversations in text-based peer-to-peer mental health support. *Nature Machine Intelligence, 5*(1), 46–57. DOI: 10.1038/s42256-022-00593-2

Vial, T., & Almon, A. (2023). Artificial intelligence in mental health therapy for children and adolescents. *JAMA Pediatrics, 177*(12), 1251–1252. DOI: 10.1001/jamapediatrics.2023.4212 PMID: 37843842

# Compilation of References


Abbas, S. R., Abbas, Z., Zahir, A., & Lee, S. W. (2024). Federated learning in smart healthcare: A comprehensive review on privacy, security, and predictive analytics with IoT integration. *Sensors (Basel)*, *24*(3), 868. DOI: 10.3390/s24030868 PMID: 38339586

Abbou, B., Kessel, B., Ben Natan, M., Gabbay-Benziv, R., Dahan Shriki, D., Ophir, A., Goldschmid, N., Klein, A., Roguin, A., & Dudkiewicz, M. (2024). When all computers shut down: The clinical impact of a major cyber-attack on a general hospital. *Frontiers in Digital Health*, *6*, 1321485. Advance online publication. DOI: 10.3389/fdgth.2024.1321485 PMID: 38433989

Abdul Razak, M. S., Nirmala, C. R., Sreenivasa, B. R., Lahza, H., & Lahza, H. F. M. (2023). A survey on detecting healthcare concept drift in AI/ML models. *Frontiers in Artificial Intelligence*, *5*, 955314. DOI: 10.3389/frai.2022.955314 PMID: 37139355

Abdulwahab, L. O. (2026a). Designing Inclusive and Economically Sustainable Health Reforms in the Digital Era: A Phygital Approach to Equity, Efficiency, and Engagement. In Phygital Insights on National Health Reform: Economics, Marketing, and Leadership (pp. 191–232). IGI Global Scientific Publishing. https://www.igi-global.com/chapter/designing-inclusive-and-economically-sustainable-health-reforms-in-the-digital-era/409192

Abdulwahab, L. O. (2026b). Governing Health Equity: The Political Economy of Public Health Investment and Access in the Global South. In The Political Economy of Global Healthcare Industries: States, Markets, and Power (pp. 117–158). IGI Global Scientific Publishing. https://www.igi-global.com/chapter/governing-health-equity/404997

Abdulwahab, L. O. (2026c). Health System Sustainability and Labor Market Participation in an Aging Workforce: Economic Implications and Policy Options. In The Economics of an Aging Workforce: Challenges, Opportunities, and Policy Perspectives (pp. 245–288). IGI Global Scientific Publishing. https://www.igi-global.com/chapter/health-system-sustainability-and-labor-market-participation-in-an-aging-workforce/409708

Abdulwahab, L. O., & Azam, H. (2026). Platform Work in Europe's Green and Care Economies: Regulatory Pathways for Sustainability, Social Protection, and Fair Work. In Regulating the Gig Economy in the European Union: Challenges, Innovations, and Global Impacts (pp. 99–124). IGI Global Scientific Publishing. https://www.igi-global.com/chapter/platform-work-in-europes-green-and-care-economies/395612

Abikoye, B. E., Akinwunmi, T., Adelaja, A. O., Umeorah, S. C., & Ogunsuji, Y. M. (2024). Real-time financial monitoring systems: Enhancing risk management through continuous oversight. *GSC Advanced Research and Reviews*, *20*(1), 465–476. DOI: 10.30574/gscarr.2024.20.1.0287

Abubakari, P. (2024). *Human factors matter: the intersection of cybersecurity governance, and culture in risk management of critical infrastructure*. Pepperdine University.

Abut, S., Okut, H., Zackula, R., & Kallail, K. J. (2023). Deep neural networks and applications in medical research. In *Artificial intelligence*. IntechOpen., DOI: 10.5772/intechopen.112371

Addisu, E. G., Yirga, T. G., Yirga, H. G., & Yehuala, A. D. (2025). Transfer learning-based hybrid VGG16-machine learning approach for heart disease detection with explainable artificial intelligence. *Frontiers in Artificial Intelligence*, *8*, 1504281. DOI: 10.3389/frai.2025.1504281 PMID: 40070809

Adeniran, A. A., Onebunne, A. P., & William, P. (2024). Explainable AI (XAI) in healthcare: Enhancing trust and transparency in critical decision-making. *World Journal of Advanced Research and Reviews*, *23*(3), 2447–2658. DOI: 10.30574/wjarr.2024.23.3.2936

Adibi, A., Xu, C., Ji, Z., Kaur, J., Chen, W., Healey, E., Nuwagira, B., Ye, W., Woollard, G., Xu, M., Cui, H. T., Xi, J., Chang, T., Bikia, V., Zhang, N., Noori, A., Yuan, X., Hossain, M. B., Frank, H. A., . . . Jabbour, S. (2025). Recent advances, applications and open challenges in machine learning for health: Reflections from research roundtables at ML4H 2024 symposium. *arXiv*. https://doi.org//arxiv.2502.06693DOI: 10.48550

Agapito, G., & Cannataro, M. (2023). An overview on the challenges and limitations using cloud computing in healthcare corporations. *Big Data and Cognitive Computing*, *7*(2), 68. DOI: 10.3390/bdcc7020068

Ahmadi, A., & RabieNezhad Ganji, N. (2023). AI-driven medical innovations: Transforming healthcare through data intelligence. [IJBLS]. *International Journal of BioLife Sciences*, *2*(2), 132–142.

Ahmed, A., Xi, R., Hou, M., Shah, S. A., & Hameed, S. (2023). Harnessing big data analytics for healthcare: A comprehensive review of frameworks, implications, applications, and impacts. *IEEE Access : Practical Innovations, Open Solutions*, *11*, 112891–112928. DOI: 10.1109/ACCESS.2023.3323574

Ahouanmenou, S., Van Looy, A., & Poels, G. (2022). Information security and privacy in hospitals: A literature mapping and review of research gaps. *Informatics for Health & Social Care*, *48*(1), 30–46. DOI: 10.1080/17538157.2022.2049274 PMID: 35300555

Akbar, W., Ullah, M., Hussain, T., Haq, M. I. U., Ullah, I., Adhikari, D., & Khan, R. (2024). Cybersecurity Challenges and Strategies for Safe Artificial General Intelligence. In *Future Tech Startups and Innovation in the Age of AI* (pp. 209–236). CRC Press.

Akhai, S., & Abbass, M. (2025). Smart Manufacturing for Better Healthcare: Integrating 3D Printing, Robotics, and IoT. In Singh, S. P., Jain, D. K., & Debayle, J. (Eds.), *Healthcare Recommender Systems*. Springer., DOI: 10.1007/978-3-031-80056-6_16

Akinnagbe, O. B. (2024). Human-AI collaboration: Enhancing productivity and decision-making. *International Journal of Education Management and Technology*, *2*(3), 387–417. DOI: 10.58578/ijemt.v2i3.4209

Akmal, I., Khan, H., Khushnood, A., Zulfiqar, F., & Shahbaz, E. (2024). An efficient artificial intelligence (Al) and blockchain-based security strategies for enhancing the protection of low-power loT devices in 5G networks. *Spectrum of engineering sciences, 2*(3), 528-586.

Al Qudah, A. M., Al-haddad, L., & Aljabali, A. (2025). Combatting medical corruption: A global review of root causes, consequences, and evidence-based interventions. *International Journal of Innovative Research and Scientific Studies*, *8*(2), 968–985. DOI: 10.53894/ijirss.v8i2.5397

Alanazi, M. M. F., Almutairi, S., Alarjani, N., Alghaylan, M. Y. A., Aljawhari, M. S. M., & Alkhulaifi, A. A. S. (2024). Advancements in AI-driven diagnostic radiology: Enhancing accuracy and efficiency. *International Journal of Health Sciences*, *8*(S1), 737–749. DOI: 10.53730/ijhs.v8nS1.14928

Alevizos, L., & Dekker, M. (2024). Towards an AI-enhanced cyber threat intelligence processing pipeline. *Electronics (Basel)*, *13*(11), 2021. DOI: 10.3390/electronics13112021

Alghamdi, S., Mehmood, R., Alqurashi, F. A., & Alzahrani, A. (2025). Paving the Roadmap for XAI and IML in Healthcare: Data-Driven Discoveries and the FIXAIH Framework. *IEEE Access : Practical Innovations, Open Solutions*, *13*, 174393–174427. DOI: 10.1109/ACCESS.2025.3616353

Alhidaifi, S. M., Asghar, M. R., & Ansari, I. S. (2024). A survey on cyber resilience: Key strategies, research challenges, and future directions. *ACM Computing Surveys*, *56*(8), 1–48. DOI: 10.1145/3649218

Almadani, B., Kaisar, H., Thoker, I. R., & Aliyu, F. (2025). A systematic survey of distributed decision support systems in healthcare. *Systems*, *13*(3), 157. DOI: 10.3390/systems13030157

Almaiah, M. A., Saqr, L. M., Al-Rawwash, L. A., Altellawi, L. A., Al-Ali, R., & Almomani, O. (2024). Classification of Cybersecurity Threats, Vulnerabilities and Countermeasures in Database Systems. *Computers, Materials & Continua*, *81*(2), 3189–3220. DOI: 10.32604/cmc.2024.057673

Almotairi, A. H., Alswegi, F. H., Almutairi, M., Almotiry, F. S. F., Rakhimi, M. N. H. A., Aljamily, A. H. M., Aldosari, N. M. M., & Alaoufi, R. Y. (2022). A review in the application of artificial intelligence in many medical sectors. *Journal of Population Therapeutics and Clinical Pharmacology = Journal de la Thérapeutique des Populations et de la Pharmacologie Clinique*. Advance online publication. DOI: 10.53555//jptcp.v29i04.5772

Alotaibi, B. (2025). *A Review of Resilient IoT Systems: Trends*. Challenges, and Future Directions.

Alowais, S. A., Alghamdi, S. S., Alsuhebany, N., Alqahtani, T., Alshaya, A. I., Almohareb, S. N., Aldairem, A., Alrashed, M., Bin Saleh, K., Badreldin, H. A., Al Yami, M. S., Al Harbi, S., & Albekairy, A. M. (2023). Revolutionizing healthcare: The role of artificial intelligence in clinical practice. *BMC Medical Education*, *23*(1), 689. DOI: 10.1186/s12909-023-04698-z

Al-Qahtani, L. A. S., Alsomali, M. M., Al-Hadad, A. M., Alfaraj, Z. A., Almutairi, S. T., Al-Anazi, T. A., Alshehri, S. A., Al-Fifi, N. J., & Alharbi, S. F. (2025). FACTORS AFFECTING THE INTEGRATION OF ELECTRONIC HEALTH RECORD WORKFLOWS AMONG NURSES, MIDWIVES, MEDICAL SECRETARIES, AND HEALTH INFORMATICS SPECIALISTS IN RIYADH HOSPITALS. Scientific Culture, 11(3.1), 565–574. DOI: 10.5281/zenodo.11032569

Alraizza, A., & Algarni, A. (2023). Ransomware Detection Using Machine Learning: A Survey. *Big Data and Cognitive Computing*, *7*(3), 143. DOI: 10.3390/bdcc7030143

Alsabah, M., Naser, M. A., Albahri, A. S., Albahri, O. S., Alamoodi, A. H., Abdulhussain, S. H., & Alzubaidi, L. (2025). A comprehensive review on key technologies toward smart healthcare systems based IoT: Technical aspects, challenges and future directions. *Artificial Intelligence Review*, *58*(11), 343. DOI: 10.1007/s10462-025-11342-3

Alvarez-Melis, D., & Jaakkola, T. S. (2018). On the robustness of interpretability methods. ICML Workshop on Human Interpretability in Machine Learning. https://arxiv.org/abs/1806.08049

American Hospital Association (AHA). (2024). A look at 2024's health care cybersecurity challenges. https://www.aha.org/news/aha-cyber-intel/2024-10-07-look-2024s-health-care-cybersecurity-challenges

American Hospital Association. (2025). Report: Health care had most reported cyberthreats in 2024. AHA News. https://www.aha.org/news/headline/2025-05-12-report-health-care-had-most-reported-cyberthreats-2024

Amin, M. S., Ahmad, S., & Loh, W. K. (2025). Federated learning for Healthcare 5.0: A comprehensive survey, taxonomy, challenges, and solutions. *Soft Computing*, *29*(2), 673–700. DOI: 10.1007/s00500-025-10508-z

Amugongo, L. M., Kriebitz, A., Boch, A., & Lütge, C. (2025). Operationalising AI ethics through the agile software development lifecycle: A case study of AI-enabled mobile health applications. *AI and Ethics*, *5*(1), 227–244. DOI: 10.1007/s43681-023-00331-3

Anderson, J., Ross, A., Back, J., Duncan, M., Snell, P., Hopper, A., & Jaye, P. (2020). Beyond 'find and fix': Improving quality and safety through resilient healthcare systems. *International Journal for Quality in Health Care : Journal of the International Society for Quality in Health Care*, *32*(3), 204–211. DOI: 10.1093/intqhc/mzaa007 PMID: 32108882

Annie Silviya, S. H., Hilda Jerlin, C. M., Anirudh, G., Indresh Kumar, E., Renuka Devi, S., & Dilli Babu, M. (2025). Enhancing Host-Based Intrusion Detection: A NEAT-Optimized Ensemble Learning Approach. Int. Conf. Next Gener. Comput. Syst.: Intell. Syst. Sustain. Dev., ICNGCS - Conf. Proc. 2025 International Conference on Next Generation Computing Systems: Intelligent System for Sustainable Development, ICNGCS 2025 - Conference Proceedings. DOI: 10.1109/ICNGCS64900.2025.11183188

Ansari, M. T. J., Al-Zahrani, F. A., Pandey, D., & Agrawal, A. (2020). A fuzzy TOPSIS based analysis toward selection of effective security requirements engineering approach for trustworthy healthcare software development. *BMC Medical Informatics and Decision Making*, *20*(1), 236. DOI: 10.1186/s12911-020-01209-8

Ardagna, C. A., Cremonini, M., De Capitani di Vimercati, S., & Samarati, P. (2008). A privacy-aware access control system. *Journal of Computer Security*, *16*(4), 369–397. DOI: 10.3233/JCS-2008-0328

Argaw, S., Bempong, N., Eshaya-Chauvin, B., & Flahault, A. (2019). The state of research on cyberattacks against hospitals and available best practice recommendations: A scoping review. *BMC Medical Informatics and Decision Making*, *19*(1), 10. DOI: 10.1186/s12911-018-0724-5 PMID: 30634962

Arora, S., Rai, M., & Gupta, M. (2024). Importance of industry 5.0 in understanding emotional intelligence. In *Human-Machine Collaboration and Emotional Intelligence in Industry 5.0* (pp. 205–219). IGI Global Scientific Publishing., DOI: 10.4018/979-8-3693-6806-0.ch011

Asan, O., Bayrak, A. E., & Choudhury, A. (2020). Artificial intelligence and human trust in healthcare: Focus on clinicians. *Journal of Medical Internet Research*, *22*(6), e15154. DOI: 10.2196/15154

Ashrafi, E., Mosadeghrad, A. M., & Arab, M. (2025). Analysis of administrative health policies in healthcare organizations. *Journal of Health Administration*, *28*(1), 56–75. DOI: 10.61882/jha.28.1.56

Aslan, Ö., Aktuğ, S. S., Ozkan-Okay, M., Yilmaz, A. A., & Akin, E. (2023). A comprehensive review of cyber security vulnerabilities, threats, attacks, and solutions. *Electronics (Basel)*, *12*(6), 1333. DOI: 10.3390/electronics12061333

Athinaiou, M. (2022). *Model-based Management of Cyber Resiliency for Healthcare Systems* University of Brighton]. Ausaf, H., & Khan, M. Threats by Artificial Intelligence to Human Health and Human Existence.

Bajpai, A. (2023). Advancing healthcare through artificial intelligence: Innovations at the intersection of AI and medicine. *Journal of Propulsion Technology*, *44*(2). Advance online publication. DOI: 10.52783/tjjpt.v44.i2.131

Bala, I., Pindoo, I., Mijwil, M. M., Abotaleb, M., & Yundong, W. (2024). Ensuring security and privacy in Healthcare Systems: A Review Exploring challenges, solutions, Future trends, and the practical applications of Artificial Intelligence. *Jordan Medical Journal*, *58*(3).

Baniecki, H., & Biecek, P. (2024). Adversarial attacks and defenses in explainable artificial intelligence: A survey. *Information Fusion*, *107*, 102303. DOI: 10.1016/j.inffus.2024.102303

Barbieri, C., Neri, L., Stuard, S., Mari, F., & Martín-Guerrero, J. D. (2023). From electronic health records to clinical management systems: How the digital transformation can support healthcare services. *Clinical Kidney Journal*, *16*(11), 1878–1884. DOI: 10.1093/ckj/sfad168 PMID: 37915897

Barik, K., Misra, S., Fernandez-Sanz, L., & Koyuncu, M. (2023). RONSI: A framework for calculating return on network security investment. *Telecommunication Systems*, *84*(4), 533–548. DOI: 10.1007/s11235-023-01039-9

Ben Fekih, R., & Lahami, M. (2020). Application of BCT in Healthcare: A Comprehensive Study. In Jmaiel, M., Mokhtari, M., Abdulrazak, B., Aloulou, H., & Kallel, S. (Eds.), Lecture Notes in Computer Science: Vol. 12157. *The Impact of Digital Technologies on Public Health in Developed and Developing Countries. ICOST 2020*. Springer., DOI: 10.1007/978-3-030-51517-1_23

Bhushan, S., & Dixit, S. (2024). Explainable AI for Shaping Adoption of Artificial Intelligence. Asian Conf. Intell. Technol., ACOIT. 2024 Asian Conference on Intelligent Technologies, ACOIT 2024. DOI: 10.1109/ACOIT62457.2024.10939416

Bhuyan, S., Kabir, U., Escareno, J., Ector, K., Palakodeti, S., Wyant, D., Kumar, S., Levy, M., Kedia, S., Dasgupta, D., & Dobalian, A. (2020). Transforming healthcare cybersecurity from reactive to proactive: Current status and future recommendations. *Journal of Medical Systems*, *44*(5), 98. DOI: 10.1007/s10916-019-1507-y PMID: 32239357

Bienefeld, N., Keller, E., & Grote, G. (2024). Human-AI teaming in critical care: A comparative analysis of data scientists' and clinicians' perspectives on AI augmentation and automation. *Journal of Medical Internet Research*, *26*, e50130. DOI: 10.2196/50130 PMID: 39038285

Biggio, B., Fumera, G., & Roli, F. (2013). Security evaluation of pattern classifiers under attack. *IEEE Transactions on Knowledge and Data Engineering*, *26*(4), 984–996. DOI: 10.1109/TKDE.2013.57

Bi, W. L., Hosny, A., Schabath, M. B., Giger, M. L., Birkbak, N. J., Mehrtash, A., Allison, T., Arnaout, O., Abbosh, C., Dunn, I. F., Mak, R. H., Tamimi, R. M., Tempany, C. M., Swanton, C., Hoffmann, U., Schwartz, L. H., Gillies, R. J., Huang, R. Y., & Aerts, H. J. W. L. (2019). Artificial intelligence in cancer imaging: Clinical challenges and applications. *CA: a Cancer Journal for Clinicians*, *69*(2), 127–157. DOI: 10.3322/caac.21552 PMID: 30720861

Boonen, T. J., Feng, Y., & Tong, Z. (2025). Cybersecurity investments and cyber insurance purchases in a non-cooperative game. *ASTIN Bulletin*, *55*(2), 426–448. DOI: 10.1017/asb.2024.40

Brohi, S., & Mastoi, Q.-U.-A. (2025). AI Under Attack: Metric-Driven Analysis of Cybersecurity Threats in Deep Learning Models for Healthcare Applications. *Algorithms*, *18*(3), 157. Advance online publication. DOI: 10.3390/a18030157

Butani, J. B. (2026). AI-Based Zero Trust Security Models for Cloud Computing. Commun. Comput. Info. Sci., 2669 CCIS, 509–518. DOI: 10.1007/978-3-032-07373-0_37

Cadet, E., Etim, E. D., Essien, I. A., Ajayi, J. O., & Erigha, E. D. (2021). The role of reinforcement learning in adaptive cyber defense mechanisms. *International Journal of Multidisciplinary Research and Growth Evaluation*, *2*(2), 544–559. DOI: 10.54660/.IJMRGE.2021.2.2.544-559

Carayon, P. (2006). Human factors of complex sociotechnical systems. *Applied Ergonomics*, *37*(4), 525–535. DOI: 10.1016/j.apergo.2006.04.011

Cascella, M., Cascella, A., Monaco, F., & Shariff, M. N. (2023). Envisioning gamification in anesthesia, pain management, and critical care: Basic principles, integration of artificial intelligence, and simulation strategies. *Journal of Anesthesia, Analgesia and Critical Care*, *3*(1), 33. DOI: 10.1186/s44158-023-00118-2 PMID: 37697415

Chakkaravarthy, A. P., & Jaganathan, D. (2025). Intersecting AI and Medicine for Improved Care and Administrative Efficiency. In Ali, O., Amini, A., & Al-Ahmad, A. (Eds.), *Intersecting AI and Medicine for Improved Care and Administrative Efficiency* (pp. 39–58). IGI Global., DOI: 10.4018/979-8-3373-1772-4.ch002

Chakraborty, S. (2025). Beyond ETL: How AI Agents Are Building Self-Healing Data Pipelines. *Journal of Computer Science and Technology Studies*, *7*(3), 741–756. DOI: 10.32996/jcsts.2025.7.3.81

Chatterjee, I., Das, K. C., & Mukherjee, K. (2024). Revolutionizing innovations and impact of artificial intelligence in healthcare. *International Journal for Multidisciplinary Research*, *6*(3), 19333. Advance online publication. DOI: 10.36948/ijfmr.2024.v06i03.19333

Chatzikou, M., Latsou, D., Apostolidis, G., Billis, A., Charisis, V., Rigas, E. S., Bamidis, P. D., & Hadjileontiadis, L. (2025). Economic Evaluation of Artificially Intelligent (AI) Diagnostic Systems: Cost Consequence Analysis of Clinician-Friendly Interpretable Computer-Aided Diagnosis (ICADX) Tested in Cardiology, Obstetrics, and Gastroenterology, from the HosmartAI Horizon 2020 Project. *Healthcare (Basel)*, *13*(14), 1661. Advance online publication. DOI: 10.3390/healthcare13141661 PMID: 40724686

Chauhan, B. V., Vedrtnam, A., Wyche, K. P., & Verma, S. (2025). Review on Artificial Intelligence in the Environmental Monitoring. *Prospects of Artificial Intelligence in the Environment*, 29-60.

Chavan, R., & Shabadi, S. (2025). Cyber Security in Healthcare. In Mahalle, P. N., Shinde, G. R., Wasatkar, N. N., & Anerao, P. R. (Eds.), *Industry 5.0 for Society 5.0: Advancing Medical IoT and Smart Healthcare* (pp. 165–175). Bentham Science Publishers., DOI: 10.2174/9798898810450125010011

Chehri, A., Fofana, I., & Yang, X. (2021). Security risk modeling in smart grid critical infrastructures in the era of big data and artificial intelligence. *Sustainability (Basel)*, *13*(6), 3196. DOI: 10.3390/su13063196

Chen, C., Gong, X., Liu, Z., Jiang, W., Goh, S. Q., & Lam, K.-Y. (2024). Trustworthy, responsible, and safe ai: A comprehensive architectural framework for ai safety with challenges and mitigations. *arXiv preprint arXiv:2408.12935*.

Chen, Y., & Esmaeilzadeh, P. (2024). Generative AI in medical practice: In-depth exploration of privacy and security challenges. *Journal of Medical Internet Research*, *26*, e53008. DOI: 10.2196/53008 PMID: 38457208

Chen, Y.-M., Hsiao, T.-H., Lin, C.-H., & Fann, Y. C. (2025). Unlocking precision medicine: Clinical applications of integrating health records, genetics, and immunology through artificial intelligence. *Journal of Biomedical Science*, *32*(1), 16. DOI: 10.1186/s12929-024-01110-w PMID: 39915780

Cho, A., Cha, C., & Baek, G. (2024). Development of an artificial Intelligence–Based tailored mobile intervention for nurse burnout: Single-Arm trial. *Journal of Medical Internet Research*, *26*, e54029. DOI: 10.2196/54029 PMID: 38905631

Chong, W. F., Feng, R., Hu, H., & Zhang, L. (2025). Cyber risk assessment for capital management. *The Journal of Risk and Insurance*, *92*(2), 424–471. DOI: 10.1111/jori.12504

Choudhury, A. (2022). Toward an ecologically valid conceptual framework for the use of artificial intelligence in clinical settings. *JMIR Human Factors*, *9*(2), e35421. Advance online publication. DOI: 10.2196/35421 PMID: 35727615

Choudhury, P., & Goel, P. (2025). Interface of Artificial Intelligence with Conventional Biostatistics in Healthcare Research. In *Methods in Molecular Biology* (Vol. 2952, pp. 411–428). Humana Press Inc., DOI: 10.1007/978-1-0716-4690-8_22

Cihan, S., Yılmaz, N., Ozsoy, A., & Beyan, O. D. (2025). A systematic review of the blockchain application in healthcare research domain: Toward a unified conceptual model. *Medical & Biological Engineering & Computing*, *63*(5), 1319–1342. DOI: 10.1007/s11517-024-03274-x PMID: 39789305

Cinar, A. B., & Bilodeau, S. (2024). Incorporating AI into the inner circle of emotional intelligence for sustainability. *Sustainability (Basel)*, *16*(15), 6648. DOI: 10.3390/su16156648

Corbin, C. K., Maclay, R., Acharya, A., Mony, S., Punnathanam, S., Thapa, R., Kotecha, N., Shah, N. H., & Chen, J. H. (2023). DEPLOYR: A technical framework for deploying custom real-time machine learning models into the electronic medical record. *Journal of the American Medical Informatics Association : JAMIA*, *30*(9), 1532–1542. DOI: 10.1093/jamia/ocad114 PMID: 37369008

Coventry, L., & Branley, D. (2018). Cybersecurity in healthcare: A narrative review of trends, threats and ways forward. *Maturitas*, *113*, 48–52. DOI: 10.1016/j.maturitas.2018.04.008 PMID: 29903648

Creed, T. A., Salama, L., Slevin, R., Tanana, M., Imel, Z., Narayanan, S., & Atkins, D. C. (2022). Enhancing the quality of cognitive behavioral therapy in community mental health through artificial intelligence generated fidelity feedback (Project AFFECT): A study protocol. *BMC Health Services Research*, *22*(1), 1177. DOI: 10.1186/s12913-022-08519-9 PMID: 36127689

Cresswell, K., & Sheikh, A. (2017). Organizational issues in the implementation and adoption of health information technology innovations: An interpretative review. *International Journal of Medical Informatics*, *86*, 1–14. DOI: 10.1016/j.ijmedinf.2015.09.012 PMID: 23146626

CTIIC / Office of the Director of National Intelligence. (2024). Ransomware attacks surge in 2023; attacks on the healthcare sector nearly double. https://www.dni.gov/files/CTIIC/documents/products/Ransomware_Attacks_Surge_in_2023.pdf

Daga, E., & Groth, P. (2024). Data journeys: Explaining AI workflows through abstraction. *Semantic Web*, *15*(4), 1057–1083. DOI: 10.3233/SW-233407

Dailah, H. G., Koriri, M., Sabei, A., Kriry, T., & Zakri, M. (2024, December). Artificial intelligence in nursing: technological benefits to nurse's mental health and patient care quality. In *Healthcare* (Vol. 12, No. 24, p. 2555). MDPI. https://doi.org/DOI: 10.3390/healthcare12242555

Daly, S. J., Hearn, G., & Papageorgiou, K. (2025). Sensemaking with AI: How trust influences Human-AI collaboration in health and creative industries. *Social Sciences & Humanities Open*, *11*, 101346. Advance online publication. DOI: 10.1016/j.ssaho.2025.101346

Das, P., Gupta, I., & Mishra, S. (2024). Artificial intelligence driven cybersecurity in digital healthcare frameworks. In Gupta, D., & Hassanien, A. E. (Eds.), *Securing Next-Generation Connected Healthcare Systems: Artificial Intelligence Technologies* (pp. 213–228). Elsevier., DOI: 10.1016/B978-0-443-13951-2.00002-7

Davahli, M. R., Karwowski, W., Fiok, K., Wan, T., & Parsaei, H. R. (2021). Controlling safety of artificial intelligence-based systems in healthcare. *Symmetry*, *13*(1), 102. DOI: 10.3390/sym13010102

De Morais Rodrigues, L. E., Santos, G. N., Bonamigo, A., Garza-Reyes, J. A., Calado, R. D., & Santos, A. B. (2025). Empirical Evaluation of the Emergency Care Ecosystem Using Artificial Intelligence for Decision-Makers' Support. IEEE Int. Conf. Ind. Appl., INDUSCON - Proc., 1012–1018. DOI: 10.1109/INDUSCON66435.2025.11241784

Department of Health and Human Services, Office for Civil Rights. (2024). Cybersecurity resources for HIPAA-regulated entities. https://csrc.nist.gov/files/pubs/sp/800/66/r2/final/docs/sp800-66r2-cybersecurity-resources.pdf

Devi, M.M Syamala Devi. (2024). Artificial intelligence in medicine. *International Journal for Multidisciplinary Research*, *6*(1), 12490. Advance online publication. DOI: 10.36948/ijfmr.2024.v06i01.12490

Dey, D. N. C. (2024). Harmonizing the threads of well-being: AI (artificial intelligence), spirituality, healthcare, and management. *Spirituality, Healthcare, And Management* (April 24, 2024). DOI: 10.2139/ssrn.5002655

Dhinakaran, D., Kumar, N. J., & Ponnuviji, N. (2025). Safeguarding confidentiality and privacy in cloud-enabled healthcare systems with spectrasafe encryption and dynamic k-anonymity algorithm. *Expert Systems with Applications, 279*, 127584. DOI: 10.1016/j.eswa.2025.127584

Dhingra, S., Raut, R. D., Yadav, V. S., Cheikhrouhou, N., & Naik, B. K. R. (2025). Blockchain adoption challenges in the healthcare sector: A waste management perspective. *Operations Management Research : Advancing Practice Through Research, 18*(2), 518–536. DOI: 10.1007/s12063-023-00413-9 PMID: 40625400

Di Martino, B., Rak, M., Ficco, M., Esposito, A., Maisto, S. A., & Nacchia, S. (2018). Internet of things reference architectures, security and interoperability: A survey. *Internet of Things : Engineering Cyber Physical Human Systems, 1*, 99–112. DOI: 10.1016/j.iot.2018.08.008

Dlamini, Z., Miya, T. V., Hull, R., Molefi, T., Khanyile, R., & de Vasconcellos, J. F. (2023). Society 5.0: Realizing Next-Generation Healthcare. In Dlamini, Z. (Ed.), *Society 5.0 and Next Generation Healthcare*. Springer., DOI: 10.1007/978-3-031-36461-7_1

Dotsenko, T., & Kuzmenko, M. (2023). Cyber fraud as a threat to the sustainable development of the health care system: A systematic bibliometric analysis. *Stalyi rozvytok ekonomiky*. https://doi.org/DOI: 10.32782/2308-1988/2023-47-7

Doukas, N. (2025). Reliability-based design optimization for cyber survivability. In *Reliability Assessment and Optimization of Complex Systems* (pp. 363–411). Elsevier. DOI: 10.1016/B978-0-443-29112-8.00029-3

Dupont, B. (2019). The cyber-resilience of financial institutions: Significance and applicability. *Journal of Cybersecurity, 5*(1), tyz013. DOI: 10.1093/cybsec/tyz013

Dupont, B., Côté, A.-M., Savine, C., & Décary-Hétu, D. (2019). The ecology of trust among hackers. *Global Crime, 17*(2), 129–151. DOI: 10.1080/17440572.2016.1157480

Dzindolet, M. T., Pierce, L. G., Beck, H. P., & Dawe, L. A. (2024). From trust in automation to trust in AI in healthcare: A 30-year longitudinal review and an interdisciplinary framework. PMC. https://pmc.ncbi.nlm.nih.gov/articles/PMC12562135/

Ehrenfeld, J. M. (2017). WannaCry, cybersecurity and health information technology: A time to act. *Journal of Medical Systems, 41*(10), 104. DOI: 10.1007/s10916-017-0752-1 PMID: 28540616

El Arab, R. A., & Al Moosa, O. A. (2025). Systematic review of cost effectiveness and budget impact of artificial intelligence in healthcare. *NPJ Digital Medicine, 8*(1), 548. Advance online publication. DOI: 10.1038/s41746-025-01722-y PMID: 40858882

Elhaddad, M., & Hamam, S. (2024). AI-driven clinical decision support systems: An ongoing pursuit of potential. *Cureus, 16*(4), e57728. DOI: 10.7759/cureus.57728 PMID: 38711724

Ellahham, S., Ellahham, N., & Simsekler, M. C. E. (2020). Application of artificial intelligence in the health care safety context: Opportunities and challenges. *American Journal of Medical Quality : The Official Journal of the American College of Medical Quality, 35*(4), 341–348. DOI: 10.1177/1062860619878515 PMID: 31581790

Emma, O., & Harri, F. (2023). Integrating Cybersecurity Measures into Data Governance Policies for Content Management.

Esmaeilzadeh, P. (2022). Benefits and concerns associated with blockchain-based health information exchange (HIE): A qualitative study from physicians' perspectives. *BMC Medical Informatics and Decision Making, 22*(1), 80. DOI: 10.1186/s12911-022-01815-8 PMID: 35346176

Esther, D. (2025). Securing Sensitive Health Data in AI Pipelines.

European Parliament & Council of the European Union. (2024). Regulation (EU) 2024/1689 — Artificial Intelligence Act. Official Journal of the European Union. https://eur-lex.europa.eu/legal-content/EN/TXT/?uri=CELEX:32024R1689

European Parliament and Council. (2016). *Regulation (EU) 2016/679 (General Data Protection Regulation).* Official Journal of the European Union.

European Parliament and Council. (2022). *Directive (EU) 2022/2555 on measures for a high common level of cybersecurity across the Union (NIS2 Directive).* Official Journal of the European Union.

Ewoh, P., & Vartiainen, T. (2024). Vulnerability to cyberattacks and sociotechnical solutions for health care systems: Systematic review. *Journal of Medical Internet Research, 26*, e46904. DOI: 10.2196/46904 PMID: 38820579

Ewoh, P., Vartiainen, T., & Mantere, T. (2025). Sociotechnical cybersecurity framework for securing health care from vulnerabilities and cyberattacks: Scoping review. *Journal of Medical Internet Research, 27*, e75584. DOI: 10.2196/75584 PMID: 40838797

Fahim, Y. A., Hasani, I. W., Kabba, S., & Ragab, W. M. (2025). Artificial intelligence in healthcare and medicine: Clinical applications, therapeutic advances, and future perspectives. *European Journal of Medical Research, 30*(1), 848. DOI: 10.1186/s40001-025-03196-w PMID: 40988064

Farahat, M. A., Darwish, A., & Hassanien, A. E. (2023). The Implication of Metaverse in the Traditional Medical Environment and Healthcare Sector: Applications and Challenges. In Hassanien, A. E., Darwish, A., & Torky, M. (Eds.), *The Future of Metaverse in the Virtual Era and Physical World. Studies in Big Data* (Vol. 123). Springer., DOI: 10.1007/978-3-031-29132-6_7

Fatima, I., Grover, V., Khan, I. R., Ahmad, N., & Yadav, A. (2023). Artificial intelligence in medical field. *EAI Endorsed Transactions on Pervasive Health and Technology*, *9*. Advance online publication. DOI: 10.4108/eetpht.9.4713

FAVINO. R., CONTE, N., DE, M. A., GARCIA, M. E., MONTANARI, E., PAGANINI, A., SANGIORGI, M., & SFALAGKIARIS, C. E. (2025). Emerging risks and opportunities for EU internal security stemming from new technologies.

Feki, I., Ammar, S., Kessentini, Y., & Philip, K. (2023). Federated learning for IoMT applications: A standardization and benchmarking framework. *IEEE Communications Magazine*, *61*(6), 36–42. DOI: 10.1109/MCOM.001.2200055

Felix, E. A., & Lee, S. P. (2019). Systematic literature review of preprocessing techniques for imbalanced data. *IET Software*, *13*(6), 479–496. DOI: 10.1049/iet-sen.2018.5193

Ferdous, J., Islam, R., Mahboubi, A., & Islam, M. Z. (2025). A novel technique for ransomware detection using image based dynamic features and transfer learning to address dataset limitations. *Scientific Reports*, *15*(1), 32342. Advance online publication. DOI: 10.1038/s41598-025-17647-1 PMID: 40897752

Ferguson, J. (2025). The human element: Ethical guardrails for AI in modern medicine. *The American Journal of Cosmetic Surgery*, *42*(3), 149–154. DOI: 10.1177/07488068251359686

Finlayson, S. G., Bowers, J. D., Ito, J., Zittrain, J. L., Beam, A. L., & Kohane, I. S. (2019). Adversarial attacks on medical machine learning. *Science*, *363*(6433), 1287–1289. DOI: 10.1126/science.aaw4399 PMID: 30898923

Folorunso, A., Wada, I., Samuel, B., & Mohammed, V. (2024). Security compliance and its implication for cybersecurity. *World Journal of Advanced Research and Reviews*, *24*(01), 2105–2121. DOI: 10.30574/wjarr.2024.24.1.3170

Forescout Technologies. (2024). Ransomware in healthcare: The NHS example and what the future holds. https://www.forescout.com/blog/ransomware-in-healthcare-the-nhs-example-and-what-the-future-holds/

Fotis, F. (2024). Economic Impact of Cyber Attacks and Effective Cyber Risk Management Strategies: A light literature review and case study analysis. *Procedia Computer Science*, *251*, 471–478. DOI: 10.1016/j.procs.2024.11.135

Furrow, B. R. (2020). The limits of current AI in health care: Patient safety policing in hospitals. *Ne. UL Rev.*, *12*, 1.

Gajula, M. (2025). Empowering Healthcare Professionals: The Role of Cloud-Native Data Engineering in Human-AI Collaboration. *Journal of Computer Science and Technology Studies*, *7*(4), 417–426. DOI: 10.32996/jcsts.2025.7.4.50

Gambetti, A., Han, Q., Shen, H., & Soares, C. (2025). A survey on human-centered evaluation of explainable AI methods in clinical decision support systems. arXiv preprint arXiv:2502.09849.

García-Pérez, A., Cegarra-Navarro, J., Sallos, M., Martínez-Caro, E., & Chinnaswamy, A. (2022). Resilience in healthcare systems: Cyber security and digital transformation. *Technovation*, *121*, 102583. DOI: 10.1016/j.technovation.2022.102583

George, A. S., George, A. H., & Baskar, T. (2024). Artificial intelligence and the future of healthcare: Emerging jobs and skills in 2035. *Partners Universal Multidisciplinary Research Journal*, *1*(1), 1–21. DOI: 10.5281/zenodo.11176554

Gerke, S., Minssen, T., Cohen, G., & Tobia, K. P. (2025). Ethical and legal considerations in healthcare AI: Innovation and policy for safe and fair use. *Royal Society Open Science*, *12*(5), 241873. Advance online publication. DOI: 10.1098/rsos.241873 PMID: 40370601

Ghafur, S., Kristensen, S., Honeyford, K., Martin, G., Darzi, A., & Aylin, P. (2019). A retrospective impact analysis of the WannaCry cyberattack on the NHS. *NPJ Digital Medicine*, *2*(1), 98. DOI: 10.1038/s41746-019-0161-6 PMID: 31602404

Ghosh, O., Kumar, B., & Roy, P. K. (2025). Role of AI in revolutionizing clinical care. In Tariq, M. U. (Ed.), *Emerging Multisector Applications of AI and IoT* (pp. 69–102). IGI Global., DOI: 10.4018/979-8-3373-4332-7.ch003

Gill, A. Y., Saeed, A., Rasool, S., Husnain, A., & Hussain, H. K. (2023). Revolutionizing healthcare: How machine learning is transforming patient diagnoses. *Journal of Wood Science*, *2*(10), 1638–1652. DOI: 10.58344/jws.v2i10.449

Giordano, C., Brennan, M., Mohamed, B., Rashidi, P., Modave, F., & Tighe, P. (2021). Accessing artificial intelligence for clinical decision-making. *Frontiers in Digital Health*, *3*, 645232. Advance online publication. DOI: 10.3389/fdgth.2021.645232 PMID: 34713115

Goh, E., Bunning, B., Khoong, E. C., Gallo, R. J., Milstein, A., Centola, D., & Chen, J. H. (2025). Physician clinical decision modification and bias assessment in a randomized controlled trial of AI assistance. *Communications Medicine*, *5*(1), 59. DOI: 10.1038/s43856-025-00781-2 PMID: 40038550

Gomez, C., Unberath, M., & Huang, C.-M. (2024). Human-AI collaboration is not very collaborative yet: A taxonomy of interaction patterns in AI-assisted decision making. *Frontiers of Computer Science*. Advance online publication. DOI: 10.3389/fcomp.2024.1521066

Graves, M., & Compson, J. (2024, October). Compassionate AI for moral decision-making, health, and well-being. In *Proceedings of the AAAI/ACM Conference on AI, Ethics, and Society* (Vol. 7, No. 1, pp. 520-533). https://doi.org/DOI: 10.1609/aies.v7i1.31655

Gundu, T. (2024). Learn, unlearn and relearn: Adaptive cybersecurity culture model. International Conference on Cyber Warfare and Security

Gyrard, A., Tabeau, K., Fiorini, L., Kung, A., Senges, E., De Mul, M., Giuliani, F., Lefebvre, D., Hoshino, H., Fabbricotti, I., Sancarlo, D., D'Onofrio, G., Cavallo, F., Guiot, D., Arzoz-Fernandez, E., Okabe, Y., & Tsukamoto, M. (2023). Knowledge engineering framework for IoT robotics applied to smart healthcare and emotional well-being. *International Journal of Social Robotics*, *15*(3), 445–472. DOI: 10.1007/s12369-021-00821-6 PMID: 34804257

Habbal, A., Ali, M. K., & Abuzaraida, M. A. (2024). Artificial Intelligence Trust, risk and security management (AI trism): Frameworks, applications, challenges and future research directions. *Expert Systems with Applications*, *240*, 122442. DOI: 10.1016/j.eswa.2023.122442

Hammad, M., Panaousis, M., Ali, H., & Khan, W. A. (2026). Industry 4.0 in Pharmaceuticals: A New Era of Smart Manufacturing. In *Smart Manufacturing Blueprint: Navigating Industry 4.0 Across Diverse Sectors. Springer Series in Advanced Manufacturing*. Springer., DOI: 10.1007/978-3-032-00214-3_6

Hanumantharaju, R., Pradeep Kumar, D., Sowmya, B. J., Siddesh, G. M., Shreenath, K. N., & Srinivasa, K. G. (2021). Enabling Technologies for Fog Computing in Healthcare 4.0: Challenges and Future Implications. In Tanwar, S. (Ed.), *Fog Computing for Healthcare 4.0 Environments. Signals and Communication Technology*. Springer., DOI: 10.1007/978-3-030-46197-3_7

He, J., Baxter, S. L., Xu, J., Xu, J., Zhou, X., & Zhang, K. (2019). The practical implementation of artificial intelligence technologies in medicine. Nature Medicine, 25(1), 30–36. PubMed

Health Service Executive (2021). Conti cyber attack on the HSE: A report by PricewaterhouseCoopers. Published December 2021.

Herath, H., Herath, H., Madhusanka, B., & Guruge, L. (2024). Data protection challenges in the processing of sensitive data. In *Data Protection: The Wake of AI and Machine Learning* (pp. 155–179). Springer. DOI: 10.1007/978-3-031-76473-8_8

Hernandez, J. P. T. (2024). Compassionate care with autonomous AI humanoid robots in future healthcare delivery: A multisensory simulation of next-generation models. *Biomimetics*, *9*(11), 687. DOI: 10.3390/biomimetics9110687 PMID: 39590259

He, X., Zheng, X., & Ding, H. (2023). Existing barriers faced by and future design recommendations for direct-to-consumer health care artificial intelligence apps: Scoping review. *Journal of Medical Internet Research*, *25*, e50342. DOI: 10.2196/50342 PMID: 38109173

He, Y., Xin, T., & Luo, C. (2025). Enhancing Cybersecurity Investment with FAIR-ROSI: A Responsible Cybersecurity Approach to Digital Society. *Information Systems Frontiers*. Advance online publication. DOI: 10.1007/s10796-025-10625-y PMID: 42206284

He, Y., Zhang, J., Shan, H., & Wang, G. (2024). Survey on adversarial attack and defense for medical image analysis: Methods and challenges. *ACM Computing Surveys*. Advance online publication. DOI: 10.1145/3702638

Higgins, O., Chalup, S. K., & Wilson, R. L. (2024). Artificial Intelligence in nursing: Trustworthy or reliable? *Journal of Research in Nursing : JRN*, *29*(2), 143–153. DOI: 10.1177/17449871231215696 PMID: 39070561

Hinder, F., Vaquet, V., & Hammer, B. (2024). One or two things we know about concept drift — A survey on monitoring in evolving environments. *Frontiers in Artificial Intelligence*, *7*, 1330257. DOI: 10.3389/frai.2024.1330257 PMID: 38962502

HOSSAINESRAT ZAHAN SNIGDHASHOHONI MAHABUB. (2023). AI-Driven Data Optimization: Automating Cleaning, Feature Engineering, and Augmentation for Superior Machine Learning Performance in Digital Health Care System. *Journal of Computer Science and Technology Studies*, *5*(4), 218–228. DOI: 10.32996/jcsts.2023.5.4.23

Hudson, J. (2024). Artificial Intelligence and Cybersecurity Integration: Modern Database Techniques for Securing AI Models.

Ibrahim, A. M., Zoromba, M. A., Abousoliman, A. D., Zaghamir, D. E. F., Alenezi, I. N., Elsayed, E. A., & Mohamed, H. A. H. (2025). Ethical implications of artificial intelligence integration in nursing practice in arab countries: Literature review. *BMC Nursing*, *24*(1), 159. DOI: 10.1186/s12912-025-02798-3 PMID: 39934834

Igwe-Nmaju, C., & Anadozie, C. (2022). Commanding digital trust in high-stakes sectors: Communication strategies for sustaining stakeholder confidence amid technological risk. *World Journal of Advanced Research and Reviews*, *15*(3), 609–630. DOI: 10.30574/wjarr.2022.15.3.0920

Ilori, O., Lawal, C. I., Friday, S. C., Isibor, N. J., & Chukwuma-Eke, E. C. (2022). Cybersecurity auditing in the digital age: A review of methodologies and regulatory implications. *Journal of Frontiers in Multidisciplinary Research*, *3*(1), 174–187. DOI: 10.54660/.IJFMR.2022.3.1.174-187

Islam, S., Basheer, N., Papastergiou, S., Ciampi, M., & Silvestri, S. (2025). Intelligent dynamic cybersecurity risk management framework with explainability and interpretability of AI models for enhancing security and resilience of digital infrastructure. *Journal of Reliable Intelligent Environments*, *11*(3), 12. DOI: 10.1007/s40860-025-00253-3 PMID: 40656511

Ispahany, J., Islam, M., Islam, M. Z., & Khan, M. A. (2024). Ransomware Detection Using Machine Learning: A Review, Research Limitations and Future Directions. *IEEE Access : Practical Innovations, Open Solutions*, *12*, 68785–68813. DOI: 10.1109/ACCESS.2024.3397921

Issa, W. B., Shorbagi, A., Alshorman, A., Rababa, M., Majed, K. A., Radwan, H., Raffat, F. A., Al-Yateem, N., Mottershead, R., Abdelrahim, D. N., Hijazi, H., Khasawneh, W., Ibrahim, A., Abbas, N., & Fakhry, R. (2024). Shaping the future: Perspectives on the integration of artificial intelligence in health profession education. *Research Square*. https://doi.org/DOI: 10.21203/rs.3.rs-4396289/v1

Jabarulla, M. Y., & Lee, H.-N. (2021). A blockchain and artificial intelligence-based, patient-centric healthcare system for combating the COVID-19 pandemic: Opportunities and applications. Healthcare

Jalali, M., & Kaiser, J. (2018). Cybersecurity in hospitals: A systematic, organizational perspective. *Journal of Medical Internet Research*, *20*(5), e10059. DOI: 10.2196/10059 PMID: 29807882

Jalali, M., Razak, S., Gordon, W., Perakslis, E., & Madnick, S. (2019). Health care and cybersecurity: Bibliometric analysis of the literature. *Journal of Medical Internet Research*, *21*(2), e12644. DOI: 10.2196/12644 PMID: 30767908

Javed, H., El-Sappagh, S., & Abuhmed, T. (2024). Robustness in deep learning models for medical diagnostics: security and adversarial challenges towards robust AI applications. Artificial Intelligence Review, 58(1), 12.

Jia, J., & Zhao, S. (2025). Ethical and legal governance of generative AI in Chinese healthcare. *Journal of Multidisciplinary Healthcare*, *5405*, 5405–5419. Advance online publication. DOI: 10.2147/JMDH.S541271 PMID: 40917542

Jiang, J. X., Ross, J. S., & Bai, G. (2025). Ransomware Attacks and Data Breaches in U.S. Health Care Systems. *JAMA Network Open*, *8*(5), e2510180. DOI: 10.1001/jamanetworkopen.2025.10180 PMID: 40366661

Jonas, D., Maria, E., Widiasari, I. R., Rahardja, U., & Wellem, T. (2024). Design of a tam framework with emotional variables in the acceptance of health-based iot in indonesia. *ADI Journal on Recent Innovation*, *5*(2), 146–154. DOI: 10.34306/ajri.v5i2.1005

Jourdain, D. (2026). Cybersecurity for Interventional Radiologists: A Clinical Imperative for Protecting Patient Data and Imaging Systems. *Journal of Vascular and Interventional Radiology*, *37*(3), 107920. Advance online publication. DOI: 10.1016/j.jvir.2025.107920 PMID: 41270935

Journal, H. I. P. A. A. (2025). The biggest healthcare data breaches of 2024. https://www.hipaajournal.com/biggest-healthcare-data-breaches-2024/

Juang, W.-C., Hsu, M.-H., Cai, Z.-X., & Chen, C.-M. (2022). Developing an AI-assisted clinical decision support system to enhance in-patient holistic health care. *PLoS One*, *17*(10), e0276501. DOI: 10.1371/journal.pone.0276501 PMID: 36315554

Kamel Boulos, M. N., Wilson, J. T., & Clauson, K. A. (2018). Geospatial blockchain: Promises, challenges, and scenarios in health and healthcare. *International Journal of Health Geographics*, *17*(1), 25. DOI: 10.1186/s12942-018-0144-x PMID: 29973196

Kashyap, V. R., Bhushan, B., Farhaoui, Y., & Alkhayyat, A. (2025). Digital Twin Robots for Securing IoT Based Healthcare 4.0 Application: Key Technologies, Integration Trends and Recent Advancement. In Sharma, R., & Jeon, G. (Eds.), *Data Analytics for Smart Robotics and Its Applications. Intelligent Systems Reference Library* (Vol. 272). Springer., DOI: 10.1007/978-3-031-87697-4_3

Kaul, D., & Khurana, R. (2021). AI to detect and mitigate security vulnerabilities in APIs: Encryption, authentication, and anomaly detection in enterprise-level distributed systems. *Eigenpub Review of Science and Technology*, *5*(1), 34–62.

Kaushik, K., Khan, A., Kumari, A., Sharma, I., & Dubey, R. (2024). Ethical considerations in AI-based cybersecurity. In *Next-generation cybersecurity: AI, ML, and Blockchain* (pp. 437-470). Springer. DOI: 10.1007/978-981-97-1249-6_19

Kaviani, S., Khokhar, A. A., & Sharifzadeh, M. (2022). Adversarial attacks and defenses on AI in medical imaging informatics: A survey. *Neurocomputing*, *492*, 278–307. DOI: 10.1016/j.neucom.2022.04.051

Kavitha, N., Nivethitha, T., Deebanchakkarawarthi, G., & Shakthipriya, P. (2025). Transforming Healthcare: Unleashing the Power of Artificial Intelligence of Things (AIoT). In Rajasekaran, A. S., Al-Turjman, F., & Suganyadevi, S. (Eds.), *AIoT: Artificial Intelligence of Things* (pp. 99–129). CRC Press., DOI: 10.1201/9781003482338-5

Khan, M. Z., Naeem, M. S., Khalid, S., Gill, Z., Ali, H., Iqbal, S., Shahid, S., Sulman, A., Awan, A., & Kharl, H. A. A. (2026). AI-GUIDED QSAR, MOLECULAR DYNAMICS, AND PHARMACOPHORE MODELING. *PharmA AI: Revolutionizing Drug Discovery and Healthcare with Artificial Intelligence*.

Khan, A. A., Laghari, A. A., Baqasah, A. M., Bacarra, R., Alroobaea, R., Alsafyani, M., & Alsayaydeh, J. A. J. (2025). BDLT-IoMT—a novel architecture: SVM machine learning for robust and secure data processing in Internet of Medical Things with blockchain cybersecurity. *The Journal of Supercomputing*, *81*(1), 271. DOI: 10.1007/s11227-024-06782-7

Khan, A. A., Shaikh, A. K., Alroobaea, R., Baqasah, A. M., Alsafyani, M., Alsufyani, H., & Laghari, A. A. (2025). Blockchain-enabled secure Internet of Medical Things (IoMT) architecture for multi-modal data fusion in precision cancer diagnosis and continuous monitoring. *Journal of Cloud Computing (Heidelberg, Germany)*, *14*(1), 58. DOI: 10.1186/s13677-025-00775-4

Kharl, H. A. A. (2026). *PharmA AI: Revolutionizing Drug Discovery and Healthcare with Artificial Intelligence*. IBH Publisher.

Khurana, P., Narula, S., Tiwari, N., Kapoor, R., & Arora, M. (2024). Mapping the cybersecurity research: A comprehensive bibliometric analysis. *International Journal of Experimental Research and Review*, 46, 016. https://doi.org/DOI: 10.52756/ijerr.2024.v46.016

Kim, Y. J., Park, Y. S., & Park, S.-P. (2026). Enhancing data governance through transparency: An empirical study of the data trust model. *Technological Forecasting and Social Change*, *225*, 124551. Advance online publication. DOI: 10.1016/j.techfore.2026.124551

Kleinrichert, D. (2024). Empathy: An ethical consideration of AI & others in the workplace. *AI & Society*, *39*(6), 2743–2757. DOI: 10.1007/s00146-023-01831-w

KnowBe4 (2023). Hacked healthcare: A global crisis in cybersecurity. https://www.knowbe4.com/hubfs/Global-Healthcare-Report-and-Timeline-EN_US.pdf

Komaragiri, S., Alla, S., Duvall, T., Karahan, S., Bheesetty, N., & Chattu, V. (2025). A governance-centric framework for strengthening healthcare cybersecurity: A systems perspective. *International Conference on Cyber Warfare and Security*. https://doi.org/DOI: 10.34190/iccws.20.1.3374

Konnoth, C. (2024). AI and data protection law in health. In Solaiman, B., & Cohen, I. G. (Eds.), *Research Handbook on Health, AI and the Law*. Edward Elgar Publishing., DOI: 10.4337/9781802205657.ch07

Koppel, R., Smith, S., Blythe, J., & Kothari, V. (2015). Workarounds to computer access in healthcare settings. *Studies in Health Technology and Informatics*, *208*, 287–291.

Kruegel, C., Kirda, E., Mutz, D., Robertson, W., & Vigna, G. (2005). Automating mimicry attacks using static binary analysis. USENIX Security Symposium

Kumari, A., Kumar, P., & Golyan, A. (2024). Introduction of Blockchain for Biomedical and Healthcare System. In Kumar, P., & Kumari, A. (Eds.), *Blockchain for Biomedical Research and Healthcare. Interdisciplinary Biotechnological Advances*. Springer., DOI: 10.1007/978-981-97-4268-4_1

Kumari, M., Gupta, M., & Ved, C. (2021). Blockchain in Pharmaceutical Sector. In Namasudra, S., & Deka, G. C. (Eds.), *Applications of Blockchain in Healthcare. Studies in Big Data* (Vol. 83). Springer., DOI: 10.1007/978-981-15-9547-9_8

Kusumadewi, S., & Miladiyah, I. (2023). Do clinical decision support systems improve patient safety? *Indonesian Journal of Electrical Engineering and Computer Science*, *30*(3), 1748. DOI: 10.11591/ijeecs.v30.i3.pp1748-1761

Kwon, J., & Johnson, M. E. (2018). Meaningful healthcare security. *Management Information Systems Quarterly*, *42*(4), 1043–A1047. DOI: 10.25300/MISQ/2018/13580

Latif, R. M. A., Mamarasulov, S., Farhan, M., Ullah, F., & Ahmad, J. (2026). Explainability of AI in Multimedia Security: Bridging the Gap between Complexity and Trust. In Srivastava, V. K., Khare, P., Awasthi, D., & Garg, L. (Eds.), *Multimedia And Multimodal Intelligence For Sustainable Development* (pp. 1–22). CRC Press., DOI: 10.1201/9781003634522-1

Lee, J., Kim, J., Jeong, H., & Lee, K. (2025). A Machine Learning-Based Ransomware Detection Method for Attackers' Neutralization Techniques Using Format-Preserving Encryption. *Sensors (Basel), 25*(8), 2406. DOI: 10.3390/s25082406 PMID: 40285096

Leenen, J. P. L., Hiemstra, P., Ten Hoeve, M. M., Jansen, A. C. J., van Dijk, J. D., Vendel, B., Versteeg, G., Hakvoort, G. A., & Hettinga, M. (2025). Exploring the complex nature of implementation of Artificial intelligence in clinical practice: An interview study with healthcare professionals, researchers and Policy and Governance Experts. PLOS Digital Health, 4(5 May). DOI: 10.1371/journal.pdig.0000847

Levin, C., Naimi, E., & Saban, M. (2024). Evaluating GenAI systems to combat mental health issues in healthcare workers: An integrative literature review. *International Journal of Medical Informatics, 191*, 105566. DOI: 10.1016/j.ijmedinf.2024.105566 PMID: 39079316

Li, J.. (2025). Analysis of LockBit 3.0 and its infiltration into Advanced's infrastructure crippling NHS services. arXiv:2308.05565.

Lindgren, H. (2025). Emerging roles and relationships among humans and interactive AI systems. *International Journal of Human-Computer Interaction, 41*(17), 10595–10617. DOI: 10.1080/10447318.2024.2435693

Lin, J., Yu, W., Zhang, N., Yang, X., Zhang, H., & Zhao, W. (2017). A survey on internet of things: Architecture, enabling technologies, security and privacy, and applications. *IEEE Internet of Things Journal, 4*(5), 1125–1142. DOI: 10.1109/JIOT.2017.2683200

Loscocco, P. A., Smalley, S. D., Muckelbauer, P. A., Taylor, R. C., Turner, S. J., & Farrell, J. F. (1998). The inevitability of failure: The flawed assumption of security in modern computing environments. In Proceedings of the 21st national information systems security conference

Lundberg, S. M., & Lee, S. I. (2017). A unified approach to interpreting model predictions. *Advances in Neural Information Processing Systems, 30*, 4765–4774.

Lysaght, T., Lim, H. Y., Xafis, V., & Ngiam, K. Y. (2019). AI-assisted decision-making in healthcare. *Asian Bioethics Review, 11*(3), 299–314. DOI: 10.1007/s41649-019-00096-0 PMID: 33717318

Mackey, T. K., Kuo, T. T., & Gummadi, B.. (2019). 'Fit-for-purpose?' – challenges and opportunities for applications of BCT in the future of healthcare. *BMC Medicine, 17*, 68. DOI: 10.1186/s12916-019-1296-7 PMID: 30914045

Mahajan, H. B. (2022). Emergence of Healthcare 4.0 and Blockchain into Secure Cloud-based Electronic Health Records Systems: Solutions, Challenges, and Future Roadmap. *Wireless Personal Communications, 126*(3), 2425–2446. DOI: 10.1007/s11277-022-09535-y

Malerbi, F. K., Nakayama, L. F., Dychiao, R. G., Ribeiro, L. Z., Villanueva, C., Celi, L. A., & Regatieri, C. V. (2023). Digital education for the deployment of artificial intelligence in health care. *Journal of Medical Internet Research, 25*, e43333. Advance online publication. DOI: 10.2196/43333 PMID: 37347537

Mandava, R., Vellela, S. S., Gorintla, S., Dalavai, L., Malathi, N., & Haritha, K. (2025). Evaluating the Impact of Explainable AI on User Trust in Financial Decision-Support Systems. Int. Conf. Comput. Robot., Test. Eng. Eval., ICCRTEE. International Conference on Computational Robotics, Testing and Engineering Evaluation, ICCRTEE 2025. DOI: 10.1109/ICCRTEE64519.2025.11052919

Mandl, K. D., Gottlieb, D., & Mandel, J. C. (2024). Integration of AI in healthcare requires an interoperable digital data ecosystem. *Nature Medicine, 30*(3), 631–634. DOI: 10.1038/s41591-023-02783-w PMID: 38291298

MarketsandMarkets. (2025). Artificial intelligence in healthcare market — global forecast to 2030. https://www.marketsandmarkets.com/Market-Reports/artificial-intelligence-healthcare-market-54679303.html

Marron, J. A. (2024). *Implementing the health insurance portability and accountability act (HIPAA) security rule*. National Institute of Standards and Technology., DOI: 10.6028/NIST.SP.800-66r2

Mastrantonas, A., Kokkas, P., Chatzopoulos, A., Papoutsidakis, M., Stergiou, C., Vairis, A., & Kanetaki, Z. (2024). Identifying the effects of Industry 4.0 in the pharmaceutical sector: Achieving the sustainable development goals. *Discover Sustainability, 5*(1), 460. DOI: 10.1007/s43621-024-00716-2

Mbacop, T. L., De La Cruz, E., Nadella, G. S., Le, H., De La Cruz, A. M., & Oni, O. (2025). Exploring Cybersecurity Challenges, Strategies, and Implications in Healthcare: A Qualitative Study. IEEE Integr. STEM Educ. Conf., ISEC. 2025 15th IEEE Integrated STEM Education Conference, ISEC 2025. DOI: 10.1109/ISEC64801.2025.11147260

Mendes, J. M. (2025). Reimagining healthcare education through nurturing AI-driven innovation. *BMC Medical Education, 25*(1), 1644. DOI: 10.1186/s12909-025-08254-9 PMID: 41291684

Meng, N., Nagy, S., Yao, D., Zhuang, W., & Argoty, G. A. (2018). Secure coding practices in java: Challenges and vulnerabilities. Proceedings of the 40th International Conference on Software Engineering, Mennella, C., Maniscalco, U., De Pietro, G., & Esposito, M. (2024). Ethical and regulatory challenges of AI technologies in healthcare: A narrative review. *Heliyon, 10*(4). Naeem, M. S., Ahmed, S., Sulman, A., Usman, S., Farooq, M. A., Talha, M., Awan, A., Afzal, Z., Khan, M. Z., & Hanif, A. Role of Medicinal Plants in the Management of Metabolic Disorders: Mechanisms, Efficacy, and Therapeutic Prospects.

Micheal, D. (2025). Comprehensive Survey of Security Techniques in the Post-Digital Era: From Intrusion Detection to Blockchain-Based Assurance Models.

MITRE Corporation. (2024). MITRE ATT&CK framework v14: Enterprise matrix ransomware techniques. https://attack.mitre.org/

Mitsea, E., Drigas, A., & Skianis, C. (2024). Artificial intelligence, immersive technologies, and neurotechnologies in breathing interventions for mental and emotional health: A systematic review. *Electronics (Basel), 13*(12), 2253. DOI: 10.3390/electronics13122253

Moral-Munoz, J. A., Herrera-Viedma, E., Santisteban-Espejo, A., & Cobo, M. J. (2020). Software tools for conducting bibliometric analysis in science: An up-to-date review. *El Profesional de la Información, 29*(1). Advance online publication. DOI: 10.3145/epi.2020.ene.03

Morley, J., Morton, C. E., Karpathakis, K., Taddeo, M., & Floridi, L. (2021). Towards a framework for evaluating AI systems for health. SSRN *Electronic Journal.* https://doi.org/DOI: 10.2139/ssrn.3826358

Morrow, E., Zidaru, T., Ross, F., Mason, C., Patel, K. D., Ream, M., & Stockley, R. (2023). Artificial intelligence technologies and compassion in healthcare: A systematic scoping review. *Frontiers in Psychology, 13*, 971044. DOI: 10.3389/fpsyg.2022.971044 PMID: 36733854

Moussa, F. Z., & Zine-Dine, K. (2025). The impact of cyber-attacks on cybersecurity investment game model. *Chaos, Solitons, and Fractals, 200,* 117040. Advance online publication. DOI: 10.1016/j.chaos.2025.117040

Mukherjee, P., & Singh, D. (2020). The Opportunities of Blockchain in Health 4.0. In Rosa Righi, R., Alberti, A., & Singh, M. (Eds.), *BCT for Industry 4.0. Blockchain Technologies*. Springer., DOI: 10.1007/978-981-15-1137-0_8

Musa, A., & Abdulfatai, A. O. (2024). Artificial intelligence for secured cybersecurity in emerging healthcare systems. In A. L. Imoize, C. Meshram, J. B. Awotunde, Y. Farhaoui, & D.-T. Do (Eds.), Cybersecurity in Emerging Healthcare Systems (pp. 203–240). Institution of Engineering and Technology. DOI: 10.1049/PBHE064E_ch7

Naeem, M. S., Naeem, M., Mehmood, M., Sulman, A. A., & Kharl, H. A. A. (2026). MACHINE LEARNING IN FORMULATION OPTIMIZATION AND PROCESS CONTROL. *PharmA AI: Revolutionizing Drug Discovery and Healthcare with Artificial Intelligence.*

Nair, S., & Saha, S. (2023). Advancements in cyber security and information systems in healthcare from 2004 to 2022: A bibliometric analysis. *2023 International Conference on Intelligent Systems, Advanced Computing and Communication (ISACC)*, 1–6. https://doi.org/DOI: 10.1109/ISACC56298.2023.10084049

Naiseh, M., Al-Thani, D., Jiang, N., & Ali, R. (2023). How the different explanation classes impact trust calibration: The case of clinical decision support systems. *International Journal of Human-Computer Studies*, *169*, 102941. DOI: 10.1016/j.ijhcs.2022.102941

Namli, T., Anıl Sınacı, A., Gönül, S., Herguido, C. R., Garcia-Canadilla, P., Muñoz, A. M., Esteve, A. V., & Ertürkmen, G. B. L. (2024). A scalable and transparent data pipeline for AI-enabled health data ecosystems. *Frontiers in Medicine*, *11*, 1393123. DOI: 10.3389/fmed.2024.1393123 PMID: 39139784

National Institute of Standards and Technology. (2023). Artificial intelligence risk management framework (AI RMF 1.0) (NIST AI 100-1). DOI: 10.6028/NIST.AI.100-1

National Institute of Standards and Technology. (2024). Cybersecurity Framework 2.0. *NIST CSWP*, *29*. Advance online publication. DOI: 10.6028/NIST.CSWP.29

National Institute of Standards and Technology. (2024). Post-quantum cryptography standards: FIPS 203, FIPS 204, FIPS 205. https://csrc.nist.gov/projects/post-quantum-cryptography

Ndabu, T., Mulgund, P., Sharman, R., & Singh, R. (2021). Perceptual gaps between clinicians and technologists on health IT errors. *JMIR Human Factors*, *8*(1). Advance online publication. DOI: 10.2196/21884 PMID: 33544089

Ngo, C., & Wright, C. B. (2024). EFFECTIVE INTEGRATION OF COMMERCIAL AND OPERATIONAL RISKS. Proc. Bienn. Int. Pipeline Conf. IPC, 5. DOI: 10.1115/IPC2024-134036

Nifakos, S., Chandramouli, K., Nikolaou, C. K., Papachristou, P., Koch, S., Panaousis, E., & Bonacina, S. (2021). Influence of human factors on cyber security within healthcare organisations: A systematic review. *Sensors (Basel)*, *21*(10), 3523. DOI: 10.3390/s21155119 PMID: 34372354

Nikolaev, A. A. (2025). An integrative model for health technology assessment: Perspectives for the Russian healthcare system. *Health Care of the Russian Federation*, *69*(5), 416–422. DOI: 10.47470/0044-197X-2025-69-5-416-422

Nobanee, H., Alodat, A., Bajodah, R., Al-Ali, M., & Darmaki, A. (2023). Bibliometric analysis of cybercrime and cybersecurity risks literature. *Journal of Financial Crime*, *30*(6), 1736–1754. Advance online publication. DOI: 10.1108/JFC-11-2022-0287

Noor, I., Mahmood, S., Aslam, M., Iqbal, S., Naeem, M. S., Shafaqat, M., Sulman, A., Awan, A., Aamir, H., & Kharl, A. (2026). AI ALGORITHMS AND TOOLS FOR PHARMACEUTICAL APPLICATIONS. *PharmA AI: Revolutionizing Drug Discovery and Healthcare with Artificial Intelligence*.

Noor, F., Bano, S., Shafiq, M., & Iqbal, M. W. (2025). Unveiling explainable AI in healthcare: Current trends, challenges, and future directions. *Wiley Interdisciplinary Reviews. Data Mining and Knowledge Discovery*, *15*(2), e70018. Advance online publication. DOI: 10.1002/widm.70018

Nunez Migliorisi, T. N. (2025). Healthcare Data Breaches: Diving in the Dark. Lect. Notes Networks Syst., 1424 LNNS, 587–602. DOI: 10.1007/978-3-031-92605-1_36

Oke, F., Bolaji, O., & Umakor, M. (2025). Building AI-ready infrastructure for U.S. healthcare: A product management perspective. *World Journal of Advanced Research and Reviews*, *27*(2), 588–603. DOI: 10.30574/wjarr.2025.27.2.2892

Okolo, C. T., Kamath, S., Dell, N., & Vashistha, A. (2021). "It cannot do all of my work": Community health worker perceptions of AI-enabled mobile health applications in rural India. Proceedings of the 2021 CHI conference on human factors in computing systems, Pellino, I. M., & Pellino, G. (2015). Consequences of defensive medicine, second victims, and clinical-judicial syndrome on surgeons' medical practice and on health service. *Updates in Surgery*, *67*(4), 331–337.

Onatuyeh, E. A., Oghorodi, D., Okpako, E. A., Ojei, E., Osakwe, G., Chinedu, N. B., Okoh, S. K., Odu, V. C., Chinedu, P. U., & Nwankwo, W. (2025). CYBERSECURITY AND BUSINESS SURVIVAL IN NIGERIA: BUILDING CUSTOMER'S TRUST. *African Journal of Applied Research*, *11*(1), 786–813. DOI: 10.26437/ajar.v11i1.882

Onur, D., & Özbakır, Ç. (2025). Pediatrics 4.0: The Transformative Impacts of the Latest Industrial Revolution on Pediatrics. *Health Care Analysis : HCA : Journal of Health Philosophy and Policy*. Advance online publication. DOI: 10.1007/s10728-025-00536-z PMID: 40690134

Orabi, M. M., Emam, O., & Fahmy, H. (2025). Adapting security and decentralized knowledge enhancement in federated learning using BCT: Literature review. *Journal of Big Data*, *12*, 55. DOI: 10.1186/s40537-025-01099-5

Oriaro, S., & Mishra, S. (2025). Improving cybersecurity through explainable artificial intelligence: A systematic literature review. *Issues in Information Systems*, *26*(3), 387–400. DOI: 10.48009/3_iis_2025_2025_131

Ouanes, K., & Farhah, N. (2024). Effectiveness of AI in clinical decision support systems and care delivery. *Journal of Medical Systems*, *48*(1), 74. DOI: 10.1007/s10916-024-02098-4 PMID: 39133332

Papadopoulos, I., & Lazzarino, R. (2024). Developing, delivering, and evaluating an online course on socially assistive robots in culturally competent and compassionate healthcare: A sequential multiphase, mixed-method study. *Digital Health*, *10*, 20552076241271792. DOI: 10.1177/20552076241271792 PMID: 39493631

Papadopoulos, P., Soflano, M., Chaudy, Y., Adejo, W., & Connolly, T. (2022). A systematic review of rule-based clinical decision support systems. *Health Technology (Hong Kong)*, *12*(4), 713. DOI: 10.1007/s12553-022-00672-9

Parise, G., Parise, L., Allegri, M., De Marco, A., & Anthony, M. A. (2020). Operational resilience of hospital power systems in the digital age. *IEEE Transactions on Industry Applications*, *57*(1), 94–100. DOI: 10.1109/TIA.2020.3032941

Park, S. H., & Langlotz, C. P. (2025). Crucial role of understanding in human-AI interaction for clinical adoption. *Korean Journal of Radiology*, *26*(4), 287. DOI: 10.3348/kjr.2025.0071 PMID: 40015562

Paul, J., Lim, W. M., O'Cass, A., Hao, A. W., & Bresciani, S. (2021). Scientific procedures and rationales for systematic literature reviews (SPAR-4-SLR). *International Journal of Consumer Studies*, *45*(4), O1–O16. DOI: 10.1111/ijcs.12695

Pemmasani, P. K., & Abd Nasaruddin, M. A. (2022). Strengthening public sector data governance: Risk management strategies for government organizations. *International Journal of Modern Computing*, *5*(1), 108–118.

Peng, M. L., Wickersham, J. A., Altice, F. L., Shrestha, R., Azwa, I., Zhou, X., Halim, M. A. A., Ikhtiaruddin, W. M., Tee, V., Kamarulzaman, A., & Ni, Z. (2022). Formative evaluation of the acceptance of HIV prevention artificial intelligence chatbots by men who have sex with men in Malaysia: Focus group study. *JMIR Formative Research*, *6*(10), e42055. DOI: 10.2196/42055 PMID: 36201390

Pfitzner, B., Steckhan, N., & Arnrich, B. (2021). Federated learning in a medical context: A systematic literature review. *ACM Transactions on Internet Technology*, *21*(2), 1–38. DOI: 10.1145/3412357

Pichan, A., Lazarescu, M., & Soh, S. T. (2018). Towards a practical cloud forensics logging framework. *Journal of Information Security and Applications*, *42*, 18–28. DOI: 10.1016/j.jisa.2018.07.008

Posso, R., & Altmann, J. (2025). Trust and Trust-Building Policies to Support Cybersecurity Information Sharing: A Systematic Literature Review. Lect. Notes Comput. Sci., 15358 LNCS, 212–228. DOI: 10.1007/978-3-031-81226-2_19

Pratama, I., Widyantara, I., Linawati, L., & Gunantara, N. (2025). Bibliometric analysis of AI-based prototype proposal for user security awareness in healthcare. *JOIV: International Journal on Informatics Visualization*, *9*(3), 982. Advance online publication. DOI: 10.62527/joiv.9.3.3319

Prateek, M., & Rathore, S. P. S. (2025). Clinical validation of AI disease detection Models—An overview of the clinical validation process for AI disease detection models, and how they can be validated for accuracy and effectiveness. *AI in Disease Detection: Advancements and Applications*, 215-237.

Preston, K. (2024). Bridging the gap: how human factors can support the development of AI technology in healthcare.

Quinn, C. (2025). Generative Ai. In *Clinical Practice: A Physician's Guide To Transforming Medicine*. World Scientific. DOI: 10.1142/9789819822218_0001

Qureshi, A. S.. (2024). Advancing healthcare systems: A tri-tier architecture using data communication, AI data generative and regulation and compliance standards. *Expert Systems: International Journal of Knowledge Engineering and Neural Networks*. Advance online publication. DOI: 10.1111/exsy.13742

Radanliev, P., De Roure, D., Maple, C., Nurse, J. R., Nicolescu, R., & Ani, U. (2024). AI security and cyber risk in IoT systems. *Frontiers in Big Data*, *7*, 1402745. DOI: 10.3389/fdata.2024.1402745

Rahimi, A. K., Pienaar, O., Ghadimi, M., Canfell, O. J., Pole, J. D., Shrapnel, S., van der Vegt, A., & Sullivan, C. (2024). Implementing AI in hospitals to achieve a learning health system. *Journal of Medical Internet Research*, *26*, e49655. Advance online publication. DOI: 10.2196/49655 PMID: 39094106

Raj, A., & Prakash, S. (2024). Privacy preservation of the internet of medical things using blockchain. *Health Services and Outcomes Research Methodology*, *24*(1), 112–139. DOI: 10.1007/s10742-023-00306-1

Ranjitsingh, L. M., & Rao, T. S. (2025). Establish legal and regulatory standards for the testing and validation of AI systems to ensure their reliability and safety in operational environments. *International Journal of System Assurance Engineering and Management*, *16*(10), 3338–3353. DOI: 10.1007/s13198-025-02865-7

Ransomware Task Force. (2021). Combating ransomware: A comprehensive framework for action. Institute for Security and Technology. https://securityandtechnology.org/ransomwaretaskforce/

Ranwala, R. A. D. L. M. K., & Andrade, A. Q. (2025). Enhancing AI Clinical Decision Support Trust: Design Workshop Insights from General Practitioners. *Studies in Health Technology and Informatics*, *329*, 593–597. DOI: 10.3233/SHTI250909 PMID: 40775927

Rao, T. R., Mitra, P., Bhatt, R., & Goswami, A. (2019). The big data system, components, tools, and technologies: A survey. *Knowledge and Information Systems*, *60*(3), 1165–1245. DOI: 10.1007/s10115-018-1248-0

Rattanapong, P., Sukma, N., & Darakorn Na Ayuthaya, S. (2025). Determinants of cybersecurity investment in ASEAN organizations: An integrated structural equation modeling approach. *Frontiers in Communications and Networks*, *6*, 1594554. Advance online publication. DOI: 10.3389/frcmn.2025.1594554

Razavi, H., . . .. (2023). Entropy sharing in ransomware: bypassing entropy-based detection of cryptographic operations. Sensors. https://pmc.ncbi.nlm.nih.gov/articles/PMC10934942/

Reddy, S., Fox, J., & Purohit, M. P. (2019). Artificial intelligence-enabled healthcare delivery. *Journal of the Royal Society of Medicine*, *112*(1), 22–28. DOI: 10.1177/0141076818815510 PMID: 30507284

Rejeb, A., Treiblmaier, H., Rejeb, K., & Zailani, S. (2021). Blockchain research in healthcare: A bibliometric review and current research trends. *Journal of Data, Information and Management*, *3*(2), 109–124. DOI: 10.1007/s42488-021-00046-2

Reuben, J. S., Meiri, H., & Arien-Zakay, H. (2024). AI's pivotal impact on redefining stakeholder roles in healthcare. *Frontiers in Digital Health*, *6*. Advance online publication. DOI: 10.3389/fdgth.2024.1458811 PMID: 39564581

Ribeiro, M. T., Singh, S., & Guestrin, C. (2016). "Why should I trust you?": Explaining the predictions of any classifier. Proceedings of the 22nd ACM SIGKDD International Conference on Knowledge Discovery and Data Mining, 1135–1144. DOI: 10.1145/2939672.2939778

Richardson, N., Kothapalli, S., Onteddu, A. R., Kundavaram, R., & Talla, R. R. (2023). AI-Driven Optimization Techniques for Evolving Software Architecture in Complex Systems. *ABC Journal of Advanced Research*, *12*(2), 71–84. DOI: 10.18034/abcjar.v12i2.783

Riggi, J. (2024). A look at 2024's health care cybersecurity challenges. American Hospital Association. https://www.aha.org/news/aha-cyber-intel/2024-10-07-look-2024s-health-care-cybersecurity-challenges

Rongali, S. K. (2025). AI-Powered Threat Detection in Healthcare Data. Int. Conf. Artif. Intell. Mach. Vis., AIMV. 2025 International Conference on Artificial Intelligence and Machine Vision, AIMV 2025. DOI: 10.1109/AIMV66517.2025.11203733

Saadeh, M., Janhonen, J., de Beer, E. S., Castelyn, C., & Hoffman, D. N. (2025). Automation complacency in medical decision-making. *AI and Ethics*, *5*(6), 5783–5793. Advance online publication. DOI: 10.1007/s43681-025-00825-2

Sahiner, B., Chen, W., Lu, L., Ko, Y., & Hung, L. Y. (2023). Strategies for detecting and mitigating dataset shift in machine learning for health predictions. *Journal of Biomedical Informatics*. Advance online publication. DOI: 10.1016/j.jbi.2025.104818

Sahinoglu, M. (2016). *Cyber-risk informatics: Engineering evaluation with data science*. John Wiley & Sons. DOI: 10.1002/9781119087540

Sajid, S. Nazir, Mohd., & Aijaz, M. (2025). Beyond Severity: Tactical Risk Scoring for Healthcare Vulnerabilities. Int. Conf. Multidiscip. Res. Innov. Eng., MRIE, 427–432. DOI: 10.1109/MRIE66930.2025.11156632

Salahuddin, Z., Woodruff, H. C., Chatterjee, A., & Lambin, P. (2021). Transparency of deep neural networks for medical image analysis. *Computers in Biology and Medicine*, *140*, 105111. DOI: 10.1016/j.compbiomed.2021.105111 PMID: 34891095

Salih, A., Galazzo, I. B., Raisi-Estabragh, Z., Petersen, S., Menegaz, G., & Radeva, P. (2024). A perspective on explainable artificial intelligence methods: SHAP and LIME. *Advanced Intelligent Systems*. Advance online publication. DOI: 10.1002/aisy.202400304

Samajdar, S. S., Chatterjee, R., Mukherjee, S., Dey, A. K., Saboo, B., Pal, J., Joshi, S., & Chatterjee, N. (2025). Artificial intelligence in healthcare: Current trends and future directions. *Current Medical Issues*, *23*(1), 53–60. DOI: 10.4103/cmi.cmi_93_24

Santos, A. R., Sampaio, F., Londral, A. R., & Perelman, J. (2025). Mapping methodologies for economic assessment of digital health technologies: A scoping review protocol. *BMJ Open*, *15*(7), e099933. Advance online publication. DOI: 10.1136/bmjopen-2025-099933 PMID: 40750290

Santos, A. R., von Hafe, F., Sampaio, F., Londral, A. R., & Perelman, J. (2025). Mapping Methodologies for Economic Evaluation of Digital Health Technologies: A Scoping Review. *Value in Health : The Journal of the International Society for Pharmacoeconomics and Outcomes Research*. Advance online publication. DOI: 10.1016/j.jval.2025.09.012 PMID: 41015334

Sarker, I. H., Janicke, H., Mohammad, N., Watters, P., & Nepal, S. (2023). AI potentiality and awareness: a position paper from the perspective of human-AI teaming in cybersecurity. International Conference on Intelligent Computing & Optimization, Sharma, N., & Kaushik, P. (2025). Integration of AI in healthcare systems—A discussion of the challenges and opportunities of integrating AI in healthcare systems for disease detection and diagnosis. *AI in Disease Detection: Advancements and Applications*, 239-263.

Sarker, M. (2023). Assessing the integration of AI technologies in enhancing patient care delivery. *Journal of Knowledge Learning and Science Technology*, *2*(2), 338–351. DOI: 10.60087/jklst.vol2.n2.p351

Schmidt, A.. (2023). Effective ransomware detection using entropy estimation of files for cloud services. *Sensors (Basel)*, *23*(6), 3023. DOI: 10.3390/s23063023 PMID: 36991730

Schwarzschild, A., Goldblum, M., Gupta, A., Dickerson, J. P., & Goldstein, T. (2021). Just how toxic is data poisoning? a unified benchmark for backdoor and data poisoning attacks. International Conference on Machine Learning, Shandilya, S. K., Datta, A., Kartik, Y., & Nagar, A. (2024). Navigating the regulatory landscape. In *Digital Resilience: Navigating Disruption and Safeguarding Data Privacy* (pp. 127-240). Springer.

Security, I. B. M. (2023). Cost of a data breach report 2023. IBM Corporation. https://www.ibm.com/reports/data-breach

Sezgin, E. (2024). Redefining virtual assistants in health care: The future with large language models. *Journal of Medical Internet Research*, *26*, e53225. DOI: 10.2196/53225 PMID: 38241074

Shafrin, J., Kim, J., Cohen, J. T., Garrison, L. P., Goldman, D. A., Doshi, J. A., Krieger, J., Lakdawalla, D. N., Neumann, P. J., Phelps, C. E., Whittington, M. D., & Willke, R. (2024). Valuing the Societal Impact of Medicines and Other Health Technologies: A User Guide to Current Best Practices. *Forum for Health Economics & Policy*, *27*(1), 29–116. DOI: 10.1515/fhep-2024-0014 PMID: 39512185

Sharma, P. (2024). Enhancing Cyber Resilience: Development, Challenges, and Strategic Insights in Cyber Security Report Websites using Artificial Inteligence.

Sharma, P., Gounder, M., & Kumar, K. (2024). Mastering Feature Engineering: Unlocking the Art of Data Transformation for Enhanced Predictive Modeling with Neural Networks. International Conference on Data Science and Applications, Sloan, R., & Warner, R. (2017). *Unauthorized access: The crisis in online privacy and security*. Taylor & Francis.

Sharma, A., Lin, I. W., Miner, A. S., Atkins, D. C., & Althoff, T. (2023). Human–AI collaboration enables more empathic conversations in text-based peer-to-peer mental health support. *Nature Machine Intelligence*, *5*(1), 46–57. DOI: 10.1038/s42256-022-00593-2

Sheikh, A., & Cresswell, K. (2018). Addressing the human aspects of EHR-enabled health system change. *Journal of the American Medical Informatics Association : JAMIA*, *25*(3), 225–226. DOI: 10.1093/jamia/ocx152

Shneiderman, B. (2020). Bridging the gap between ethics and practice: Guidelines for reliable, safe, and trustworthy human-centered AI systems. [TiiS]. *ACM Transactions on Interactive Intelligent Systems*, *10*(4), 1–31. DOI: 10.1145/3419764

Shukla, A. (2025). AI for Healthcare Security: The Intersection of Innovation and Resilience. Commun. Comput. Info. Sci., 2404 CCIS, 109–127. DOI: 10.1007/978-3-031-85558-0_6

Siddiqi, S., Masud, T. I., Nishtar, S., Peters, D. H., Sabri, B., Bile, K. M., & Jama, M. A. (2009). Framework for assessing governance of the health system in developing countries: Gateway to good governance. *Health Policy (Amsterdam)*, *90*(1), 13–25. DOI: 10.1016/j.healthpol.2008.08.005

Siddiq, M. (2021). Integration of machine learning in clinical decision support systems. *Eduvest*, *1*(12), 1579–1591. DOI: 10.59188/eduvest.v1i12.809

Sindiramutty, S. R., Jhanjhi, N. Z., & Khan, N. A. (2025). AI in healthcare safeguarding patient privacy and confidentiality. In Hussain, K. (Ed.), *Vulnerabilities Assessment and Risk Management in Cyber Security* (pp. 369–404). IGI Global., DOI: 10.4018/979-8-3693-6135-1.ch015

Sinha, S., & Lee, Y. M. (2024). Challenges with developing and deploying AI models and applications in industrial systems. *Discover Artificial Intelligence*, *4*(1), 55. DOI: 10.1007/s44163-024-00151-2

Sirbu, C. L., & Mercioni, M. A. (2024). Fostering Trust in AI-Driven Healthcare: A Brief Review of Ethical and Practical Considerations. Int. Symp. Electron. Telecommun., ISETC - Conf. Proc. 2024 16th International Symposium on Electronics and Telecommunications, ISETC 2024 - Conference Proceedings. DOI: 10.1109/ISETC63109.2024.10797264

Slack, D., Hilgard, S., Jia, E., Singh, S., & Lakkaraju, H. (2020). Fooling LIME and SHAP: Adversarial attacks on post hoc explanation methods. Proceedings of the AAAI/ACM Conference on AI, Ethics, and Society, 180–186. DOI: 10.1145/3375627.3375830

Snigdha, E. Z., Jalil, M. S., Dahwal, F. M., Saeed, M., Mehedy, M. T. J., & Hasan, S. K. (2025). Cybersecurity in Healthcare IT Systems: Business Risk Management and Data Privacy Strategies. *The American Journal of Engineering and Technology*, *7*(03), 163–184. DOI: 10.37547/tajet/Volume07Issue03-15

Sobb, T., Moustafa, N., & Turnbull, B. (2025). Responsible resilience in cyber–physical–social systems: A new paradigm for emergent cyber risk modeling. *Future Internet*, *17*(7), 282. DOI: 10.3390/fi17070282

Sokol, K., Fackler, J. C., & Vogt, J. E. (2025). Artificial intelligence should support clinical reasoning. *npj. Digital Medicine*, *8*(1), 345. DOI: 10.1038/s41746-025-01725-9 PMID: 40494886

Sommer, R., & Paxson, V. (2010). Outside the closed world: On using machine learning for network intrusion detection. *Proceedings of the IEEE Symposium on Security and Privacy*, 305–316. DOI: 10.1109/SP.2010.25

Sophos. (2024). The state of ransomware in healthcare 2024. Sophos Research Report.

Sophos. (2025). The state of ransomware in healthcare 2025. Sophos Research Report.

Spear, J., Ehrenfeld, J. M., & Miller, B. J. (2023). Applications of artificial intelligence in health care delivery. *Journal of Medical Systems*, *47*(1), 121. Advance online publication. DOI: 10.1007/s10916-023-02018-y PMID: 37975946

Srijayanthi, S., & Sethukarasi, T. (2023). Design of privacy preserving model based on clustering involved anonymization along with feature selection. *Computers & Security*, *126*, 103027. DOI: 10.1016/j.cose.2022.103027

Stallings, W., & Brown, L. (2018). *Computer security: Principles and practice* (4th ed.). Pearson Education.

Stoica, I., Song, D., Popa, R. A., Patterson, D., Mahoney, M. W., Katz, R., Joseph, A. D., Jordan, M., Hellerstein, J. M., & Gonzalez, J. E. (2017). A berkeley view of systems challenges for ai. *arXiv preprint arXiv:1712.05855.*

Sudheer, S. (2024). Ransomware Attacks and Their Evolving Strategies: A Systematic Review of Recent Incidents. *Journal of Technology and Systems*, *6*(7), 32–59. DOI: 10.47941/jts.2399

Sutton, R. T., Pincock, D., Baumgart, D. C., Sadowski, D., Fedorak, R. N., & Kroeker, K. I. (2020). Overview of clinical decision support systems. *npj. Digital Medicine*, *3*(1), 17. DOI: 10.1038/s41746-020-0221-y PMID: 32047862

Székely, B. (2022). Mitigating the privacy risks of AI through privacy-enhancing technologies. *Acta Universitatis Sapientiae. Legal Studies*, *11*(2), 35–64.

Tao, H., Bhuiyan, M. Z. A., Rahman, M. A., Wang, G., Wang, T., Ahmed, M. M., & Li, J. (2019). Economic perspective analysis of protecting big data security and privacy. *Future Generation Computer Systems*, *98*, 660–671. DOI: 10.1016/j.future.2019.03.042

Tariq, M. U. (2024). Enhancing cybersecurity protocols in modern healthcare systems: Strategies and best practices. In Garcia, M. B., & de Almeida, R. P. P. (Eds.), *Transformative Approaches to Patient Literacy and Healthcare Innovation* (pp. 223–241). IGI Global., DOI: 10.4018/979-8-3693-3661-8.ch011

Ten, C.-W., Manimaran, G., & Liu, C.-C. (2010). Cybersecurity for critical infrastructures: Attack and defense modeling. *IEEE Transactions on Systems, Man, and Cybernetics. Part A, Systems and Humans*, *40*(4), 853–865. DOI: 10.1109/TSMCA.2010.2048028

Theilmann, K., Dahlem, N., Steffny, L., Podevin, D., Hartnik, J., & Greff, T. (2025). Towards Effective AI in Healthcare: Identifying Success Factors and the Potential of Human-in-the-Loop. IFIP Advances in Information and Communication Technology, 755 IFIPAICT, 173–188. DOI: 10.1007/978-3-031-96239-4_13

Thesmar, D., Sraer, D., Pinheiro, L., Dadson, N., Veliche, R., & Greenberg, P. (2019). Combining the power of artificial intelligence with the richness of healthcare claims data: Opportunities and challenges. *PharmacoEconomics*, *37*(6), 745–752. DOI: 10.1007/s40273-019-00777-6

Thiyagarajan, A., . . .. (2025). The role of artificial intelligence in safeguarding patient privacy in healthcare systems. PMC. https://pmc.ncbi.nlm.nih.gov/articles/PMC12244842/

Tick, A., & Szabo-Harka, N. (2024). Analysis of Information Security in a Corporate Environment-a Human Perspective. IEEE World Symp. Appl. Mach. Intell. Informatics, SAMI - Proc., 469–474. DOI: 10.1109/SAMI60510.2024.10432889

Topol, E. J. (2019). High-performance medicine: The convergence of human and artificial intelligence. *Nature Medicine*, *25*(1), 44–56. DOI: 10.1038/s41591-018-0300-7 PMID: 30617339

U.S. Food and Drug Administration. (2021). Artificial intelligence/machine learning (AI/ML)-based software as a medical device (SaMD) action plan. https://www.fda.gov/media/145022/download

UcedaVelez. T., & Morana, M. M. (2015). Risk centric threat modeling: Process for attack simulation and threat analysis. Wiley.

Ueda, D., Kakinuma, T., Fujita, S., Kamagata, K., Fushimi, Y., Ito, R., Matsui, Y., Nozaki, T., Nakaura, T., Fujima, N., Tatsugami, F., Yanagawa, M., Hirata, K., Yamada, A., Tsuboyama, T., Kawamura, M., Fujioka, T., & Naganawa, S. (2023). Fairness of artificial intelligence in healthcare. *Japanese Journal of Radiology*, *42*(1), 3–15. DOI: 10.1007/s11604-023-01474-3 PMID: 37540463

Uma, S. (2023). Blockchain and AI: Disruptive Digital Technologies in Designing the Potential Growth of Healthcare Industries. In Rai, B. K., Kumar, G., & Balyan, V. (Eds.), *AI and Blockchain in Healthcare. Advanced Technologies and Societal Change*. Springer., DOI: 10.1007/978-981-99-0377-1_9

United Kingdom NHS. (2017). WannaCry ransomware attack spreads worldwide. BMJ / PMC. https://pmc.ncbi.nlm.nih.gov/articles/PMC5461132/

Vadillo, J., Santana, R., & Lozano, J. A. (2025). Adversarial attacks in explainable machine learning: A survey of threats against models and humans. *Wiley Interdisciplinary Reviews. Data Mining and Knowledge Discovery*, *15*(1), e1567. Advance online publication. DOI: 10.1002/widm.1567

van Eck, N. J., & Waltman, L. (2010). Software survey: VOSviewer, a computer program for bibliometric mapping. *Scientometrics*, *84*(2), 523–538. DOI: 10.1007/s11192-009-0146-3 PMID: 20585380 van Kessel, R., Ranganathan, S., Anderson, M., McMillan, B., & Mossialos, E. (2024). Exploring potential drivers of patient engagement with their health data through digital platforms: A scoping review. *International Journal of Medical Informatics, 189*, 105513. Advance online publication. DOI: 10.1016/j.ijmedinf.2024.105513 PMID: 38851132

Vardas, E. P., Marketou, M., & Vardas, P. (2025). Medicine, healthcare and the AI act. *European Heart Journal. Digital Health, 6*(4), 833–839. DOI: 10.1093/ehjdh/ztaf041 PMID: 40703136

Varnosfaderani, S. M., & Forouzanfar, M. (2024). The role of AI in hospitals and clinics. *Bioengineering (Basel, Switzerland), 11*(4), 337. DOI: 10.3390/bioengineering11040337 PMID: 38671759

Varri, D. B. S. V. (2025). Human-AI collaboration in healthcare security.

Vasilica, B.-V., Anton, F. D., Mocanu, S., & Chiriac, B. N. (2025). Implementation and Evaluation of a Zero-Trust Security Model in Distributed Industrial Networks. Proc. - Int. Conf. Control Syst. Comput. Sci., CSCS, 243–250. DOI: 10.1109/CSCS66924.2025.00044

Veriti Research. (2025). Healthcare ransomware statistics 2025. Cobalt / Veriti Analysis. https://www.cobalt.io/blog/healthcare-data-breach-statistics

Verma, P., Newe, T., O'Mahony, G. D., Brennan, D., & O'Shea, D. (2025). Towards a Unified Understanding of Cyber Resilience: A Comprehensive Review of Concepts, Strategies, and Future Directions. *IEEE Access : Practical Innovations, Open Solutions*. Advance online publication. DOI: 10.1109/ACCESS.2025.3551887

Vial, T., & Almon, A. (2023). Artificial intelligence in mental health therapy for children and adolescents. *JAMA Pediatrics, 177*(12), 1251–1252. DOI: 10.1001/jamapediatrics.2023.4212 PMID: 37843842

Vitacca, M., Giardini, A., Gazzi, L., & Vitacca, M. (2022). Hidden biases in clinical decision-making. *Monaldi Archives for Chest Disease*. Advance online publication. DOI: 10.4081/monaldi.2022.2339 PMID: 36069639

Wachter, R. M., & Pronovost, P. J. (2009). Balancing "no blame" with accountability in patient safety. *The New England Journal of Medicine, 361*(14), 1401–1406. DOI: 10.1056/NEJMsb0903885

Waheed, H., Waheed, F., Ashiq, E., Afzal, A., Sarosh, A., Maqbool, W., Sulman, A., Awan, A., & Kharl, H. A. A. (2026). INTRODUCTION TO ARTIFICIAL INTELLIGENCE AND MACHINE LEARNING IN PHARMACY. *PharmA AI: Revolutionizing Drug Discovery and Healthcare with Artificial Intelligence*.

Wang, B., Sun, F., & Luan, Y. (2024). Comparison of the effectiveness of different normalization methods for metagenomic cross-study phenotype prediction under heterogeneity. *Scientific Reports, 14*(1), 7024. DOI: 10.1038/s41598-024-57670-2 PMID: 38528097

Wang, L., Zhang, Z., Wang, D., Cao, W., Zhou, X., Zhang, P., Liu, J., Fan, X., & Tian, F. (2023). Human-centered design of AI clinical decision systems. *Frontiers of Computer Science, 5*. Advance online publication. DOI: 10.3389/fcomp.2023.1187299

Wang, Z., Ma, J., Wang, X., Hu, J., Qin, Z., & Ren, K. (2022). Threats to training: A survey of poisoning attacks and defenses on machine learning systems. *ACM Computing Surveys, 55*(7), 1–36. DOI: 10.1145/3538707

Wasif, N. (2024). *Enhancing Cloud Security with AI-Driven Data Pipelines for Robust Infrastructure Protection: A Guide to Meeting HIPAA*. IAM, and SOX Compliance.

Wasserman, L., & Wasserman, Y. (2022). Hospital cybersecurity risks and gaps: Review (for the non-cyber professional). *Frontiers in Digital Health, 4*, 86222. DOI: 10.3389/fdgth.2022.862221 PMID: 36033634

Wen, H. (2024). Human-AI collaboration for enhanced safety. In *Methods in Chemical Process Safety* (Vol. 8, pp. 51–80). Elsevier.

Whig, P., Aggarwal, A., Ganeshan, V., Modhugu, V. R., & Bhatia, A. B. (2024). AI for Secure and Resilient Cyber-Physical Systems. In *Artificial Intelligence Solutions for Cyber-Physical Systems* (pp. 40–63). Auerbach Publications. DOI: 10.1201/9781032694375-2

Williams, C., Watson, T., Bryant, I., Mahrra, J., Miller, W. D., Fonash, P. M., Badillo, B., Abrams, M., Nagarajan, A., & Sood, A. (2012). Resilient cyber ecosystems. *Crosstalk, 25*(5).

Williamson, S. M., & Prybutok, V. (2024). Balancing privacy and progress: A review of privacy challenges, systemic oversight, and patient perceptions in AI-driven healthcare. *Applied Sciences (Basel, Switzerland), 14*(2), 675. DOI: 10.3390/app14020675

Wosny, M. (2025). Understanding the Root Causes of Healthcare Professionals' Frustration with Digital Tools. *Studies in Health Technology and Informatics, 323*, 344–348. DOI: 10.3233/SHTI250109 PMID: 40200506

Wu, W.-T., Chao, Y.-W., Lin, T.-K., Huang, C.-K., & Hsieh, P.-H. (2025). Economic evaluation of AI-assisted technologies in healthcare: A systematic review. *Journal of Food and Drug Analysis, 33*(4), 487–500. DOI: 10.38212/2224-6614.3570 PMID: 41525195

Yoon, S., Goh, H., Lee, P. C., Tan, H. C., Teh, M. M., Lim, D. S. T., Kwee, A., Chandran, S., Carmody, D., Swee, D. S., Tan, S. Y. T., Wong, A. J.-W., Choo, C. H., Wee, Z., & Bee, Y. M. (2024). AI-enabled prescription advisory tool study. *JMIR Human Factors, 11*. Advance online publication. DOI: 10.2196/50939 PMID: 38869934

Yuman, Y., Goyal, S. B., Rajawat, A. S., Kumar, M., Shankar, A., Alhayan, F., & Basheer, S. (2025). A blockchain-based solution for enhancing the efficiency and security of healthcare knowledge management systems in the era of industry 4.0. *Wireless Networks*, *31*(2), 983–1004. DOI: 10.1007/s11276-024-03770-w

Zakiyah, N., Marulin, D., Alfaqeeh, M., Puspitasari, I. M., Lestari, K., Lim, K. K., & Fox-Rushby, J. (2024). Economic Evaluations of Digital Health Interventions for Patients With Heart Failure: Systematic Review. *Journal of Medical Internet Research*, *26*, e53500. Advance online publication. DOI: 10.2196/53500 PMID: 38687991

Zbrzezny, A. M., & Grzybowski, A. E. (2023). Deceptive tricks in artificial intelligence: Adversarial attacks in ophthalmology. *Journal of Clinical Medicine*, *12*(9), 3266. DOI: 10.3390/jcm12093266 PMID: 37176706

Zeb, S., Abbasi, N., & Fahad, M. (2024). AI in healthcare: Revolutionizing diagnosis and therapy. *International Journal of Multidisciplinary Sciences and Arts*, *3*(3), 118–128. DOI: 10.47709/ijmdsa.v3i3.4546

Zhang, Z., Al Hamadi, H., Damiani, E., Yeun, C. Y., & Taher, F. (2022). Explainable artificial intelligence applications in cyber security: State-of-the-art in research. *IEEE Access : Practical Innovations, Open Solutions*, *10*, 93104–93139. DOI: 10.1109/ACCESS.2022.3204051

Zhao, L., Wu, X., Li, J., & Tong, H. (2025). Economics of Cybersecurity Investment and Information Sharing: Firm Decision Making Under Policy Constraints. *Systems*, *13*(2), 83. Advance online publication. DOI: 10.3390/systems13020083

# About the Contributors

**Hanh Le** is a dedicated researcher, Full Stack Software Developer, and manager of a software development team. She holds a Ph.D. in Information Technology and a Master's degree in Computer Science. Her research interests include artificial intelligence (AI), software development, data analytics, data science, and cloud computing. Dr. Le's work focuses on leveraging AI and data-driven technologies to enhance decision-making and optimize software systems across industries such as healthcare, law enforcement, and retail. With expertise in both front-end and back-end development, she designs object-oriented, database-driven applications and values interdisciplinary collaboration to drive innovation and discovery.

***

**Lawal Abdulwahab Olamilekan** is a dedicated academic with a PhD in Economics from the Universiti Brunei Darussalam, School of Business and Economics (AACSB-accredited). He holds a Master's degree in Health Economics and a Bachelor's in Economics Education from Taraba State University, Nigeria. His research interests span natural resource economics, health economics, development, and macroeconomics, particularly in Africa and emerging economies. With over six years of academic experience, he has taught and supervised students across Nigeria, Somalia, Somaliland, and Brunei. His teaching expertise covers economics, management, and public health, while his research contributions include conference papers, journal articles, and book chapters. Lawal's proficiency in quantitative and qualitative methodologies, coupled with his advanced skills in econometric modelling and using software such as Stata, SPSS, and EViews, instills confidence in his technical abilities. He is a member of the World Economics Association and the Institute of Chartered Economists of Nigeria. His active engagement in collaborative research that bridges health policy, governance, and economic development to provide evidence-based insights for sustainable growth is truly inspiring.

**Anorgul Ashirova** is working as an Associate Professor at the Department of General Professional Sciences, Mamun University, Khiva, Uzbekistan

**Andi Asrifan**, S.Pd., M.Pd. is a senior lecturer in the Doctoral Program in English Language Education at the Graduate School of Universitas Negeri Makassar (UNM), Indonesia (unm.ac.id). With a Doctor of Education in English Language Education, he has demonstrated a consistent commitment to advancing research in English as a Foreign Language (EFL), digital pedagogy, and the integration of artificial intelligence (AI) in language instruction. Dr. Asrifan previously served as Head of the Institute for Cooperation and International Affairs at Universitas Muhammadiyah Sidenreng Rappang and continues to collaborate across academic institutions, both nationally and internationally, actively. Over the past two years, Dr. Asrifan has led several research initiatives focused on AI-driven curriculum development, bilingual education in Southeast Asia, and digital parenting in urban Indonesia. He is frequently invited as a keynote speaker at international conferences and serves as a reviewer and editorial board member for various Scopus-indexed journals. His publications have appeared in high-impact outlets and span the disciplines of education, linguistics, and cultural studies.

**Shaik Johny Basha** working as Assistant Professor in the Department of CSE, SRM University-AP, Andhra Pradesh. His research interests are Security, Internet of Things and Data Science.

**Yarmanova Yulduz Burievna** is an academic professional in the Department of Primary Education at Karshi State University, Karshi, Uzbekistan. She is actively engaged in teaching, curriculum development, and pedagogical research related to primary and elementary education. Her academic interests focus on innovative teaching methodologies, learner-centered education, and the integration of modern educational technologies to enhance foundational learning outcomes. She contributes to academic discussions through scholarly activities and collaborative initiatives aimed at improving teacher education and classroom practices. Yarmanova Yulduz Burievna is committed to advancing quality education through research-informed instruction and continuous professional development.

**Amanpreet Kaur** is a researcher with interests in corporate governance, financial risk management, cybersecurity, and digital transformation. Her research focuses on emerging interdisciplinary areas such as healthcare cybersecurity, governance frameworks, and technology-driven risk management. She has conducted bibliometric and systematic literature studies to identify research trends and knowledge structures in evolving academic domains. Her recent work explores the integration of governance, risk, and technology paradigms in financial and healthcare systems.

**Nurhajar Patinrosi** is a lecturer in Islamic Educational Management at the Faculty of Tarbiyah and Teacher Training, UIN Palopo, Indonesia. She obtained her Bachelor's degree in English Education and a Master's degree in Islamic Educational Management. She has teaching experience in multiple study programs, including English Education and Islamic Educational Management. In addition to her teaching role, she serves as the Coordinator of English Language Development at the Language Development Unit. Her research interests include higher education management, the internationalization of Islamic higher education, climate and environmental education, and educational policy. She has actively participated in international conferences and academic forums and is currently engaged in ongoing research and scholarly publications in the field of education.

**Sabyasachi Pramanik** is a professional IEEE member. He obtained a PhD in Computer Science and Engineering from Sri Satya Sai University of Technology and Medical Sciences, Bhopal, India. Presently, he is an Associate Professor, Department of Computer Science and Engineering, Haldia Institute of Technology, India. He has many publications in various reputed international conferences, journals, and book chapters (Indexed by SCIE, Scopus, ESCI, etc). He is doing research in the fields of Artificial Intelligence, Data Privacy, Cybersecurity, Network Security, and Machine Learning. He also serves on the editorial boards of several international journals. He is a reviewer of journal articles from IEEE, Springer, Elsevier, Inderscience, IET and IGI Global. He has reviewed many conference papers, has been a keynote speaker, session chair, and technical program committee member at many international conferences. He has authored a book on Wireless Sensor Network. He has edited 8 books from IGI Global, CRC Press, Springer and Wiley Publications.

**Sahabuddin**, M.Pd. is a permanent lecturer in the Department of Sports Coaching Education, Faculty of Sports Science and Health, Universitas Negeri Makassar, Indonesia. He earned his bachelor's degree in Sports Coaching Education from IKIP Ujung Pandang, his master's degree in Physical Education and Sports from Universitas Negeri Makassar, and his doctoral degree in Sports Education from Universitas Negeri Jakarta. His teaching and research expertise include sports coaching science, badminton, volleyball, physical conditioning, training theory, multilateral athlete development, sports testing and measurement, physiotherapy, sports massage, and injury prevention. He has authored and edited several academic books in sports science, physical education, research methodology, and coaching models. In addition to his academic work, he actively participates in professional training and certifications related to sports therapy, health psychology, and holistic healing. He is also the founder of Cakra Education Science and Holistic Therapy Foundation in Makassar, established in 2022.

**Keshav Sinha** was born in Dhanbad, India, in 1991. He received a B.E. Degree in Computer Science and Engineering from Sri Chandrasekharendra Saraswathi Viswa Mahavidyalaya, Kanchipuram, India, in 2013 and an M.E. Degree in Software Engineering from the Birla Institute of Technology, Mesra, India, in 2016. He completed a PhD in cryptography and network security from Birla Institute of Technology, Mesra, India, in 2022. He is an assistant professor specializing in Cryptography and Network Security. His research focuses on developing a secure environment for multimedia transmission. He has contributed to soft computing, humanities, and social and cyber policy and published numerous papers in conferences and journals. His work aims to bring flexibility and innovation to the computer science society.

**L.Sumalatha** has over 18 years of teaching experience in Computer Science & Engineering Department at University College of Engineering Kakinada. Currently she is the Director for Industry Institute Interaction Placements & Skill Development, Chairman Board of Studies for Computer Science & Engineering, Chief Coordinator SDC, DMC Coordinator (i/c). She is a 'University Innovation Fellow – Stanford University, CA, USA', Research Lead of AI Platoon research group with leading india. ai- AI & Deep Learning research initiative. She is the president for Institute of Innovation Council associated with MHRDs Innovation Council.

**Duggineni Veeraiah** received the Ph.D. degree from Jawaharlal Nehru Technological University Kakinada (JNTUK), India, in 2017. He is currently a Professor and the Head of the Department, SMD at Lakireddy Bali Reddy College of Engineering (Autonomous), Mylavaram, Andhra Pradesh, India. He has authored more than 40 publications in reputed journals and conferences and has executed multiple funded projects. His research interests include machine learning, data science, security in cloud and IoT environments, and deep learning-based intrusion detection.

# Index

## H



## I



## N



## P



## R



## S



## T



## W

## Z

www.ingramcontent.com/pod-product-compliance
Lightning Source LLC
LaVergne TN
LVHW080903300926
849162LV00003B/530